HEALTH AND HUMAN DEVELOPMENT

RURAL CHILD HEALTH

INTERNATIONAL ASPECTS

Health and Human Development

Joav Merrick, Series Editor

Adolescent Behavior Research: International Perspectives
Joav Merrick and Hatim A. Omar
2007. ISBN: 1-60021-649-8

Complementary Medicine Systems: Comparison and Integration
Karl W. Kratky
2008. ISBN: 978-1-60456-475-4

Pain in Children and Youth
Patricia Schofield and Joav Merrick
2008. ISBN: 978-1-60456-951-3

Behavioral Pediatrics, 3rd Edition
Donald E. Greydanus, Dilip R. Patel, Helen D. Pratt and Joseph L. Calles, Jr.
2009. ISBN: 978-1-60692-702-1

Behavioral Pediatrics, 3rd Edition
Donald E. Greydanus, Dilip R. Patel, Helen D. Pratt and Joseph L. Calles, Jr.
2009. ISBN: 978-1-60876-630-7 (E-book)

Health and Happiness from Meaningful Work: Research in Quality of Working Life
Søren Ventegodt and Joav Merrick
2009. ISBN: 978-1-60692-820-2

Obesity and Adolescence: A Public Health Concern
Hatim A. Omar, Donald E. Greydanus, Dilip R. Patel and Joav Merrick
2009. ISBN: 978-1-60456-821-9

Poverty and Children: A Public Health Concern
Alexis Lieberman and Joav Merrick
2009. ISBN: 978-1-60741-140-6

Living on the Edge: The Mythical, Spiritual, and Philosophical Roots of Social Marginality
Joseph Goodbread
2009. ISBN: 978-1-60741-162-8

Challenges in Adolescent Health: An Australian Perspective
David Bennett, Susan Towns, Elizabeth Elliott and Joav Merrick (Editors)
2009. ISBN: 978-1-60741-616-6

Challenges in Adolescent Health: An Australian Perspective
David Bennett, Susan Towns, Elizabeth Elliott and Joav Merrick (Editors)
2009. ISBN: 978-1-61668-240-8 (E-book)

Alcohol-Related Cognitive Disorders: Research and Clinical Perspectives
Leo Sher, Isack Kandel and Joav Merrick
2009. ISBN: 978-1-60741-730-9

Alcohol-Related Cognitive Disorders: Research and Clinical Perspectives
Leo Sher, Isack Kandel and Joav Merrick
2009. ISBN: 978-1-60876-623-9 (E-book)

Advances in Environmental Health Effects of Toxigenic Mold and Mycotoxins- Volume 1
Ebere Cyril Anyanwu
2010. ISBN: 978-1-60741-953-2

Children and Pain
Patricia Schofield and Joav Merrick (Editors)
2009. ISBN: 978-1-60876-020-6

Child Rural Health: International Aspects
Erica Bell and Joav Merrick (Editors)
2010. ISBN: 978-1-60876-357-3

Conceptualizing Behavior in Health and Social Research: A Practical Guide to Data Analysis
Said Shahtahmasebi and Damon Berridge
2010. ISBN: 978-1-60876-383-2

Chance Action and Therapy. The Playful Way of Changing
Uri Wernik
2010. ISBN: 978-1-60876-393-1

Adolescence and Chronic Illness. A Public Health Concern
Hatim Omar, Donald E. Greydanus, Dilip R. Patel and Joav Merrick (Editors)
2010. ISBN: 978-1-60876-628-4

Adolescence and Sports
Dilip R. Patel, Donald E. Greydanus, Hatim Omar and Joav Merrick (Editors)
2010. ISBN: 978-1-60876

International Aspects of Child Abuse and Neglect
Howard Dubowitz and Joav Merrick (Editors)
2010. ISBN: 978-1-60876-703-8

Positive Youth Development: Evaluation and Future Directions in a Chinese Context
Daniel T.L. Shek, Hing Keung Ma and Joav Merrick (Editors)
2010. ISBN: 978-1-60876-830-1

Positive Youth Development: Evaluation and Future Directions in a Chinese Context
Daniel T.L. Shek, Hing Keung Ma and Joav Merrick (Editors)
2010. ISBN: 978-1-61668-376-4 (E-book)

Positive Youth Development: Implementation of a Youth Program in a Chinese Context
Daniel T.L Shek, Hing Keung Ma and Joav Merrick (Editors)
2010. ISBN: 978-1-61668-230-9

Pediatric and Adolescent Sexuality and Gynecology: Principles for the Primary Care Clinician
Hatim A. Omar, Donald E. Greydanus, Artemis K. Tsitsika, Dilip R. Patel and Joav Merrick (Editors)
2010. ISBN: 978-1-60876-735-9

Understanding Eating Disorders: Integrating Culture, Psychology and Biology
Yael Latzer, Joav Merrick and Daniel Stein (Editors)
2010. ISBN: 978-1-61668-261-3.

Advanced Cancer Pain and Quality of Life
Edward Chow and Joav Merrick (Editors)
2010. ISBN: 978-1-61668-207-1

Social and Cultural Psychiatry Experience from the Caribbean Region
Hari D. Maharajh and Joav Merrick (Editors)
2010. ISBN: 978-1-61668-506-5

Social and Cultural Psychiatry Experience from the Caribbean Region
Hari D. Maharajh and Joav Merrick (Editors)
2010. ISBN: 978-1-61728-088-7 (E-book)

Bone and Brain Metastases: Advances in Research and Treatment
Arjun Sahgal, Edward Chow and Joav Merrick (Editors)
2010. ISBN: 978-1-61668-365-8

Bone and Brain Metastases: Advances in Research and Treatment
Arjun Sahgal, Edward Chow and Joav Merrick (Editors)
2010. ISBN: 978-1-61728-085-6 (E-book)

Environment, Mood Disorders and Suicide
Teodor T. Postolache and Joav Merrick (Editors)
2010. ISBN: 978-1-61668-505-8

HEALTH AND HUMAN DEVELOPMENT

RURAL CHILD HEALTH

INTERNATIONAL ASPECTS

ERICA BELL
AND
JOAV MERRICK
EDITORS

Nova Biomedical Books
New York

For permission to use material from this book please contact us:
Telephone 631-231-7269; Fax 631-231-8175
Web Site: http://www.novapublishers.com

LIBRARY OF CONGRESS CATALOGING-IN-PUBLICATION DATA

Rural child health : international aspects / editors, Erica Bell and Joav Merrick.
p. ; cm. -- (Health and human development series)
Includes bibliographical references and index.
ISBN 978-1-60876-357-3 (hardcover)
1. Rural children--Health and hygiene. I. Bell, Erica, Dr. II. Merrick, Joav, 1950- III. Series: Health and human development series.
[DNLM: 1. Rural Health. 2. Adolescent. 3. Child. 4. Rural Health Services. 5. World Health. WA 390 R948045 2009]
RJ101.R87 2009
618.92--dc22

2009036328

Published by Nova Science Publishers, Inc. ✝ New York

CONTENTS

FOREWORD

Throughout the years, health research has focused mostly on urban and inner city subjects for various reasons. That focus has made our understanding of the health aspects of rural populations around the world less than adequate. In the past decade, more attention has been paid to rural areas and their health-related problems than ever before. However, it is still much less than the attention given urban centers. The fact that most universities and academic research centers are primarily located in urban areas has contributed to the dearth of studies. This is even more noticeable for child and adolescent health issues, despite the fact that in many areas of the world, rural health statistics regarding children and adolescents are more grim than those of urban areas. Adolescent morbidity and mortality worldwide continues to be the result of risk-taking behaviors and is mostly preventable. Accidents, homicide, suicide, teen pregnancy, sexually transmitted diseases, substance abuse and eating disorders are leading the way. In Kentucky in the United States for example, youth suicide rates are almost twice as high in some rural areas than those in the metropolitan areas.

In order to imrove this situation, much work needs to be done to address the health care needs of rural populations while taking into account cultural, ethnic and geographic differences.

This present book on "Child rural health. International aspects" edited by Erica Bell and Joav Merrick, two prominent authors and scientists, is dedicated to the health aspects of rural populations. This book addressess rural health care issues affecting people from childhood to geriatric age. It also provides unique aspects from various regions of the world. I feel that this will be a great resource for anyone working with rural populations anywhere and am confident that many training programs will add it prominently to their library. I know I will.

Hatim A Omar, MD
Professor of Pediatrics and Obstetrics/Gynecology
Director of Adolescent Medicine and Young Parent programs
Kentucky Clinic
University of Kentucky
Lexington, Kentucky, United States of America
E-mail: haomar2@uky.edu

INTRODUCTION

Erica Bell, PhD and Joav Merrick, MD, MMedSci, DMSc

University Department of Rural Health, University of Tasmania, Tasmania, Australia, National Institute of Child Health and Human Development, Office of the Medical Director, Division for Mental Retardation, Ministry of Social Affairs, Jerusalem, Israel and Kentucky Children's Hospital, University of Kentucky, Lexington, United States

RURAL CHILD HEALTH

Rural child health can be defined quite differently depending on the areas of practice, policy and research involved. Different definitions of rurality apply in different countries, depending on the purpose of those definitions, such as the allocation of government funding. What we do know is that rural child health is a concept that involves communities that are located away from major urban centres. These communities often have more limited resources, health infrastructure, workforce shortages, particular demographics and relatively poorer health outcomes (1). As one of the most vulnerable groups within these already often disadvantaged communities, rural children and adolescents face particular health challenges. This is so increasingly in a global community now facing cataclysmic events brought about by climate change and global economic meltdown, which are predicted to impose further great hardships on rural communities. For example, rural communities are likely to see the increasing effects of drought, new diseases and conditions brought about by climate change, displacements caused by peoples fleeing climate change, and other events that will require new styles of health and allied health practice and policy (2).

The rural health sector has developed a distinctive research literature, as well as professional organisations representing rural practitioners, medical education and training programs, as well as distinctive curriculum documents (3). There has been increasing recognition among policy-makers, practitioners and researchers that, for example, indigenous communities require styles of health and allied health practice that is responsive to the distinctive cultural contexts of indigenous people and their traditional lifestyles. In many countries these developments have helped position rural and remote communities to better deal with the health challenges of the new millennium.

THE CHALLENGES IN PRACTICE, POLICY AND RESEARCH

However, there is much work to be done in the area of rural child health. First, we need to develop our understandings of rural child health practice. It is known that, even in developed countries where government funding has made rural and remote health a major priority, many health and allied health professionals continue to be ill-prepared for the demands of rural practice (4). It is not simply that rural practice places particular demands on the health practitioner's clinical skills in a context in which large city hospitals may be far away. Rural practice also places new demands on the practitioner's repertoire of non clinical skills. For example, consideration of definitions of rural practice developed in countries such as Canada, the United Kingdom and Australia suggests they involve distinctive teamwork and communication skills, as well as ethical understandings (5-7). It follows that child and adolescent healthcare in rural communities also places a particular impost on the rural health professional's clinical and non clinical skills.

Second, we need to develop understandings of how to make policy work better for children and adolescents in rural communities. Health policy is an emerging discipline, led by the innovative work of Huw Davies and Sandra Nutley in the United Kingdom (8). The Blair government has developed a number of useful models of evidence-based health policy-making as part of its drive to modernise the public sector (9). However, in many developed and developing countries alike, high quality health policy-making continues to be an elusive goal. Too much health policy is made without good quality information about the particular health needs of rural children and adolescents. The reasons for this can range from free market ideology to lack of good quality information about rural communities. The consequences, however, continue to be poorer quality outcomes for these children and adolescents.

The third related challenge that faces us in improving outcomes in rural child health lies in research. There is an urgent need to develop the existing body of research on the needs of rural and remote children and adolescents. Research in rural communities represents particular challenges. Such research often involves small numbers, which make classical experimental designs difficult to implement. Further, the research participants can be difficult to engage for ethical, practical and cultural reasons. Finally, the research questions and methods often have to engage with complex challenges, such as chronic disease, which have causal conditions that lie not only in health, but also education, transport and welfare. In a context in which health often reinforces a gold standard of research that privileges big-*N* classical statistic methods in clinical experimental designs, research into rural child health runs the risk of being marginalised as a poor relation of biomedical research. The result is that those few researchers who are engaged with the particular needs of rural child health can often struggle to find forums (or grants) for their research that offer appropriate recognition. This serves to further hamper good quality health policy and practice for rural children and adolescents.

THE AIM OF THIS BOOK

In this context, this book offers an opportunity to reflect on the special needs of rural children and adolescents. It aims to contribute to the work of those researchers around the globe who have recognised that if we are to make a difference to rural child health internationally and in our respective countries, we must build a body of evidence that can better serve policy and practice for our rural communities.

Readers of this book will note that the papers published are about diverse subjects. However, they all share a focus on the particular practical and policy-making needs of rural and remote children and adolescents. They also share an interest in understanding health from a multi-disciplinary perspective. This means that they are about engaging with the contextual complexity facing policy-makers for, and practitioners in, rural communities. Accordingly, we commend this book to all those who want to stimulate new knowledge and international collaborations in rural child health.

REFERENCES

[1] Walker JH. Health informatics in action: Rural and remote health. In: Whetton S, eds. Health informatics: A socio-technical perspective. Melbourne, VIC: Oxford Univ Press; 2005:219-41.

[2] MacCracken M. Prospects for future climate change and the reasons for early action. J Air Waste Manag Assoc 2008;58(6):735-86.

[3] Smith J, Hays R, Sen Gupta T. Is rural medicine a separate discipline? Aust J Rural Health 2004;(12):67-72.

[4] Smith D. Barriers facing junior doctors in rural practice. Rural Remote Health 2005;5:348.

[5] ACRRM. ACRRM Primary Curriculum for Rural and Remote Medicine (Edition 3). 2007 [online]. Australian College of Rural and Remote Medicine. Available at: http://www.acrrm.org. au/main. asp?NodeID=90. Accessed 3 July, 2008

[6] Rourke J, Frank JR. Implementing the CanMEDS physician roles in rural specialist education: the multi-speciality community training network. Rural Remote Health 2005;5:406.

[7] Prime RD Ltd. Map of competencies for rural and remote healthcare. Bristol: Skills for Health, 2004.

[8] Davies H, Nutley S, Smith P. Introducing evidence-based policy and practice in public services. In: Davies H, Nutley S, Smith P, eds. What works? Evidence based policy and practice in public services. Bristol: Policy Press, 2000:1-11.

[9] Government Chief Social Researcher's Office. Magenta Book: Guidance Notes on Policy Evaluation. 1997 [online]. Cabinet Office. Available at: http://www.nationalschool.gov.uk/policyhub/magenta_book/index.asp. Accessed 21 May, 2008

Section One:
Holistic Approaches to Rural Child Health

In: Rural Child Health: International Aspects
Editors: Erica Bell and Joav Merrick

ISBN: 978-1-60876-357-3

Chapter 1

QUALITY OF LIFE AND ADOLESCENTS IN RURAL KENTUCKY

Hatim A Omar, MD, FAAP*[*1], Søren Ventegodt, MD, MMedSci, EU-MSc-CAM[2,3,4,5,6] and Joav Merrick, MD, MMedSci, DMSc[1,7,8]

[1]Kentucky Children's Hospital, University of Kentucky, Lexington, United States of America

[2]The Quality of Life Research Center, Copenhagen, Denmark

[3]Research Clinic for Holistic Medicine, Copenhagen, Denmark

[4]Nordic School of Holistic Medicine, Copenhagen, Denmark

[5]Scandinavian Foundation for Holistic Medicine, Sandvika, Norway

[6]Interuniversity College, Graz, Austria

[7]National Institute of Child Health and Human Development, Jerusalem, Israel

[8]Office of the Medical Director, Division for Mental Retardation, Ministry of Social Affairs, Jerusalem, Israel

In many rural areas in Kentucky, adolescents lack the basic assets for a good quality of life, such as having caring adults, a safe place and useful activities after school. In this chapter we analyze data from middle and high school students referred to a comprehensive school based health promotion center (SBHPC). From August 2006 to February 2008, a total of 382 students (200 female, 182 male, aged 12-18 years) were referred to the SBHPC for help. Only two (0.5%) students had two parents living with them and 12 (3.1%) had safe, organized after school activities. 19.9% of the total were suicidal, 27.2% used drugs, 44% smoked, 26.7% used alcohol, 45% were depressed, 29.3% had conduct problems, 37.4% had school problems, 43% were overweight, 50% lacked safety procedures (seat belts, access to guns) and 17.5% had other mental health

* Correspondence: Professor Hatim Omar, MD, FAAP, Director of Adolescent Medicine and Young Parent programs, J422 Kentucky Clinic, Department of Pediatrics, Kentucky Children's Hospital, University of Kentucky College of Medicine, Lexington, KY 40536 United States. Tel. 859-323-6426 ext. 311; Fax. 859-257-7706; E-mail: haomar2@uky.edu

problems. Conclusions: Poor quality of life is a major factor leading to negative outcomes in rural adolescents.

INTRODUCTION

Adolescent mortality and morbidity is directly related to risk taking behaviors. Leading causes include accidents, homicide and suicide. Many protective factors contribute to reduction of risk taking behaviors. Factors such as having two parents or at least one supportive adult, access to a safe place for interaction with others and having a useful afterschool activity with adult supervision contibute to improved quality of life and thus decreased risk taking behaviors (1-5). When adolescents have good quality of life, they tend to be more productive and less likely to take major risks, which in turn lead to decreased morbidity and mortality. Rural areas of Kentucky have mostly white population, high unemployment and increased rate of divorce, possession of fire arms and drug abuse. In this study we evaluated the quality of life of adolescents in a rural area of the state in order to understand causes of higher rates of risk taking behaviors and poor outcome results.

OUR STUDY

In August of 2006, we established the School Based Health Promotion Center (SBHPC) in a rural county of Kentucky. This center is operating from the area Board of Education Building and serves adolescents in the school system from 6th to 12th grade. Teachers, school counselors, parents, local health care providers and the court system in the area refer students to the SBHPC for evaluation and intervention. Students who exhibit risk taking behaviors, violate the law or are at risk for failing school are referred. For this study, we analysed data from middle and high school students referred to the SBHPC between August 2006-February 2008. Simple percentages were calculated for demographics and risk taking behaviors and compared with the data on the state level. Although Kentucky ranks among the top states in regards to health care provision for children and adolescents (6), Kentucky adolescents have higher than the national average rates of risk taking behaviors and poor outcomes (7).

FINDINGS

During the study period, a total of 382 students with an age range of 12-18 years were referred to the SBHPC. All were white/caucasian, 200 (52%) were females and 182 (48%) were males. Only two students (0.5%) had two biological parents living with them and only 12 (3.1%) had safe, organized afterschool activities. Results regarding risk taking behaviors compared with the data on the state levels are shown in table 1. Data for state wide results were obtained from the Kentucky youth risk behavior survey (YRBS) (7).

Table 1. Outcome measures at the SBHPC and the State of Kentucky (YRBS)

Outcome	SBHPC Students	KY YRBS
Smoking (daily)	44%	21.1%
Regular alcohol use	26.7%	11.3%
Regular marijuana use	27.2%	16.4%
Depression	45%	29.4%
Suicidal plan	19.9%	11.9%
Conduct problems	29.3%	13.7%
Obese/overweight	43%	17%
Other mental health problems	17.5%	11.2%
Physical/Sexual abuse	26.7%	13%

DISCUSSION

The results of this study showed much higher rates of risk taking behaviors among the rural adolescents evaluated in the SBHPC. It also shows extremely high percentage of lack of protective factors, such as supportive parents or other adults, lack of a safe place for after school activities or even the availability of such activities altogether. Adolescents who have access to supportive parenting, safe schools and productive activities (1-5) are more likely to have better outcomes and less risk taking behaviors.

Many adolescents in rural areas live in single parent homes and are exposed to higher rates of physical and sexual abuse, violence, access to fire arms and drug use than their urban counter parts. Poverty levels are also high in these areas and many families are multiple generations of wellfare reciepients that lack the culture of hard work and self reliance. Many of these teens have nothing to do after school, which results in their activities usually replaced by peer groups getting together for smoking, dinking alcohol, usind illicit drugs and high risk sexual activity. The combination of these factors, contibutes to increased levels of depression, poor self esteem and suicidality.

This study is very limited, because of the small number of participants included, retrospective nature of the study and lack of actual control. However, the results are still adequate to show that poor quality of life as assessed by lack of caring adults, safe place and availability of after school activities may be a significant factor leading to poor outcomes in rural adolescents.

ACKNOWLEDGMENTS

Thanks to Eva Stone, licensed nurse practiotioner, without whose help none of this study would have been possible.

REFERENCES

[1] Sesma AJr, Roehlkepartain EC. Unique strengths, shared strengths: Developmental assets among youth of color. Search Inst Insights Evid 2003;1(2):1–13.

[2] Lerner RM, Benso PL, eds. Developental assets and asset-building communities: Implications for research, policy, and practice. New York: Kluwer/Plenum, 2003:19-43.

[3] Scales PC, Leffert N. Developmental assets: A synthesis of the scientific research on adolescent development, 2nd ed. Minneapolis: Search Inst, 2004.

[4] Center for Disease Control and Prevention. Improving the health of adolescents and young adults: A guide for states and communities. Atlanta, GA: CDC, 2004

[5] US Department of Health and Human Services Healthy people 2010: Understanding and improving health and objectives for improving health, 2nd ed. Washington, DC: US Gov Printing office, 2000.

[6] Shea KK, Davis K, Schor EL. US variations in child health system performance: A state scorecard. Commonwealth Fund Publ 2008;1140. www.commonwealthfund.org

[7] Eaton DK, Kann L, Kinchen S, Shanklin S, Ross J, et al. Youth risk behavior surveillance United States, 2007. MMWR Surveill Summ 2008;57(4):1-131.

In: Rural child health: International aspects
Editors: Erica Bell and Joav Merrick

ISBN: 978-1-60876-357-3

Chapter 2

HOME ENVIRONMENT AS A DETERMINANT OF PSYCHOLOGICAL HARDINESS AMONG CREATIVE INDIAN ADOLESCENTS

Jagpreet Kaur**, PhD, MSc, MEd, PGDCA and Kulwinder Singh, PhD, MPhil, MA, BSc

Depatment of Education,
Punjabi University, Patiala, India

The role of psychological hardiness in stress reduction and enhancing self-esteem and social competence, as well as life-satisfaction including success has been documented in a varied manner by Western researchers. In a similar vein, the present investigation is an attempt to study home environment as a determinant of psychological hardiness in a random sample of 1,011 Indian adolescents through descriptive method of research. The results of the study revealed creative adolescents to be more hardy than their non-creative counterparts. Further, the adolescents having higher levels of control, protectiveness, conformity, reward, nurturance and permissiveness were more hardy than their counterparts with lower level of these home environment dimensions. Further, creative adolescents with more protectiveness and permissiveness component of home environment were found to be more hardy than their counterparts having low level of these home environment dimensions. The results of the study emphasize upon the improvement of home environment in terms of parental control, conformity, reward and nurturance for enhancing psychological hardiness and creativity among adolescents.

INTRODUCTION

Psychological hardiness - as a combination of adaptive personality traits that allows one to overcome stressful life-events - has emerged as an important variable in psychological researches in the previous two decades. Kobasa (1) proposed hardiness as a personality style that is a source of positive resistance to the debilitating effects of stressful life events on

* Correspondence: Lecturer Jagpreet Kaur, PhD, MSc, MEd, PGDCA, Department of Education, Arts Block no 5, Punjabi University, Patiala (PB), 147002 India. E-mail: jagpreetmahal@yahoo.com

health. The hardy personality is a constellation of three important personality traits: commitment, control and challenge, Hardy persons tend to have dedication to a purpose, a sense of control over events and tend to perceive events as facilitating in all life situations. Kobasa et al (2) presented hardy persons "as having considerable curiosity and tending to find their experiences interesting and meaningful. They believe they can be influential through what they imagine, say and do. They accept change to be the norm, and regard it as the key to development". Hardiness is thus considered as the measure of one's tendency to make relationship with oneself and one's outside world through a process of understanding conditions around oneself and about capacity to survive and excel in different life situations. Maddi et al (3) found that apparently, people who have the courage (hardiness) to simultaneously favor involvement with others and events (commitment), keep trying to influencing the outcomes going on around them (control), and emphasize learning from their experiences, whether positive or negative (challenge), have more fulfilling, satisfying, resilient and remarkable lives.

Psychological hardiness among adolescents has been studied by researchers in varied manner. Hannah and Morrisey (4) reported a highly significant negative relationship between age and hardiness, when school grade was taken into account. Further, female subjects were found to be high hardy than the male subjects. Wiebe (5) found that high hardy subjects perceived the stressor as less threatening, responded to the stressor with more positive affect

Shepperd and Kashani (6) indicated that adolescents high in either commitment or control experienced fewer somatic problems than their counterparts. Hoblit (7) in a study on 101 adolescents reported that hardiness and family support exerted significant effects psychological health. Sansone et al (8) indicated that hardiness reflected a productive approach to the amount of stress experienced in one's environment that is independent of neuroticism. Maddi et al (9) supported the conceptualization of hardiness as "vigorous mental health". Further, hardiness appeared to be the pervasive aspect of personality reflecting a general tendency, which involves showing psychological health, extroversion, openness, and conscientiousness. Baramee and Blegen (10) found a significant relationship of hardiness with student effort, clinical learning environment and student- faculty relationship among Thai nursing graduates.

McCall (11) observed that hardy individuals expressed lower levels of perceived stress throughout their development. Amat (12) reported that adjustment scores and hardiness scores of male and female international students were not significantly different. Results also indicated that western international students were hardier that non-western international students.

Bartone et al (13) found that special forces course graduates (US Army) were significantly higher in psychological hardiness, as compared to non-graduates. Psychological hardiness appears to be an important individual characteristic associated with stress tolerance and successful performance in highly demanding occupations.

While looking into hardiness among adolescents vis-à-vis social and psychological factors, it may be noted that hardiness among gifted, especially the creative ones along with home environment is a neglected area and hence needs to be studied. In this chapter our objectives were:

- To study psychological hardiness among school-going adolescents in relation to creativity.
- To study psychological hardiness among school-going adolescents in relation to home environment.
- To study psychological hardiness among creative school-going adolescents in relation to home environment.

and in order to fulfill the objectives of the study, the following hypotheses were formulated:

- Creative school-going adolescents will have higher levels of psychological hardiness as compared to their non-creative counterparts.
- School-going adolescents having better home environment will have higher levels of psychological hardiness as compared to their counterparts with poor home environment.
- Creative school-going adolescents having better home environment will have higher levels of psychological hardiness as compared to their non-creative counterparts having poor home environment.

The key terms used in the study are operationally defined as under:

- Psychological hardiness is conceived as a personality-based tendency to diminish the impact of stressful life events by optimistic cognitive appraisals and decisive coping actions. It is defined as a constellation of three dispositions – control, commitment, and challenge and summation of three determining psychological hardiness.
- Creativity in the present investigation has been considered as a multidimensional attribute, differentially distributed unevenly among individuals and consisting the abilities of fluency, flexibility, originality, and expressed accordingly by respondent score on these abilities as measured by the verbal test of creative thinking by Mehdi (15). The summated scores on these abilities have been taken as composite creativity scores.
- Home environment refers to the quality and quantity of the cognitive, emotional and social support that has been available to the child within the home and note the psychological environment of home as perceived by school-going adolescents in terms of: parental attitude towards education; parental aspirations for child; parental encouragement to the education of child and general behaviour of parents in the family"; to be measured by Home Environment Inventory, developed by Misra (16) having 100 items, divided into ten dimensions namely:

    - Control (autocratic atmosphere in which many restrictions are imposed on children by the parents in order to discipline them)
    - Protectiveness (prevention of independent behaviour and prolongation of infantile care)
    - Punishment (physical as well as affective punishment to avoid the occurrence of undesirable behaviour)

- o Conformity (parents' directions, commands, or orders with which child is expected to comply by action, including to demands to work according to parents' desires and expectations)
- o Social Isolation (use of isolation from beloved persons, except family members for negative sanctions)
- o Reward (material as well as symbolic rewards to strengthen or increase the probability of desired behaviour of child in expected social conditions);
- o Deprivation of privileges (controlling children's behaviour by depriving them of their rights to seek love, respect and child care from parents, depending on child's behaviour)
- o Nurturance (existence of excessive unconditional physical and emotional attachment of parents with the child, in which parents have a keen interest in the child and love for the child)
- o Rejection (conditional love recognizing that the child has no right as a person, no right to express his feelings, no right to uniqueness and no right to become an autonomous individual, thereby meaning that parental expectations are on an authoritative principle) and
- o Permissiveness (provisions of opportunities to child to express his views freely and act according to his desires with no interference from parents, and providing and atmosphere for the child to express in his own way).

Thus, it may be summed up that total home environment refers to both positive and negative conditions, which interact with each other, either favourably or unfavourably, to determine home environment to be "better" or "poor" on these ten dimensions.

- School-going adolescents: In the present study, it refers to the adolescents studying in eleventh grade in government secondary schools of Punjab (creative and non-creative adolescents taken together).

OUR STUDY

The population of the study was the secondary school students studying in 1,151 secondary schools situated in 17 districts (now 20) in Punjab state of India. The number of schools in each district in Punjab varies from 23 in Mansa to 145 in Ludhiana. Keeping in view, the uneven location of schools in the districts, two districts each were selected randomly from three clusters of districts having highest, average and lowest number of schools. Further, selection of schools from each of these six randomly selected districts was made on random basis giving due weightage to boys and girls schools situated in urban and rural areas. A total of 44 schools were randomly selected for the conduct of the present study. A sample of 30-45 adolescents studying in eleventh grade from randomly selected 44 schools from different districts of Punjab, totaling 1,011 adolescents (male = 448 and female = 563; mean age = 17 years) was taken for assessment of creative talent, psychological hardiness and home environment.

RESEARCH TOOLS

The Psychological Hardiness Scale (14) was used for measuring psychological hardiness among adolescents. This is a 30-item scale having 17 positively worded and 13 negatively worded statements, to be responded on 5-point Likert scale: strongly agree (1), agree (2), neither agree nor disagree (3), disagree (4) and strongly disagree (5). The scale has 10 items each pertaining to challenge, control and commitment dimensions. The scoring in case of positively worded statements is from "5 to 1" from 'strongly agree' to 'strongly disagree' and vice versa in case of negatively worded statements. The range of score is 30-150 for psychological hardiness and high score is indicative of being a hardy individual.

Verbal test of creative thinking developed (15) was used to classify adolescents in terms of being creative and non-creative. The test contains certain primary traits related to divergent thinking, which seem to go with creative output. The verbal test of creative thinking consists of four activities, namely, consequences test, unusual uses test, similarity test, and product improvement test. The dimensional scores obtained from each of the test activities are fluency, flexibility and originality. The summated scores on these abilities have been taken as composite verbal creativity scores.

The Home Environment Inventory (HEI) (16) was used to measure the psycho-social climate of home as perceived by adolescents. It provides a measure of the quality and quantity of the cognitive, emotional, and social support that has been available to the child within the home. HEI contains 100 items related to 10 dimensions of home environment as mentioned above. Each dimension has ten items belonging to it. It may be mentioned that this scale has considered both positive and negative reward mechanisms to discipline the child for adult role, and higher score in each component depicts a distinctive feature – though integral part of home environment.

The inventory required pupils to tell the frequency with which a particular parent-child interaction behaviour has been observed by them in their homes i.e. he/she was requested to tell whether a particular parental behaviour (as mentioned in an item) occur as mostly, often, sometimes, least and never. There is no time-limit for this tool.

DATA COLLECTION

The investigators personally visited the schools for the purpose of data collection. The respondents were made aware about the purpose of the study and assured that the information provided by them would be kept confidential and used for research purposes only. The assessment of creative talent was done by verbal tests of creative thinking. After identification of creative and non-creative adolescents based on first and third quartile respectively (Q1 = 139 and Q3 = 171), the test of psychological hardiness and home environment inventory were administered.

FORMATION OF FACTORIAL DESIGN

The perceptions of school-going adolescents with regard to home environment, as measured with the help of Home Environment Inventory (16) provided scores on ten dimensions. The means and standard deviations obtained by students on each of these dimensions along with median and Ist (P25) and III rd quartile (P75) are provided in table 1.

Table 1. Means and SDs of scores of ten dimensions of home environment obtained by school-going adolescents

S. No.	Home Environment Component	Mean	SD	Median	P_{25}	P_{75}
1.	Control	20.87	6.01	21	17	25
2.	Protectiveness	26.72	6.28	27	23	31
3.	Punishment	26.56	5.98	27	23	30
4.	Conformity	30.94	13.07	31	27	35
5.	Social Isolation	14.32	7.01	14	9	19
6.	Reward	30.22	6.57	31	26	35
7.	Deprivation of Privileges	12.45	6.86	12	7	17
8.	Nurturance	23.61	6.4	24	20	28
9.	Rejection	12.03	6.81	12	7	17
10.	Permissiveness	18.33	5.76	18	14	22

On the basis of the Ist (P25) and III rd quartile (P75) cut points on each of these dimensions of home environment, the number of school-going adolescents was identified as given in table 2.

Table 2. Distribution of school-going adolescents on ten dimensions of home environment

S. No.	Home Environment Component(B)	Level	Total
1.	Control	Better (B_1)	269
		Poor (B_2)	294
2.	Protectiveness	Better(B_1)	278
		Poor (B_2)	292
3.	Punishment	Better(B_1)	326
		Poor (B_2)	302
4.	Conformity	Better(B_1)	277
		Poor (B_2)	281
5.	Social Isolation	Better(B_1)	275
		Poor (B_2)	277
6.	Reward	Better (B_1)	292
		Poor (B_2)	264
7.	Deprivation of Privileges	Better(B_1)	283
		Poor (B_2)	284
8.	Nurturance	Better(B_1)	275
		Poor (B_2)	293
9.	Rejection	Better(B_1)	265
		Poor (B_2)	286
10.	Permissiveness	Better(B_1)	291
		Poor (B_2)	267

These adolescents with better and poor home environment dimensions were further classified into creative and non-creative on the basis of Ist (P25) and III rd quartile (P75) cut points on creativity scores as shown in table 3.

Table 3. Description of scores of school-going adolescents on ten dimensions of home environment

S. No.	Home Environment Component(B)	Level	High Creative (A_1)	Low Creative (A_2)	Total
1.	Control	Better(B_1)	67	73	140
		Poor (B_2)	75	71	146
2.	Protectiveness	Better(B_1)	65	83	148
		Poor (B_2)	92	72	164
3.	Punishment	Better(B_1)	92	84	176
		Poor (B_2)	81	70	151
4.	Conformity	Better(B_1)	71	68	139
		Poor (B_2)	77	74	151
5.	Social Isolation	Better(B_1)	76	71	147
		Poor (B_2)	64	84	148
6.	Reward	Better (B_1)	72	76	148
		Poor (B_2)	77	62	139
7.	Deprivation of Privileges	Better(B_1)	85	74	159
		Poor (B_2)	66	85	151
8.	Nurturance	Better(B_1)	69	79	148
		Poor (B_2)	77	89	166
9.	Rejection	Better(B_1)	75	70	145
		Poor (B_2)	70	75	145
10.	Permissiveness	Better(B_1)	66	81	147
		Poor (B_2)	92	55	147

In order to study the effect of home environment in terms of its ten dimensions on psychological hardiness among creative adolescents, 2 x 2 factorial design was formulated. The distribution of creative and non-creative adolescents in terms of high/better and low/poor levels of each of the dimensions of home environment obtained on the basis of 1,011 school-going adolescents is provided in table 3. It may also be seen from table 3 that number of adolescents, as expected to have differential pattern of distribution, varied in term of being high (above P75) and low (below P25).

OUR FINDINGS

In order to test the significance of mean differences in psychological hardiness across high and low levels of creativity in relation to ten dimensions of home environment, two-way ANOVA was applied, the summary of which is presented in the table 4.

Table 4. Summary of analysis of variance (creativity x home environment): Psychological hardiness

S. No.	Source of Variation	SS	df	MS	F
1.	Creativity (A)	15219	1	15219	785.92**
	Control Component of Home Environment(B)	2130	1	2130	109.94**
	A X B	37	1	37	1.88
	Within	3817	196	19	
	Total	21022	199		
2.	Creativity (A)	15365	1	15365	446.41**
	Protectiveness Component of Home Environment (B)	2443	1	2443	70.89**
	A X B	202	1	202	5.87*
	Within	6746	196	34	
	Total	24756	199		
3.	Creativity (A)	15051	1	15051	270.13**
	Punishment Component of Home Environment (B)	130	1	130	2.33
	A X B	10	1	10	0.18
	Within	10921	196	56	
	Total	26112	199		
4.	Creativity (A)	16891	1	16891	443.08**
	Conformity Component of Home Environment (B)	3943	1	3943	103.42**
	A X B	0	1	0	0.00
	Within	7472	196	38	
	Total	28306	199		
5.	Creativity (A)	15726	1	15726	305.51**
	Social Isolation Component of Home Environment (B)	0.00	1	0.00	0.00
	A X B	33	1	33	0.64
	Within	10140	196	51	
	Total	25894	199		
6.	Creativity (A)	14792	1	14792	386.28**
	Reward Component of Home Environment (B)	2578	1	2578	67.31**
	A X B	16	1	16	0.41
	Within	7505	196	38	
	Total	24891	199		
7.	Creativity (A)	15506	1	15506	295.6**
	Deprivation of PrivilegesComponent of Home Environment (B)	43	1	43	0.82
	A X B	14	1	14	0.27
	Within	10281	196	52	
	Total	25844	199		
8.	Creativity (A)	18298	1	18298	508.42**
	Nurturance Component of Home Environment (B)	2387	1	2387	66.34**
	A X B	30	1	30	0.82
	Within	7054	196	36	
	Total	27769	199		
9.	Creativity (A)	14552	1	14552	347.43**
	Rejection Component of Home Environment (B)	37	1	37	0.88
	A X B	6	1	6	0.14
	Within	8209	196	42	
	Total	22804	199		
10.	Creativity (A)	12896	1	12896	498.13**
	Permissiveness Component of Home Environment (B)	1469	1	1469	56.74**
	A X B	212	1	212	8.20**
	Within	5074	196	26	
	Total	19651	199		

** $p < .01$, * $p < .05$

The perusal of table 4 reveals the main effect of creativity on psychological hardiness among adolescents averaged over high and low levels of each of the ten dimensions of home environment (F = 785.92, 446.41, 270.13, 443.08, 305.51, 386.28, 295.60, 508.42, 347.43, 498.13; $p < .01$) turned out to be significant. This shows that creative adolescents are significantly more hardy than their non-creative counterparts (see table 5).

Table 5. Means and SDs of psychological hardiness among adolescents in creativity x home environment factorial design

S. No.	Component of Home Environment (B)			Creativity (A)	
				Creative(A_1)	Non-creative (A_2)
1.	Control	Better (B_1)	Mean	107.92	91.37
			SD	4.69	3.97
		Poor (B_2)	Mean	102.26	84.00
			SD	4.98	3.88
2.	Protectiveness	Better (B_1)	Mean	110.20	90.66
			SD	8.51	3.77
		Poor (B_2)	Mean	101.20	85.68
			SD	5.11	5.00
3.	Punishment	Better (B_1)	Mean	103.80	86.00
			SD	7.74	6.51
		Poor (B_2)	Mean	104.96	88.06
			SD	8.96	6.35
4.	Conformity	Better (B_1)	Mean	110.14	91.70
			SD	9.34	3.74
		Poor (B_2)	Mean	101.28	82.88
			SD	4.41	5.66
5.	Social Isolation	Better (B_1)	Mean	105.88	87.38
			SD	8.54	6.02
		Poor (B_2)	Mean	105.00	88.12
			SD	7.65	6.20
6.	Reward	Better (B_1)	Mean	109.28	91.52
			SD	8.85	4.00
		Poor (B_2)	Mean	101.54	84.90
			SD	4.10	6.49
7.	Deprivation of Privileges	Better (B_1)	Mean	104.14	87.06
			SD	8.64	6.44
		Poor (B_2)	Mean	105.60	87.46
			SD	6.61	7.07
8.	Nurturance	Better (B_1)	Mean	110.26	90.36
			SD	8.14	4.29
		Poor (B_2)	Mean	102.58	84.22
			SD	6.03	4.78
9.	Rejection	Better (B_1)	Mean	103.52	86.80
			SD	6.23	6.67
		Poor (B_2)	Mean	104.72	87.32
			SD	6.81	6.16
10.	Permissiveness	Better (B_1)	Mean	108.54	90.42
			SD	6.51	3.52
		Poor (B_2)	Mean	101.06	87.06
			SD	4.12	5.64

Table 4 further shows the main effects of control, protectiveness, conformity, reward, nurturance and permissiveness dimensions of home environment on psychological hardiness among adolescents turned out to be significant (F = 109.94, 70.89, 103.42, 67.31, 66.34, 56.74; $p < .01$) showing that there are significant differences in psychological hardiness among adolescents across high and low levels of these six home environment dimensions. Further, it may be seen from table 5 that adolescents with higher level of these six home environment dimensions are significantly more hardy than their counterparts belonging to poor level of these six home environment dimensions.

The interaction effect of creativity with protectiveness and permissiveness dimensions of home environment turned out to be significant (F = 5.87; $p<.05$, 8.20; $p<.01$), meaning that significant main effect of creativity in combination with protectiveness and permissiveness dimensions of home environment are dependent upon each other to explain psychological hardiness among adolescents (see figure 1).

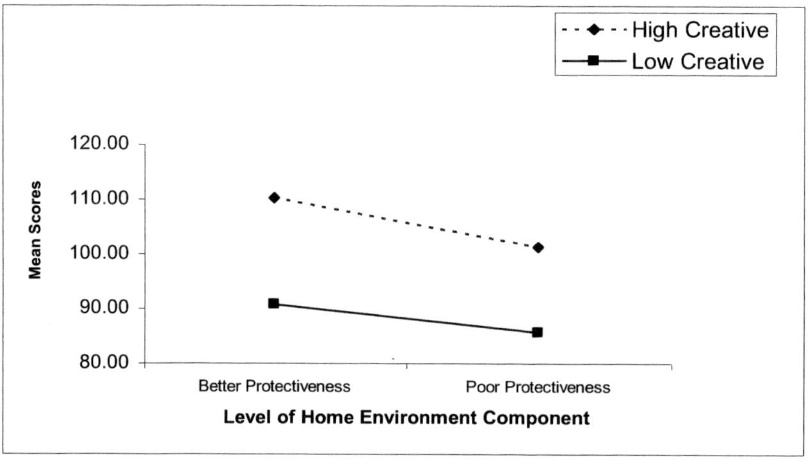

(i) Creativity x Protectiveness component of Home Environment

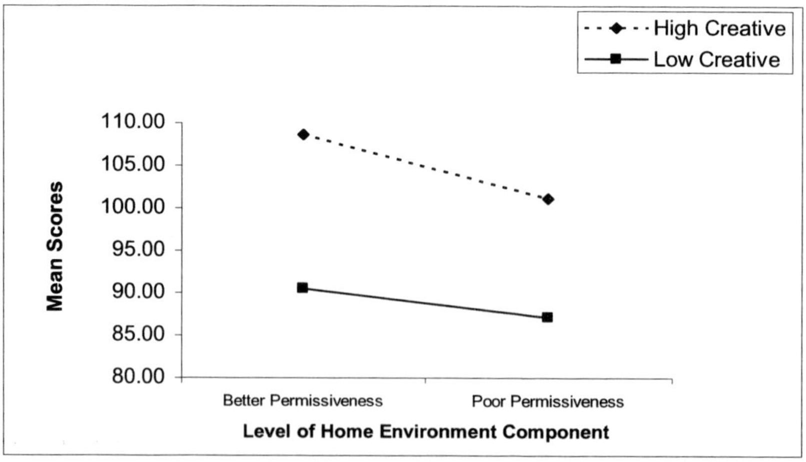

(ii) Creativity x Permissiveness component of Home Environment

Figure 1. Interactive effect of creativity and home Environment dimensions on psychological hardiness.

Also, table 5 shows that creative adolescents with higher nurturance (110.26) component of home environment have highest level of psychological hardiness as compared to their counterparts with higher control, protectiveness, punishment, conformity, social isolation, reward, deprivation of privileges, rejection and permissiveness dimensions of home environment. It may be mentioned here that non-creative adolescents with lower permissiveness component of home environment scored least on psychological hardiness. On the basis of results of the study, as reported in the preceding section, testing of hypotheses showed that:

- Since the main effect of creativity for psychological hardiness turned out to be significant, the hypothesis: "Creative school-going adolescents will have higher levels of psychological hardiness as compared to their non-creative counterparts" was accepted. Creative school-going adolescents have significantly higher level of psychological hardiness than their non-creative counterparts.
- The main effect of home environment on psychological hardiness in terms of its dimensions namely control, protectiveness, conformity, reward, nurturance and permissiveness is significant, whereas the main effect of home environment dimensions of punishment, social isolation, deprivation of privileges and rejection came out to be non-significant and hence the hypothesis: "School-going adolescents having better home environment will have higher levels of psychological hardiness as compared to their counterparts with poor home environment." was partially accepted. The results of the study revealed that school-going adolescents having higher levels of control, protectiveness, conformity, reward, nurturance and permissiveness dimensions of home environment are significantly more hardy than their counterparts having lower levels of these home environment dimensions.
- The interaction effect of creativity with home environment in terms of its ten dimensions on psychological hardiness came out to be significant for protectiveness and permissiveness dimensions of home environment only indicating that school-going adolescents with higher protectiveness and permissiveness dimensions of home environment were found to be more hardy than their counterparts having lower levels of home environment dimensions of protectiveness and permissiveness. Hence, the hypothesis: "Creative school-going adolescents having better home environment will have higher levels of psychological hardiness as compared to their non-creative counterparts having poor home environment." was partially accepted.

DISCUSSION

On the basis of the findings of the study it was found that creative adolescents possessed significantly higher level of psychological hardiness than their non-creative counterparts. Adolescents perceiving higher levels of home environment dimensions of control, protectiveness, conformity, reward, nurturance and permissiveness dimensions of home environment were significantly more hardy than their counterparts having lower levels of these home environment dimensions. The creative adolescents perceiving higher on protectiveness and permissiveness dimensions of home environment were found to be more hardy than their counterparts having lower levels of these home environment dimensions.

The results of the study revealed creative adolescents to be more hardy than their non-creative counterparts, especially when the home environment was more protective and permissive. Therefore, the creative talent at school stage need to be nurtured as the fuller use of creative and hardiness skills enhances possibilities for success and leadership for adolescents as they grow into adulthood and may help them during various dilemmas faced in life. The results are to be seen in the context of some related research evidence. Chan (17) reported hardiness to be having a direct effect on self-perceived creativity. The hardy students perceived themselves as engaging more in behaviors and activities that could be regarded as creative. Maddi et al (3) found hardiness to be correlated with innovative behavior, the correlation reaching statistical significance in case of challenge components of hardiness only. These findings support the hypothesis that the higher hardiness, the greater the likelihood of innovative, creative functioning. The results of the study suggest that the existence of hardiness encourages openness to other people and a willingness to strike out in uncharted directions.

Further, adolescents with better home environment dimensions of control, protectiveness, conformity, reward, nurturance and permissiveness were found to be hardier indicating that these home environment components contribute towards the enhancement of hardiness among adolescents. These results are in congruence with Failla and Jones (18), who found hardiness to be associated with family appraisal, social support, parental coping related to maintaining family integration, and satisfaction with family functioning. Higher satisfaction with family functioning was correlated with coping-integration, network support, functional support, and hardiness. In another study by Hoblit (19), family support was found to be an important factor in protecting health of low hardy young adolescents. Castillo (20) reported that undergraduate students high on hardiness and social support showed significantly more altruistic behaviors and family corrosion than their low hardy counterparts. Carson et al (21) found hardiness to be positively correlated with perceptions of family quality of life. However, Kaur (22) reported that the school-going adolescents with better family climate perceived significantly greater sense of control upon themselves than their counterparts with poor family climate. Thus, the findings of the present study pertaining to psychological hardiness vis-à-vis creativity and home environment have a theoretical and empirical support from the literature and these are logical and relevant to explain adolescents' development perspective for future life.

EDUCATIONAL IMPLICATIONS

In a rapidly changing world, the cultivation of a creative personality, sensitive and open to problems in his environment, is not only important, but also urgent. A special care and personalized support system is, therefore, imperative to nourish the creative potential of children by:

- Providing a stimulating environment that appeal to the child's developmental age level abilities and skills.

- Encouraging the child to experiment with the novel and unusual ideas and listening to the child's questions and comments about his or her observations.
- Relaxing and enjoying the creative process with the child for the development of creative thinking.
- Respecting the child's efforts and let them know that parents have confidence in his/her ability to do well.
- Exposing the child to a diversity of cultures, experiences, people, and ways of thinking and allowing them to see that there are different ways to think about a problem.
- Setting an example of the enjoyment of life experiences and the willingness to appreciate novel thinking processes.

So, it is suggested that hardiness training should be an important aspect of school enrichment programme and the families need to be strengthened as the hardy individuals and groups take the lead in change, show greater performance, leadership, morale, conduct, and health. Hardiness training approach can thus, help adolescents in building attitudes and managing resources, which improve the individual and can help turn adversity to advantage. Hardiness training has been used effectively with "at risk" students in college and university institutions (23-26). The retention rates have been found to increase substantially and grade point averages have also increased for those undergoing hardiness training, thus providing a benefit to both the individual and the institution (27-29). Taken together, these research findings on the effectiveness of hardiness training show a number of beneficial results that persist over time as trainees feel more self-confident, energetic, enthusiastic and more involved in the events going on around them. They have a sense of a better future for themselves. They feel more flexible, and open to whatever happens. Hardiness will help adolescents in mastering disruptive changes and conflicts in private life, which can include a range of typical living problems, or can emphasize subjects such as divorce, loneliness, marriage, addictions that include food, alcohol and drugs, or career.

Like any other research endeavor our study had a few limitations. Firstly, the population of the study was delimited to the adolescents studying in eleventh grade in government secondary schools of Punjab state of India. Also, creativity was assessed on the basis of verbal tests of creative thinking only. The secondary school students were classified with high and low levels of creative thinking on the basis of P75 and P25 cut points to be designated as creative and non-creative. The results might vary if non-verbal creativity or the summation of verbal and non-verbal creativity is taken for the identification of creative adolescents. Lastly, analytic approach to analysis i.e. analysis of variance was used in the analysis of data. In the light of these limitations of the present study, following suggestions for further research may be laid down:

- The present investigation was undertaken on secondary school boys and girls of 10+1 class. This study may be further extended to college and university students and adults.
- The sample of the present investigation included students of the same grade and approximately of the same age. The same may be expanded to cover various age and grade levels in order to make age-wise and grade-wise comparison.

- Only verbal measure of creativity was used to assess the creativity of the subjects. Non-verbal or figural creativity was not assessed. The results may vary if both verbal as well as figural measures are employed. The investigation using both types of measures, need to be designed so as to ascertain if a differential picture of the phenomenon emerges as a consequence of varying impact of both kinds of creative thinking.
- Different school systems are characterized by differential students of excellence in teaching, curricular and co-curricular activities and stimulation for creative and intellectual growth. It will be a useful research endeavor to compare adolescents from different school systems, such as government and private, Navodya and Central, and Public and Ordinary, on the phenomenon studied in this investigation.
- More socio-psychological variables can be incorporated in the research design to determine their possible influence on psychological hardiness.
- The study is conducted with normal children. Researches can be conducted in the area of special education within the groups of creative and intellectually gifted children.
- Socially disadvantaged group of students may be the focus of some researches to determine socio-psychological correlates of hardiness.
- Experimental studies may be undertaken to determine effect of certain curricular strategies and innovative methods of teaching on hardiness and creativity among school-going adolescents.

REFERENCES

[1] Kobasa, SC. Stressful life events, personality, and health: an inquiry into hardiness. J Pers Soc Psychol 1979;37:1-11.

[2] Kobasa SC, Maddi SR, Kahn S. Hardiness and health: A prospective study. J Pers Soc Psychol 1982;42:168-77.

[3] Maddi SR, Khoshaba DM, Persoci M, Lu J, Harvey R, Bleecker F. The personality construct of hardiness. J Res Pers 2002;36:72-85.

[4] Edward HT, Craig M. Correlates of psychological hardiness in Canadian adolescents. J Soc Psychol 1986;1271(4):339-44.

[5] Wiebe DJ. The role of hardiness in moderating the impact of stress. DAI (Dissertation Abstracts International)1988;50(3):1128-B.

[6] Shepperd JA, Kashani JH. The relationship of hardiness, gender, and stress to health outcomes in adolescents. J Pers 1991;59(4):747-68.

[7] Hoblit CK. Stressful events and the stress–moderating effects of hardiness and family support on adolescents' psychological health: A prospective study. DAI 1993; 54(5): 4730-B.

[8] Sansone C, Wiebe DJ, Morgan C. Self-regulating interest: The moderating role of hardiness and conscientiousness. J Per 1999; 67(4):701-33.

[9] Maddi SR, Harvey RH, Khoshaba DM, Lu JL, Persico M, Brow M. The personality construct of hardiness, III: Relationship with repression, innovativeness, authoritarianism, and performance. J Pers 2006;74(2):575-97.

[10] Baramee J, Blegen MA. New graduate perception of clinical competence: testing a causal model. Int J Nurs Stud 2003;40:389-99.

[11] McCall J. Development of hardiness III: Objective and subjective stress. Conf MU Undergrad Res Creative Achievements Forum, Columbia, MO, 2006.

[12] Amat S. An investigation of college adjustment and its relationship to hardiness. 14th Int Learning Conf, Johannesburg, SA, 2007.
[13] Bartone PT, Roland RR, Picano JJ, Williams TJ. Psychological hardiness predicts success in US army special forces candidates. Int J Selection Assess 2008;16(1):78-81.
[14] Nowack KM. Initial development and validation of a stress and health risk factor instrument. J Health Promot 1990;4:173-80.
[15] Mehdi B. Tests and manual for verbal and non-verbal tests of creative thinking. Agra: Natl Psychol Corp, 1973.
[16] Misra KS. Manual of home environment inventory. Agra: Ankur Psychol Agency, 1989.
[17] Chan DW. Self-perceived creativity, family hardiness, and emotional intelligence of Chinese gifted students in Hong Kong. J Sec Gifted Educ 2005;16(2/3):47-56.
[18] Failla S, Jones LC. Families of children with developmental disabilities: an examination of family hardiness. Res Nurs Health 1991;14(1): 41-50.
[19] Hoblit CK. Stressful events and the stress–moderating effects of hardiness and family support on adolescents' psychological health: A prospective study. DAI 1993;54(5):4730-B.
[20] Castillo SC. The relationship between hardiness, social support, family environment, and stress-related behaviors in college-age siblings of mildly handicapped children. DAI 1993;54(12):6491-B.
[21] Carson DK, Araquistain M, Ide B, Quoss B, Weigel R. Stress, strain, and hardiness as predictors of adaptation in farm and ranch families. J Child Fam Stud 1994;3(2):157-74.
[22] Kaur J. Psychological hardiness among school-going adolescents in relation to family climate. Dissertation. Patiala, India: Punjabi Univ, 2006.
[23] Maddi SR. Hardiness training at Illinois Bell Telephone. WI: Natl Wellness Inst, 1987.
[24] Rice M. The effect of structured hardiness training intervention program for stress on university women. DAI 1997;58(2):392-A.
[25] Judkins S, Furlow L. Creating a hardy work environment: can organizational policies help? Texas J Rural Health 2003;21(4):11-7.
[26] Judkins S, Reid B. Hardiness training among nurse managers: Building a healthy workplace. J Contin Educ Nurs 2006;37(5):202-7.
[27] Dillard NL. Hardiness and academic achievement. DAI 1990;52(8): 4121-B.
[28] Cozzi LM. The influence of hardiness, stress, and social support on academic achievement among urban commuter students. DAI 1991; 52(4):2339-B.
[29] Sheard M, Golby J. Hardiness and undergraduate academic study: The moderating role of commitment. Pers Individ Dif 2007;43(3): 579-88.

In: Rural child health: International aspects
Editors: Erica Bell and Joav Merrick

ISBN: 978-1-60876-357-3

Chapter 3

THE RURAL SCHOOL SUPPORT IN EARLY CHILDHOOD

Susan Johns**, *BEd, BAdVocEd, MEd (Research)
University Department of Rural Health, University of Tasmania, Launceston, Tasmania, Australia

The growing focus on early childhood intervention has seen a range of service providers enter the field. While research has been undertaken to inform the development of school-based models, very little focuses specifically on rural communities. Objective: The purpose of the study reported in this paper was to document the roles of rural schools in two Tasmanian sites in relation to the early years, and to identify factors that might influence the nature and extent of these schools' responses. The paper presents preliminary findings from the study. Study group: Interviews were conducted with three groups of participants from each site: (i) senior managers from government and non government agencies; (ii) staff from government, non government and community groups engaged in service provision, and (iii) a sample of parents of 0-4 year olds. Methods: This qualitative study uses multi-site, multi-method techniques, and a case study approach. Data were collected from three sources; interviews, written documentation, and observation. Data were analysed using NVivo data analysis software. Results: Rural schools support the early years in three main ways: service provision; brokering of services, and building capacity amongst service providers and the wider community. School activity is determined by the nature of the community and resource availability. Conclusions: By working collaboratively with other providers, rural schools contribute to the provision of a continuum of care and support for the early years. School contributions will be enhanced by an outward focus, an appreciation of the relative merits of other service providers, and dedicated funding.

---

* Correspondence: Susan Johns, PhD Candidate, University Department of Rural Health, University of Tasmania, Locked Bag 1372, Launceston, Tasmania, Australia 7250. E-mail: Susan.Johns@utas.edu.au

INTRODUCTION

Research indicates that the health and wellbeing of populations is related to community social capital, or sense of connectedness to community (1). Linked to this is the importance of family social capital (relationships between parents and children), in determining outcomes for children and youth (2,3). There is a strong and growing evidence base supporting the importance of the early years (0-4 year olds) in determining outcomes later in life across a range of indicators, including school achievement and retention, negative outcomes in terms of engagement with juvenile justice and teenage pregnancy, and unemployment (4-6). Research shows that patterns established in the early years of life are difficult to change as children develop, meaning that supports and interventions employed in the early years provide society with the best chance of improving children's life trajectories (7). A specific focus in the early years should be on reducing risk factors and enhancing protective factors (7) in order to ensure young children have attained age appropriate levels of physical, cognitive, emotional, psychological and social development by the time they begin compulsory schooling at five years of age. Sometimes this is referred to as school readiness in its broadest sense.

Ensuring school readiness means providing supports and services relating to child health and development, supporting parents to create a home environment that fosters early childhood development, and increasing the capacity of communities to support children and families. This paper is particularly concerned with the second and third areas: that is, building capacity of parents and communities to support the early years. Research identifies that positive outcomes for young children are linked to access to quality services such as childcare and preschool (8,9), as well as effective parenting and supportive neighbourhoods (9,10). Outcomes are enhanced when services and supports are strengthened and integrated (11). The evidence base provided by this research has driven a range of state, national and international strategies for the early years (see, for example, Children's Trusts in the United Kingdom; the Toronto First Duty project in Canada; the Australian government's Stronger Families and Communities Strategy 2004-2009, and various Australian state initiatives such as Families First in New South Wales, Children's Centres in South Australia, and Launching into Learning in Tasmania). Many of these strategies use schools as hubs for early childhood development and parenting, however the idea of schools as hubs or service centres is not new (12).

Some schools have been operating as hubs for many years, albeit in an informal way, and in most cases without additional funding. Until recently in Tasmania, schools wishing to provide programs for pre-kindergarten children (under four years of age) did so largely out of their own school resource package, or accessed limited-term funding from other external sources. State Department of Education funding did not begin until kindergarten, whereby each child was entitled to the equivalent of two full days per week of kindergarten. To attend kindergarten, children must reach four years of age by the end of the year prior to enrolment. Kindergartens in Tasmania are not separate entities, but operate as the first tier of primary school, generally located within the school or in some cases on an adjacent site. The extent of pre-kindergarten programs was determined by individual schools according to their priorities. Some schools provided a community playgroup; others provided a more structured pre-kindergarten program for children due to start kindergarten in the following year. Some schools offered a range of services; some offered few or no services.

In many small rural areas, the school offers the only early years' service available on site, and will most likely continue to be the focal point of early childhood activity, long after limited-term funded projects have come and gone. The extensive contributions of rural school to their communities, beyond education, is well documented (13). Research from a variety of fields such as education, management and community development, also documents factors that influence community collaborations, including the pivotal role of mediators or boundary crossers (14-16). Yet little research specifically focuses on small rural schools and the contributions they make to the early years, in the face of a range of context-specific issues such as lower population density, low socioeconomic status, inadequate or declining rural infrastructure, and geographic isolation. Similarly, less is known about the factors that influence how rural schools work collaboratively with parents of young children, and with the community more broadly. The purpose of this study is to explore early years' service provision and collaboration in rural areas.

OUR STUDY

This qualitative study uses a case study approach to investigate the nature of early childhood interventions involving schools in three small rural communities in Tasmania. Findings from two of the sites only are presented in this paper. Consistent with Creswell (17), a case study approach was determined to be appropriate because the phenomena being studied represented an entity bounded in time and place. Multiple sources of data were collected to enhance methodological triangulation (18), namely interviews, document analysis and observation. The specific objectives of the study were to document the different early childhood intervention arrangements that existed within the target communities, and to explore the impact of a range of factors on the capacity of schools and other agencies to provide these services. In line with research by Bazzoli et al (19), the overarching purpose was to assess the relations among different influencing factors, and between influencing factors, partnership processes and outcomes, rather than to map causation in terms of these variables.

Communities were defined using the Australian Bureau of Statistics category of local government areas (LGA). Rural was defined according to degree of remoteness from larger service centres using the Australian Standard Geographical Classification (ASGC) (20), with the majority of Tasmanian LGAs classified as outer regional. Small communities were determined to be LGAs with a combined population of no more than 10,000 people, as very little qualitative research on early childhood interventions has focused on communities of this size. The two LGAs featured in this paper were located in different parts of the state. Each comprised a larger population centre which was the seat of local government, together with a number of smaller population centres. Further details are provided below.

Sites were selected in consultation with a range of experts from the education, health, and community service sectors. They were selected to reflect different types and levels of early childhood activity and collaboration, and to include at least one site in which little early years' research had been undertaken previously.

Ethical approval was received from the Social Sciences Human Research Ethics Committee (Tasmania) Network in September 2006.

Data were collected from participants by semi structured, face-to-face interviews. Representatives from three groups were interviewed: (i) senior managers from relevant government and non government agencies; (ii) staff from government, non government and community groups engaged in service provision in the sites, and (iii) a sample of parents of 0-4 year olds living in each site. The parent sample was designed to include two sub groups: young parents (under 21 years) and parents of children with a developmental delay or disability. Parents were offered the option of focus group or individual interviews; all other participants were interviewed individually, or occasionally in pairs at their request. A total of 33 interviews was conducted in site 1 (four focus groups and 29 individual) and 37 in site 2 (four focus groups and 33 individual). Interviews were digitally recorded and transcribed. Transcripts were sent back to groups (i) and (ii) for validation.

Written documentation, including policy documents, strategic plans, reports and website material was collected, and participant observation notes made during visits to each site were typed up. Written documentation and participant observation notes, together with checked interview transcripts, were input into NVivo data analysis software. Data were then coded and analysed against themes from the literature as well as emerging themes. The findings presented in this paper are the result of preliminary analysis.

A limitation of the study was restricted access to parents who did not normally engage with services, despite attempts to recruit participants such as young mothers, by working with relevant community support groups and non government organisations. Also, only a small number of parents of children with a developmental delay or disability elected to participate (n=3 in site 1 and n=2 in site 2). Information about these sub groups of parents was largely derived from secondary sources (service providers).

BACKGROUND TO SITES

Site 1

This LGA has a population of 10,000. Half the population lives in the main population centre (Community 1A). This part of the LGA is classified as inner regional (20). The remainder of the population is scattered throughout the region in a number of very small centres. This part of the LGA is classified as outer regional (20). In terms of early years' services, the school configuration is as follows:

- Community 1A (two primary schools from K-6 and a high school from 7-10)
- Community 1B (district high school from K-10 with a skills centre for years 11-12, and adults)
- Communities 1C, 1D, 1E (each has a small primary school from K-6)

All schools are part of the same education administrative cluster. Community 1A is a 30 minute car trip to the nearest large service centre; the most distant community (Community 1E) is around 1.25 hours by car. Compared to the Tasmanian state average, within this site there are relatively high rates of unemployment, teenage parents, and children in the 0-4 age group, and relatively low rates of post compulsory education attainment and participation. Schools report between 50-75% of their students are receiving state government financial assistance due to low parental incomes.

Much early years' activity in the site has been externally driven, using local providers for service provision, with schools playing a key role. Since 2002, the site has been home to several large, government-funded early years' initiatives, designed to increase access to services and to facilitate service integration. Two were state government funded (departments of education, and health and human services, respectively) and one was funded by the Australian government.

Site 2

This LGA has a total population of approximately 6,000, comprised of one larger population centre (community 2A with a population of 2,100), two smaller population centres and several smaller hamlets. Nearly all the LGA is classified as outer regional, with a small percentage (6.8%) classified as remote (20). In terms of early years' services, the school configuration is as follows:

- Community 2A (district high school from K-10 plus skills centre for years 11 and 12, and adults)
- Community 2B (district high school from K-10, with provision for years 11 and 12)
- Community 2C (primary school from K-6)

An additional population centre (community 2D, population approximately 800) was included in the study, even though it is located in an adjacent LGA. Community 2D is included because it is in the same education administrative cluster, children from its primary school complete their secondary education at the district high school in community 2B, and the same early childhood service providers operate across each of Communities 2A to 2D.

The nearest large service centre is one hour by car from community 2C, and around 1.75 hours by car for the more distant communities (Communities 2A and 2D). The site has been a popular destination for retirees, from elsewhere in the state and from other Australian states. While there has traditionally been a focus on older people, the more recent influx of families with younger children has encouraged a greater focus on the provision of services for this group. Although the community represents all levels of socioeconomic status, the LGA has been identified as one of the most disadvantaged in the state, in terms of a range of indicators including inadequacy of access to services. There is also a higher than average rate of teenage pregnancies.

Early years' activity in this site has been both community driven and externally driven. School involvement across the site has been more limited than in site 1, although this is gradually changing. Site 2 is home to three government-funded early years' projects: one funded by the state department of education which is based around a model of schools as hubs, and two Australian government-funded projects, focusing on children's therapy and parent support interventions, respectively. One of the Australian government-funded projects was initiated by the community. The state department of education project was in early stages of development at the time interviews were conducted.

In both sites, lack of transport is a major problem, both within the LGA and between the LGA and the nearest large service centre. This relates to inadequate public transport infrastructure, and to the cost of owning and running a car.

OUR FINDINGS

Findings suggest that the nature and extent of school focus on the early years has developed in the context of a commitment at varying levels of the education hierarchy, including a commitment by individual schools. In site 1, a school District focus on the early years developed several years ago and provided a framework for action. The local District Superintendent, responsible for some 33 state government schools in the broader region, was a strong believer in the importance of early childhood intervention, and worked with principals in the development of a District Plan that included a focus on 0-4 year olds as one of the top five priorities. In site 2, a more recent statewide move by the state department of education to a smaller cluster structure for administrative purposes, provided for a coordinated approach to the early years. The cluster applied for and received department of education funding in 2007 to implement early years' initiatives. The proposal included the appointment of a cluster coordinator to coordinate planning and implementation of individual school initiatives, including shared professional development opportunities.

The individual rural schools in this study also demonstrated an awareness of their unique and central role in providing support to families, including those with pre school children. As a senior staff member from the district high school in community 1B notes: 'we actually support [the early years] because the range of other services is just so small'. Schools in both sites have principals and staff who are supportive of early years' initiatives, and where size permits, also have a supportive formal leadership structure in terms of a senior staff member with specific responsibility for early childhood (K-2) and early years' (pre school) initiatives. In site 1, two of the schools have a senior teacher position with a strong focus on early childhood. These people have worked with the community for some years and have extensive networks. As part of their role they actively seek opportunities for engagement with others who have expertise beyond what the school can offer. Working across multiple domains, their formal leadership positions allow them to act as mediators or boundary crossers (14, 15), accessing resources that can be used for the benefit of families and pre school children. One of these senior staff members reflects:

> "… in that [senior] role too you get to organise quite a few things and get to meet quite a few people outside of schools … and that's been particularly important in trying to access things for school and for families … you really do need to try to find a support base for people, it's not necessarily here".

Working within the context of their financial and human resource base, and management structure, rural schools in this study play three roles in supporting the early years:

- Provision of services for families
- Brokering services for families
- Building capacity amongst service providers and the wider community

SERVICE PROVISION

In site 1, all schools offer an informal community playgroup for parents and children 0-5 years. In all but one school, the playgroup is facilitated by a school staff member, usually the teacher's aide. These playgroups have been operating for some years, funded out of each school's resource package. Most of the schools also offer a school transition or pre-Kindergarten program for children due to start Kindergarten the following year. These are generally more structured than playgroup, with a stronger literacy and numeracy focus.

In site 2, the nature and extent of service provision is more varied, possibly reflecting the lack of an overarching framework for the early years until recently. Two of the schools (in Communities 2A and 2C) have only just introduced community playgroups in 2007, utilising state department of education funding for the early years, while the school in Community 2D has run a community playgroup for over twenty years, funded out of its own resource package. Playgroups are facilitated by a school staff member, either an early childhood teacher or a teacher's aide. The school in community 2B provides a venue for a parent-run community playgroup to meet each week, and has done so for a number of years, however it does not provide funds or staffing for the playgroup. In terms of school transition programs, again there is variation across the schools in this site. Schools in communities 2A, B and D have offered some form of school transition program for a number of years. The small primary school in community 2C is in the process of introducing a combined playgroup/school transition program for the first time, utilising department of education funding for the early years.

School-run community playgroups, in particular, provide socialisation opportunities for children and parents, role modelling and information for parents, and school familiarisation for children. Early screening for children with additional needs occurs informally. Community playgroups were identified by parents and service providers as important in connecting parents to each other and to the school community, and were particularly useful for those who are socially or geographically isolated. They provide a support network where you can 'chat and compare problems' with other parents. Connecting parents to community is a key part of effective parenting (1,10), leading to positive outcomes for young children. There is some evidence that school transition or pre-Kindergarten programs continue to build connections between school and parents, and to some extent between parents themselves, although they are more structured and have a stronger focus on school preparation for children. Relatively high rates of attendance by parents and children indicate that community playgroups and pre school transition programs are being well utilised, particularly in small rural areas where there are no other early years' services available on site.

It appears that availability of resources is a key factor in determining the extent to which schools are able to provide early years' services beyond the immediate school environment. In site 1, where schools did not have additional funding, most activities were located in the school. In site 2, which had just received additional early years' funding from the state department of education, there were plans to implement strategies to reach hard-to-engage and isolated parents through home visiting, outreach and mobile programs, consistent with good practice in the delivery of accessible early childhood services (21).

SERVICE BROKERING

There are examples of schools in both sites using their knowledge and resources to identify and access relevant services for families with pre school aged children. For some schools the focus has had a strong educational foundation, such as linking parents to specialist department of education services for pre school children with developmental delays and disabilities. For others, the focus is more holistic and includes relationships with a range of agencies from different sectors, which provide parent support and education, in addition to allied health and health services.

Service brokering activities ranged from provision of a venue for a visiting service or program, to referrals to therapy providers and parenting support programs, to development and implementation of a project designed to meet a specific community need. This is consistent with the range of service brokering activities identified in recent research (22). For some families, these needs may not have been met without the assistance of the school. School staff in site 1, in particular, cited examples of pre school children arriving at school with significant speech and/or other developmental delays, because parents either did not know about supports available, or did not know how to go about accessing appropriate services. Some of these families had not continued their relationship with the child health nurse beyond the first few months of their baby's life, which would have been the other most likely source of referral.

School playgroup facilitators, usually teachers' aides, play a bridging role, in terms of linking parents to the school, and to a range of other education-based and non education-based services. Playgroup parents in community 1B agreed that 'if we had any issues we'd talk to [name of facilitator] or we'd talk to [school] staff then they'd put you on the right track'. Most school playgroup facilitators have lived in the community for some years and are well known, trusted and respected. Sometimes playgroup facilitators also advocate on behalf of parents. All of these roles are consistent with brokering roles identified in the research (22,23). Like the early childhood teachers mentioned earlier, there are also indications that playgroup facilitators act as mediators or boundary crossers, because they have the trust of both parents and the school and are able to move freely between the two domains (14-16).

Beyond brokering of services for individual families, the schools in the study were also involved in brokering services and programs to benefit the child and parent population more broadly. In general, schools in site 1 were more actively involved in brokering these sorts of services than schools in site 2. This may be reflective of the nature of the community, given that at least half the schools in this site are located in very small, outlying communities with no other services. In site 1, the district high school in Community 1B , where there was no other childcare available, worked closely with the local Council and the childcare service in Community 1A to establish a family daycare centre onsite at the school. The purpose of the centre was to provide childcare so parents could undertake vocational education and training in areas such as childcare and aged care, at the school's skills centre. The service was vital given the relatively high rate of unemployment and low post compulsory education levels for the region. In a further development, a primary school in Community 1A is currently negotiating with the same childcare service to establish a similar arrangement, this time to care for young children while their parents are assisting in the school as parent helpers. This will allow the school to build stronger parent-school connections, which have been linked to better outcomes for children and youth (1,3).

In site 2, the district high school in community 2B, that also provides a venue for a parent-run community playgroup, brokered a state library-sponsored reading program for 0-4 year old children and their parents. The library funds staffing and resources, but the program is run at the school by the local Kindergarten teacher. It is held just before the parent-run community playgroup. The school made the intentional decision to run the session immediately before the community playgroup so parents and children could access both services. Had they been held on different days, transport issues, including the high cost of petrol, would have prevented a number of parents from attending both sessions.

School capacity to broker services differed, both within sites and across sites, and more detailed analysis of the factors influencing this is planned. Preliminary findings suggest that those schools most actively involved in brokering services have an extensive knowledge of services available within and outside the region, value and respect the skills and knowledge of workers from different workplaces and sectors, and are willing to access external professional expertise when needed. These findings are consistent with Polivka et al's research (24) on collaborative approaches to early interventions for children with developmental delays and disabilities, in which she established a direct link between situational factors (awareness of personnel from other agencies and awareness of the goals and services of other agencies), collaborative processes, and outcomes.

COMMUNITY CAPACITY BUILDING

There are examples of school staff, either individually or as a group, using their skills, knowledge and networks to contribute to capacity building for the early years beyond building the capacity of parents. This includes sharing their skills and knowledge formally and informally, initiating early years' services and projects to be delivered outside the school, and active involvement in joint ventures initiated by others. For example, a school playgroup facilitator was the driver of a new community playgroup that was established in a non-school setting in community 1A. She had identified a need for a playgroup in a neutral (non school) setting, to try to reach young parents and other hard-to-engage families: 'we needed a meeting place where people could come, feel comfortable and then I got their trust and could help them that way'. The playgroup was established with the initial support of the state department of education and two non government organisations (NGOs). Some two years after the playgroup was established, trust has been gradually built between some of the more marginalised parents and the facilitator, to the extent that three families had approached the facilitator over the past month seeking further assistance and support.

In site 2, staff from the school in Community 2A played a role, along with workers from the health and community service sectors, in devising and overseeing implementation of a project funded by the Australian government. The purpose of the project is to provide a mobile playgroup, including parent support and a speech, occupational and physiotherapy referral service, for families with children 0-4 years. It was developed in response to a need for parental support and increased opportunities for young children in terms of socialisation, literacy, numeracy and motor skills development.. The project is auspiced by a locally-based project worker employed by an off-site NGO experienced in children's therapy service provision. Although it has only been operating for a relatively short time, there is evidence that it is attracting some of the more isolated, hard-to-engage families, including young parents. There have also been a number of referrals of young children for therapy, as a result of early screening during the mobile playgroup sessions.

Early indications are that community capacity building in these sites is generally linked to externally-funded early childhood projects. Some of these projects have been funded by the education sector; others have involved representatives from schools assisting in the development of project proposals and implementation. This aligns with research (13) that found the education sector more broadly, and rural schools in particular, play a crucial role in community development.

DISCUSSION

The rural schools featured in this study play a key role in building family and community social capital, suggesting the potential of rural schools in early years' work. Australian initiatives that promote a schools-as-hubs model appear to be consistent with rural school practice in the two sites studied. For rural schools planning to introduce new early childhood services, it is suggested that the implementation process will be important, to ensure new programs and services do not duplicate or inadvertently replace existing community services. The relatively limited number of services available within some rural communities heightens the need for communication and collaboration between schools and other services, in an effort to build a continuum of care and support for the early years.

An inclusive approach to the early years requires a broad interpretation of the 'hub' concept, to ensure families are not marginalised by having services only operating within a school setting. The potential sphere of influence of schools is much wider than on-site service delivery, in terms of outreach, service brokering and broader community capacity building. Schools are well placed to broker services because they have an intimate knowledge of the communities in which they operate and the particular needs of families, as well as being part of a system that has both the influence and resources necessary to implement initiatives. The outreach and brokering roles of schools offer potential in terms of the early years, especially for geographically and/or socially isolated families who do not engage with other services. At the same time, of course, it is recognised that not all families feel comfortable engaging with schools, suggesting the need for schools to work with and through other local providers, such as child health nurses.

In order to explore the possibility of offering activities outside the school setting, or of collaborating with other service providers from the health, non government and community sectors, it is suggested that rural schools need to develop an outward focus and an understanding and appreciation of the work of different early childhood services and service providers. This will be influenced by a combination of factors including time, human and financial resources, the nature and level of commitment of schools to the early years, and fundamental school values and beliefs.

The issue of resourcing is ever present, and no more so than in rural schools. While small rural schools have the advantage of closeness to their communities, they are necessarily limited in terms of their resource base and small staff numbers, including the number of senior staff positions. In addition to a strong school commitment to the early years and an understanding of the holistic nature of child development, dedicated early years' funding is likely to make a significant difference to the capacity of small rural schools in particular, to address the needs of pre school children and their families.

ACKNOWLEDGMENTS

This chapter has been made possible through support provided by a Partners in Health scholarship, which is jointly funded by the Tasmanian Department of Health and Human Services, and thc Faculty of Health Science at the University of Tasmania. The researcher would also like to acknowledge support provided by her supervisors, associate professor Sue Kilpatrick and professor Bill Mulford, by providing comment on an earlier draft of this paper.

REFERENCES

[1] Putnam R. Bowling alone: The collapse and revival of American community. New York: Simon Schuster, 2000.

[2] Furstenberg FF, Hughes ME. Social capital and successful development among at-risk youth. J Marriage Fam 1995(57):580-92.

[3] Teachman JD, Paasch K, Carver K. Social capital and the generation of human capital. Soc Forces 1997; 75(4):1343-59.

[4] McCain M, Mustard F. Reversing the brain drain: Early study: Final report. Toronto: Ontario Children's Secr, 1999.

[5] Vimpani G. Health inequalities: The seeds are sown in childhood, what about the remedies? In: Eckersley R, Dixon R, Douglas B, eds. The social origins of health and well-being. Melbourne: Cambridge Univ Press, 2001:207–15.

[6] Carneiro P, Crawford C, Goodman A. Which skills matter? London: Centre Economics Educ, London School Economics, 2006.

[7] Shonkoff J, Philips D, eds. From neurons to neighborhoods: The science of early childhood development. Washington DC: Nat Acad Press, 2000.

[8] Phillipsen L, Burchinal M, Howes C, Cryer D. The prediction of quality from structural features of child care. Early Childhood Res Q 1997(12):281-303.

[9] Nelson RF. The impact of ready environments on achievement in kindergarten. J Res Childhood Educ 2005;19(3):215-21.

[10] Garbarino J, Kostelny K. Child maltreatment as a community problem. Child Abuse Negl 1992(16):445-64.

[11] Pelletier J, Corter C. Toronto first duty: Integrating Kindergarten, childcare, and parenting support to help diverse families connect to schools. Multicultural Educ 2005;13(2):30-7.

[12] Dryfoos JG. A revolution in health and social services for children, youth and families. San Francisco: Jossey-Bass, 1994.

[13] Kilpatrick S, Johns S, Mulford B, Falk I, Prescott L. More than an education: Leadership for school-community partnerships. Canberra: Rural Industries Res Dev Corp, 2002.

[14] Buxton CA, Carlone HB, Carlone D. Boundary spanners as bridges of student and school discourses in an urban science and mathematics high school. School Sci Mathemat 2005;105(6):302-12.
[15] Kilpatrick S, Auckland S, Johns S, Whelan J. Building capacity for rural health: The role of boundary crossers in coalition maturity for partnerships with external agents. In: Doyle L, Adams D, Tibbitt J, Welsh P, eds. Building stronger communities: Connecting research, policy and practice. Leicester: Nat Inst Adult Continuing Educ (NIACE), 2008:220-36.
[16] Taylor M. Communities in the lead: Power, organisational capacity and social capital. Urban Stud 2000;37(5-6):1019-35.
[17] Creswell JW. Qualitative inquiry and research design: Choosing among five traditions. Thousand Oaks, CA: Sage, 1998.
[18] Stake R. The art of case study research. Thousand Oaks, CA: Sage, 1995.
[19] Bazzoli GJ, Stein R, Alexander JA, Conrad DA, Sofaer S, Shortell SM. Public-private collaboration in health and human service delivery: Evidence from community partnerships. Milbank Q 1997; 75(4):533-61.
[20] ABS. Australian Standard Geographical Classification (ASGC), Australian Bureau of Statistics Cat No 12160 2005 [cited 2007 15 July]; Available from: http://www.abs.gov.au/AUSSTATS/abs@.nsf/Previousproducts/1216.0Contents12005?opendocument &tabname=Summary&prodno=1216.0&issue=2005&num=&view=
[21] Rogers P, Edgecombe G, Kimberley S. Evaluation of the stronger families and communities strategy 2000-2004: Early intervention – particularly in early childhood. Issues Paper. Canberra: Dept Fam Community Serv, 2004.
[22] Kilpatrick S, Fulton A, Johns S. Matching training needs and opportunities: the case for training brokers in the Australian agricultural sector. Int J Lifelong Educ 2007;26(2):209-24.
[23] Canadian Health Services Research Foundation. The theory and practice of knowledge broking in Canada's health system. Ottawa: CHSRF, 2003.
[24] Polivka B, Dresbach S, Heimlich J, Elliott M. Interagency relationships among rural early intervention collaboratives. Public Health Nurs 2001;18(5):340-9.

SECTION TWO:
DEVELOPING RURAL CHILD HEALTH POLICY

In: Rural child health: International aspects
Editors: Erica Bell and Joav Merrick

ISBN: 978-1-60876-357-3

Chapter 4

THE IMPACT OF POLICY PROCESSES ON CHILDREN'S ACCESS TO HEALTHCARE IN RURAL AUSTRALIA

Julaine Allan**, *BA (Soc Sci), BSW, M Soc Sci (Crim), PhD, Grad Dip VET Patrick Ball, BSc, MSc, PhD, MCPP(UK), FNZCP and Margaret Alston, BsocStud, Comp Allics, GradDip, MLitt, PhD

Centre for Inland Health and School of Biomedical Sciences,
Charles Sturt University, Wagga Wagga, New South Wales, Australia

Children are deserving targets of healthcare policy. However, to make a difference to children's lives, health and welfare policy goals have to be translated into services. For children and families living in small Australian rural communities, access to assistance and support from health services is dependent on the administrative and technical detail of health policy. This paper reports the findings of a case study investigating health care in two small rural towns in New South Wales. The study takes a pragmatic and practical approach to identifying the impact of policy intent on improving the health of rural children. The study identified the way policy goals are translated into practice by interviewing three distinct groups; policy makers, policy implementers and policy recipients. The research found that health policy was not well costed, implemented or available to children who lived outside regional or metropolitan areas. There were limited avenues for children, parents or health workers to influence the policy development or implementation process.

INTRODUCTION

Healthcare is an important issue on political agendas. Problems in health care access and availability will reliably cause controversy and attention resulting in rapid responses from politicians. When ill or needy children are the focus of attention the level of controversy is heightened. A common political response to topical concerns is calling for, or promising

* Correspondence: Julaine Allan, PhD, Research Fellow, Centre for Inland Health, Charles Sturt University, Locked bag 588 Wagga Wagga, NSW 2678 Australia. E-mail: juallan@csu.edu.au

action. This paper reports the findings of a project that aimed to follow the call to improve the health of rural children. The sociological action research project used community development processes to follow the policy pathway through the stages of development and implementation. The path's end is in health and welfare services provided to children and families in two small towns in rural NSW. Following an overview of health policy processes, the project method and findings are presented and the implications discussed.

Children comprise one fifth of the Australian population and are frequently the object of policy processes. Early childhood in particular is a priority area for Australian governments (1). Policy action examples include programs to develop literacy skills, support families and engage in exercise for example. Many of these programs are a direct result of changing morbidity data that demonstrates Australian children are affected by social and environmental changes occurring globally. Increasing mental health problems and rises in chronic diseases such as asthma and obesity are highlighted (2).

Chronic poor health affected 41% of children in 2004-2005 (2). Disability affected 8% of children under 15 and 15% of all children under 15 had a mental or behavioural problem. In both these categories boys were more likely to be affected than girls. Social conditions also played a part in the health of children. Sawyer et al (3) found that children in poor, non-traditional families had high rates of mental health problems and behavioural disorders. In rural areas where incomes are lower and health care access is more difficult, improving children's health is a complex problem (4).

Once a problem is on the political agenda, action becomes the responsibility of policy makers. Identifying the problem, in rural health care for example, is just the beginning of a lengthy process influenced by the electoral cycle and other competing issues (5). Policy makers must decide, within the confines of approved approaches and funding constraints, what solution(s) will quieten public debate.

Once a policy goal is developed a number of policies will follow targeting different sectors of the system it comes from. In healthcare this might include types of services provided, groups served, strategies used and locations prioritised. Jamrozik (6) notes that policy intent must be translated into administrative and technical detail that makes the policy do something to the problem.

Health policy has to consider the needs of the entire population shaping for example, minimum standards of care, promoting new treatments and prevention strategies, specifying workforce numbers, skill-mix and so on. Policy from Australian state and Federal health departments tends to be generic, that is health care focussed, in a whole-of-population approach. However, health outcomes are increasingly recognised as being the result of a combination of health services, welfare services, public policies and support strategies in times of stress. A whole-of-government approach is suggested to foster the necessary inter-sectorial action required to implement public policy (7). Partnership and collaboration between government and non-government agencies are the strategies proposed to meet the policy objectives.

The field of collaborative service provision is complicated by funding processes that impose competition policy on the non-government community service agencies designed to support people at a local level (8). This sector has a key role in providing formal services that have been identified as promoting the population's health status by raising education levels and work force participation rates, both factors in health status (9). For example, support for families with young children, education retention programs and job seeking and training services for the most disadvantaged community members are provided by community agencies.

Privatisation of all services including healthcare, is promoted and enabled by current government policies. Government rebates for taking out private health insurance are one example of encouraging support for business approaches to healthcare. However, health remains a core government function (9). While there is support for business approaches in many arenas, the legacy of the welfare state means there is an expectation of free and accessible health services in Australia (6). What the core health functions consist of, and the way they are distributed, are important questions for Australia that are echoed around the world (10).

Inland Australia is sparsely populated. Only eighteen per cent of the population live in towns and villages outside metropolitan centres and coastline (11). Many of the smaller towns have experienced population drift to regional centres or coastal areas subsequently suffering a decline in industry, employment and withdrawal of services (11,12). Limited access to general practitioners (GPs), diminishing hospital services, allied health workforce shortages, centralised support services and diminishing resource allocations have all been identified as both the cause and the result of a crisis in rural health care (13). Recognition of the crisis has resulted in political and policy attention but little concern about the impact of any action.

This project had two pragmatic and impact-focussed, policy-related objectives. The first was to clarify the policy pathway that aims to make rural Australians healthier; beginning with a policy goal and ending with the technical services delivered. The second objective was to identify the impact of the rural setting on health service policy intended to improve the health of children. The following sections of the report describe the project methodology, outline the findings relevant to the project objectives and discuss the implications of these.

OUR PROJECT

The project received approval from the Charles Sturt University Ethics in Human Research Committee (2007/140). The research project was conceived as a community development project consistent with a sociological action research approach (14). The initial research phase was a needs analysis that identified felt, expressed, normative and comparative needs for health care in rural areas (15). Within the sociological action research approach there is an aim to engage with the case study towns and implement the research findings over a period of time. Chronicling and analysing the much larger bureaucratic and government processes is a vital but under-researched part of community development and action (14).

The policy analysis was part of a case study of two rural communities in NSW. A case study approach entails an in-depth investigation of an area of interest. In this case, people and services bounded by a geographical location. The project is an instrumental case study of a bounded system (16). The aim was to identify what was similar about each case and also what was unique. Each case site was instrumental to understanding the issue of rural health and community service provision not simply the intrinsic conditions of the site (17).

The case study towns were selected because they appeared demographically similar and unremarkable in rural districts across Australia. That is, they had experienced the effects of the current long term drought, had no significant industry other than agriculture, were within one hundred kilometres of a large regional centre and had no special populations such as immigrants or Indigenous people, likely to attract specific policy attention.

Both case study towns of approximately 1,500 residents had similar profiles in the 2001 census. For example they had similar income levels, employment rates, and educational achievement. Both towns were the responsibility of the same local government and Area Health Service. Both towns had hospitals, two general practitioners, community health services and schools up to year 12. Both towns were subject to the same state and Federal health and welfare policies and service provisions. In each town children under the age of 15 were approximately 20% of the population, consistent with the national average.

Qualitative and quantitative data was collected to build a picture of each case. As well as health and community service policy analysis, the methodology included collection of available statistical data about each town and focus groups with community members including health and community workers.

Data Collection

The policy data collection involved two stages. The first stage was a desk audit that identified the available sources of support and service provision from government and non-government agencies with a clearly stated interest in the health of rural communities. Five key agencies stated in marketing material that they provided services with health related outcomes (18). One of these state agencies takes a whole-of-government approach delivering early intervention and support services to families with young children by coordinating five state government agencies (19).

The second stage of the policy analysis phase included interviews with representatives of the policy development arms of these agencies, regional managers responsible for implementing policy and local residents of the case study towns including health and welfare workers. This is set out in table 1.

Table 1. Sample and data collection

Participants	Policy goals	Policy methods	Policy input mechanisms
Policy makers 3 participants	How are policy goals identified?	How are goals put into action?	How is policy directed and changed?
Policy implementers 7 participants	What is the role of policy in allocating services?	How do you decide what needs are and where services should go?	What ways do you influence new policy or change policy?
Policy recipients 16 focus groups – 128 participants	What services are provided and how?	What service problems have you experienced? What unmet needs do you have? What is good about local services?	How do you get new or different services?

Interviews with policy makers and implementers were conducted by phone or at the participant's office. Focus groups were held with existing community groups including Rotary, CWA, mother's groups and school teachers, at their usual meeting place and time.

This included local health and community service workers. Interviews and focus groups were recorded as minutes and on a digital voice recorder. Minutes and files were transcribed into word documents. The findings of the needs analysis are reported elsewhere. This paper examines the policy processes specifically targeting children's health care.

DATA ANALYSIS

The sociological action research approach shaped the data analysis and fitted well with the pragmatic view of policy analysis (14). Strauss (20), notes that a pragmatist views the present situation as different from the past from which it has developed. This is consistent with the concept that the intent of policy could be altered during its implementation. In data analysis the approach results in exploration of the process and actions that result from ideals or concepts rather than elaboration of theory. However, discourse in the form of explanation of processes and actions, is central to the analysis.

Interview transcripts were examined and a deductive analysis was applied to the top-down approach. The intent of policy was identified from the policy maker interviews and compared with descriptions of the technical and administrative detail of implementation and subsequent impact at a regional and local level. An inductive analysis sought any participant statements that indicated the way policy mechanisms could be influenced at all levels of the process.

The findings are reported for each participant group under the subheadings of goals, methods, problems encountered and policy input processes.

OUR FINDINGS

Policy maker's goals

There is no clear and streamlined way of identifying the policy development process. Participant interviews emphasised information and support for particular action coming in from a wide variety of sources often with competing opinions. Interest groups lobby and politicians have ideas that influence policy that are not necessarily the needs of the population.

One participant noted that the current emphasis was on evidence that a particular strategy made a difference rather than developing broad policy goals:

> "Health in Australia is generally good. We have a good approach. Budget and workforce are the problems not policy development. We need new models not new policy"

When asking about the way rural conditions were considered in policy development, one participant stated:

> "You can't just go with what you think, or someone else thinks, should happen. Rural people are not special, they're just an interest group. They're no different to the homeless or people with a mental illness. The problems are the same"

Similarly, another participant noted competition between policy areas and systems that influenced the priority given to particular interest groups or issues:

> "Policy mechanisms exist within the system to prioritise different aspects of health like rural health. Consumer, clinical and government perspectives all have to be taken into account"

The way the multiple perspectives were considered could not be identified. Policy writing moved back and forward between setting goals and implementation strategies including costing. For example:

> "We can't say what should happen [in health services] without thinking about how it's going to happen"

Allocation of funding for any policy action is the end result of lobbying and consultation. For example:

> "It has to go to Treasury for the dollars to be allocated. That's when we know something can happen"

Policy maker's methods

A policy statement or directive has to be 'signed off' by political and government leaders before implementation can begin. Who signs off depends on the various department or agency and the amount of money involved. Once funding is available to implement a policy the money is given to whoever is responsible at a regional level. For example NSW Health provides funding to Area Health Services to implement policies and services as they see fit. For example:

> "The money goes to the Areas and then it's up to them"

Other agencies are more prescriptive with their funding, specifying the types of services that will be provided. However, where the services operate remains a regional decision. The funding system is complicated with the Federal government allocating money to the states for health services, but also allocating money to Federal programs that operate in the same locations as state programs. For example in NSW the Department of Aging, Disability and Health Care (DADHC) provides a range of services for children. The Federal department of Health and Aging also provides services for children and provides funding to DADHC for their services. This project could not clarify what coordination existed about what services each agency provides or where they are provided.

Problems encountered by policy makers

The most significant problem encountered by policy makers was financial. This included obtaining funding and also costing the implementation of policy, particularly if it was new or there were special conditions to be considered. For example:

> "Our biggest problem is economic analysis. We don't get proper costings. At best it's an estimate, at worst a guess"

Policy input mechanisms

A number of policy input mechanisms were identified by policy makers when they discussed lobby groups, research findings and systems mechanisms such as COAG and similar bodies. However, funding is currently tied strongly to evidence and outcomes and this limits 'soft' evaluations of community perceptions of health services that are not considered as valuable as scientific measures. For example:

> "The outcome measures have to measurable. One of ours is the size of babys' heads at birth. An increase in head circumference will indicate healthier babies through healthier pregnancies. We've done a lot of community consultation in the past to identify needs but you don't necessarily get good information, you don't create evidence"

Policy implementers goals

Policy implementers were individuals with the responsibility of distributing their funding allocation across a region and/or a range of services. Their goals were uniformly stated in participant interviews. For example:

> "We have to do the best we can with the money and within the guidelines given to us by the funding body. We have a big area to cover. I have to make best use of the resources I have, that includes funding and people on the ground to do the work"

Policy implementer's methods

Methods used by policy implementers to effectively use their funding allocations included identifying where supports for new services or strategies could come from to bolster what was already provided as well as minimising establishment costs. Any available funding opportunities were applied for to increase available resources. Policy implementers were concerned with ways of networking and sharing of resources to make use of minimal staff and services. These were often limited to certain areas and/or days of the week to stretch funding out for as long as possible.

Problems encountered

The problems encountered by policy implementers were numerous. However, they were frequently linked to trying to apply limited resources to a large area with a dispersed population. The following participant statements are two of many examples:

> "Competitive tendering means one service will run something for a whole region, sometimes half the state, on the smell of an oily rag. The most cost efficient places will get the best services and that's likely to be closest to the auspice body. We're funded to service western NSW and we can't do it. We limit most of our work to [town] because that's all we can respond to"

Service duplications and lack of coordination or communication between state and Federal funding bodies was also a problem for policy implementers. There was a concern that effort spent planning and establishing a service in an area would then be duplicated by another agency in the same area while other places would receive nothing. For example:

> "In one town it's a state funded service, in another town it's a federal funded service. They will be called different names but essentially have the same goals, client group – always families- and outcomes expected to be delivered over a huge area with one part time worker. It's pretty hit and miss"

Collaboration across sectors was often prevented by other agencies policies. For example:

> "We organised meetings with them [other agency employees] to share information and resources but they won't budge on the referral criteria"

Frequently, working in partnership across agencies resulted in additional meetings with no perceptible impact. For example:

> "We share information all the time but we're locked into service contracts set by Cabinet. There's not much room to move. If they [worker] went to all the possible meetings, they'd be serial meeting goers"

Policy input mechanisms

Policy input mechanisms noted by policy implementers included regular reporting back to funding bodies including details about budgets, community needs, service problems and outcomes and suggested changes. However the capacity to change the services or the budget was described as limited. For example:

> "We have to meet our outcomes or they will take our funding"

One participant stated that active lobbying for more resources or drawing attention to poor or inadequate services was a difficult thing to do because "you can't bite the hand that feeds you or they won't feed you".

Policy recipients goals

Policy recipients were community members in the two case study towns. The health and welfare workers living in these towns were also policy recipients. However, when talking about the delivery of services in the towns they usually referred to examples from the clients' experiences rather than their own. The main goal of policy recipients was to get a service when they needed it. Most of the time they did not know about the range of services that existed if they had not needed them and they did not know about the way services were distributed or supplied by policy guidelines. For example:

> "They've been told in Sydney their child is autistic but they haven't been told where the help might be or what it is"

Policy recipient's methods

Policy recipient's methods of adapting services for their own use seemed to vary according to their ability to advocate for themselves or have someone support them. For example:

> "We needed early intervention services so because I was on the committee I could arrange the service from [town] to come over every Monday to the pre-school and see several children. Otherwise I would have had to take time off work to take my son there every week"

Problems Encountered

Many of the problems encountered by policy recipients were related to lack of services or limited services. However, many participants stated they were lucky to have the services they could access and were unlikely to demand more. However, health and community service workers could clearly identify ongoing policy problems that they believed disadvantaged community members. For example:

> "The parents here take what they can get. If there wasn't a rule that DADHC deals with children under 5 and Health after that, some kids could have had early intervention three years ago. It's case load management not case management"

Policy input mechanisms

There were few examples of policy input mechanisms amongst policy recipients. One woman had lobbied successfully at a local level to have wheelchair ramps installed in a number of places in the town to improve her wheelchair bound son's mobility. However, other examples of policy input involved trying to identify the best policy to fit the needs of the population not vice versa. For example, a pre-school struggling with limited resources and increasingly disadvantaged parents wanted to become a long-day care centre. The change in title also came with different funding rules and allocations, staffing requirements and accreditation procedures. However, it required a substantial amount of work from the volunteer management committee and a degree of risk:

> "If we do it parents will get fee subsidies and we will get the gap so overall there will be more money in our kitty for staff and other things. But we might do the work and then a couple of families move out of town and we haven't got the numbers anyway"

Discussion

The policy pathway is difficult to follow. There was no trail from government policy documents through to services provided in the case study communities. In all of the agencies examined in this project there was no standardised number of services or type of services allocated per head of population or by identified needs of any particular population. Instead the picture developed is that the whole-of-population approach to service delivery is so badly under resourced that rural community members are wise to think they are lucky if they can readily access any service.

Competition policy drives the funding of non-government community agencies and the impact of limited resources and regional or urban auspice bodies is clearly patchy, limiting service access. However, competition is apparent throughout the policy process not just in funding allocations. Without a lobby group with evidence and a politician on-side any particular health needs are likely to be invisible. Most parents describe a lack of time and energy for high level advocacy instead relying on service providers to do what they can or restricting their lobbying to get regional service providers to come to their town rather than some other location.

The whole-of-government approach that is intended to address the structural problems linked to poor health status is also under resourced and difficult to implement. Consequently policies support short-term government funded programs with a specific population target and easily measurable outcome not related to any change in health status or life expectancy. Policy guidelines about services provided and age ranges of clients make local services inflexible. For example one state agency provides services to children under five years old and another provides services to school age children. Currently (in 2007) government funding focus is on early intervention services for children under five. However, the service that delivers this in the case study towns has staff vacancies and cannot provide a service at all. The school aged service could provide some support to families in speech pathology and occupational therapy but policy regulations prevent this. While health and welfare workers talk about bending the rules when they can see a family in need, they do it surreptiously. This strategy does not address the cause of policy problems.

The rural setting has a significant impact on policy implementation. While the policy intent is well meaning, the resources allocated to a vast area with a small population means that the intended recipients may never see the service meant for them. Without an effective adult to lobby, provide transport and come to terms with policy guidelines, children needing healthcare, other than emergency treatment, are unlikely to get it. Evidence based best practice is in the realm of fantasy for over stretched rural health and welfare workers struggling with the administrative and technical detail of policy.

CONCLUSIONS

This project's first objective; to clarify the policy pathway from goal to service delivery that aims to make rural Australians healthier was not fulfilled because the pathway was not clarified. Our documentation of this, however, demonstrates serious problems in policy implementation processes and provides an important avenue for change. Clearly the political imperative of responding to publicised need does not translate into the technical detail required for children's support such as early intervention services. Greater flexibility in funding rules, work practices and guidelines could enable collaboration between service providers and improve service delivery. However, this has to be enshrined in policy development processes rather than the current emphasis on competition.

The second objective was to identify the impact of the rural setting on health service policy intended to improve the health of children. The rural setting, with workforce shortages, small and dispersed populations and under resourced health and welfare services magnifies the effect of complex policy processes. The popular construction of children as valuable and in need of protection has limited impact on the way health care is provided, particularly to children in small rural communities.

The findings of this study indicate that political and policy attention needs to follow on through to the evaluation phase of the policy cycle rather than the development phase. A whole of government approach should begin with policy makers and be reflected in policy guidelines.

Accordingly we believe the lessons for international audiences from our rural Australian study are that political imperatives and policy intent are only the beginning of the policy pathway. Policy is affected by context and process and may not achieve the intended aim because of local conditions. Popular policy does not always equate with good outcomes particularly for vulnerable populations disengaged from the policy process such as children.

REFERENCES

[1] Aust Inst Health Welfare. A picture of Australia's children. Canberra: AIHW Cat PHE 58, 2005.

[2] ABS 2007. 4829.0.55.001 - Health of Children in Australia: A Snapshot, 2004-05 http://www.abs.gov.au/AUSSTATS/abs@.nsf/mf/4829.0.55.001/ accessed 2009 Feb 28.

[3] Sawyer M, Arney F Baghurst P, Clark JJ, Graetz BW, Kosky RJ et al. Mental health of young people in Australia. Canbarra: DoHA, 2000.

[4] AIHW 2002. Rural and urban variations in oral health. AIHW Research Unit Reearch Report 28.Urban anhttp://www.arcpoh.adelaide.edu.au/publications/report/research/ pdf_files/rr28_ urban_ rural.pdf accessed 2009 Feb 28.

[5] Prasser S. Why is it so hard for research to inform the policy process and government decision making? Aust Inst Criminal Occassional Sem Series, 2007. (Website: www.aic.gov.au).

[6] Jamrozik A. Social policy in the post-welfare state 2nd ed. Frenchs Forest: Pearson Educ, 2005.

[7] Sibthorpe B, Dixon J. Rethinking evaluation for policy action on the social origins of health and well-being. In: Eckersley R, Dixon J, Douglas B, eds. The social origins of health and well-being. Cambridge: Cambridge Univ Press, 2001:280-95.

[8] Alston M. From local to global: making social policy more effective for rural community capacity building. Aust Soc Work 2002; 55(3):214-26.

[9] Legge D. Health inequalities in the new world order. In: Eckersley R, Dixon J, Douglas B, eds. The social origins of health and well-being. Cambridge: Cambridge Univ Press, 2001:25-33

[10] OECD. The new rural paradigm: Policies and governance. Paris: OECD, Rural Policy Reviews, 2006.
[11] Salt B. The big shift: Welcome to the third Australian culture. South Yarra: Hardie Grant Books, 2001.
[12] Alston M, Kent J. Coping with a crisis: human services in times of drought. Rural Soc 2004;14(3):214-27.
[13] Allan J, Ball P, Crockett J, Alston M, Whittenbury K. It's all part of the package in rural allied health work: A pilot study of rewards and barriers in rural pharmacy and social work. Internet J Allied Health Sci July 2007;5:3.(http://ijahsp.nova.edu/)
[14] Foley S, Valenzuela A. Critical ethnography: The politics of collaboration. In: Denzin N, Lincoln Y, eds. The Sage handbook of qualitative research. 3rd edition. Thousand Oaks: Sage, 2005:217-34.
[15] Bradshaw JA. Taxonomy of social need: Problems and progress. In: McLachjan G, ed. Medical care essays on current research. Seventh Series. Oxford: Nuffield Provincial Hospitals Trust, 1972.
[16] Stake RE. The art of case study research. Thousand Oaks: Sage, 1995.
[17] Stake RE. Qualitative case studies. In: Denzin N, Lincoln Y, eds. The Sage handbook of qualitative research, 3rd ed. Thousand Oaks: Sage, 2005:443-66.
[18] Commonwealth Department of Health and Ageing http://www.health.gov.au/internet/wcms/publishing.nsf/Content/health-portout.htm accessed 2009 Feb 28.
[19] Families First http://www.familiesfirst.nsw.gov.au/public accessed 2009 Feb 28.
[20] Strauss A. Qualitative analysis for social scientists. Melbourne: Cambridge Univ Press, 1990.

In: Rural child health: International aspects
Editors: Erica Bell and Joav Merrick

ISBN: 978-1-60876-357-3

Chapter 5

'STATES OF MIND'—DEVELOPING A POLICY FRAMEWORK FOR EMERGENCY ACCOMMODATION SERVICES AND CHILDREN EXPOSED TO DOMESTIC VIOLENCE

Erica Bell**, BA (psych), MA Qual PhD
University Department of Rural Health, University of Tasmania, Tasmania, Australia

The needs of children in emergency accommodation services have been largely neglected in the research literature. This paper offers an account of a project that considered the specific needs of children aged 0-5 affected by family violence in Tasmanian Women's Immediate Emergency Accommodation (IEA) services. Specifically, it aimed to identify key elements of a best practice framework for working with children aged 0-5; identify Assessment Tools for effective responses to children aged 0-5; identify key support and links to other children's services; identify key activities and therapeutic play modules for use by Family Support Workers and Child Support Workers in Women's IEA services; describe key current early intervention activities within Women's IEA services, and identify key areas where development of services could occur. This study used a select literature review, as well as the results of formal interviews with the managers of Women's IEA accommodation services, to develop key directions for moving policy and practices forward. It offers insights into how to meet the holistic needs of these children through appropriate developments of practice, policy and research supports.

INTRODUCTION

This chapter offers an account of the outcomes of a project that aimed to consider the specific needs of children aged 0-5 affected by family violence in Tasmanian Women's Immediate Emergency Accommodation (IEA) services. Specifically, the project aimed to

* Correspondence: Erica Bell, PhD, A/Co-Director, Deputy Director, University Department of Rural Health, University of Tasmania, Private Bag 103 Hobart, Tasmania 7000 Australia, Ph: +61 (0)3 6226 7377, Mobile: +61 (0)4 3939 4141, Facsimile: +61 (0)3 6226 1952, Email: Erica.Bell@utas.edu.au

1. identify key elements of a best practice framework for working with children aged 0-5; identify Assessment Tools for effective responses to children aged 0-5;
2. identify key support and links to other children's services;
3. identify key activities and therapeutic play modules for use by Family Support Workers and Child Support Workers in Women's IEA SAAP services;
4. describe key current early intervention activities within Women's IEA SAAP services, and identify key areas where development of services could occur.

The Study

This study used a select literature review, as well as the results of formal interviews with the managers of Women's IEA SAAP accommodation services, to develop key directions for moving policy and practices forward. The research brief relating to children from the ages of 0-5 was interpreted as including women who are pregnant, so accordingly the needs of this group and the unborn child were included in the analysis of literature and SAAP practices.

The literature review the method was selective, broadly inclusive but not all-inclusive, in the following ways.

In relation to the selectiveness of the literature review for this study, the choice of material was influenced by the fact that the best practice being examined had to be relevant to crisis accommodation services. If the study had aimed to offer a framework for how to deal with each and every need of small children exposed to domestic violence, it would be a very long study indeed. The study focused very purposely on literature about domestic violence and small children as it relates to the specific research questions. This means, for example, that this study did not explore the broader literature on child development and the broad nature of interventions not specifically linked to domestic violence exposure, though that literature should not be neglected in a larger study.

Accordingly, this study did not aim to, nor could it, explore particular special issues beyond the already complex questions in the research brief, such as issues to do with domestic violence for any particular cultural group in Australian society, or special issues to do with child sexual abuse or other specialised areas of the domestic violence literature. Such special issues have already been exhaustively documented in many resources, including Australian studies that examine the needs of such groups as rural communities, families from non-English-speaking-backgrounds, gay and lesbian couples, and aboriginal communities (1). Nor did this study attempt to comprehensively answer a myriad of possible other questions about domestic violence to do with for example, the status and nature of data about its prevalence, or even the exact numbers of children in Tasmanian Women's IEA SAAP services (a recent study of service provision in Tasmania gives a figure that varies from 100% to 12% for clients presenting with dependant children to different Tasmanian services with crisis accommodation services towards the top end of those figures (2)). Figures provided by the Department of Health and Human Services reveal that in 2004-05, a total of 544 women and 850 accompanying children were accommodated at the six accommodation services providing Women's IEA in Tasmania. A further 2,336 children received support services in the wider SAAP service system during 2004-05 (NDCA Curf data 2004-05). Thus the study focused upon, and was structured by, the specific questions in the research brief.

In relation to the broad inclusiveness of the literature review for this study, it should be noted that the literature on domestic violence covers many different kinds of settings. Many important insights and evidence generalizable to Women's IEA settings would have been missed if the researcher had chosen to concentrate only on research targeting crisis accommodation. However, wherever necessary when citing best practice advice, the researcher noted the original context in which that advice was designed. Clearly, there is a difference between best practice in screening in health care settings and women's crisis accommodation settings, though the latter can benefit from knowing about research findings for the former.

Also on the subject of the inclusiveness of this study, this study included many recent reports, however, older studies that add value to understandings have not been neglected. That is, the use of 'out-of-date' references in this study helped ensure that the findings drew upon the larger body of research, not simply recent work. As noted by one leader in this field:(3) 'In our work with children of battered women, we have been wary of not "reinventing the wheel" with new intervention programs when many existing treatment strategies could be applied to this population.' (pp. 91-92)

In relation to the interviews that form the second kind of evidence used in this study, these involved six managers and staff in five of the six Women's IEA SAAP services providing crisis accommodation to women and children in Tasmania. For ethical reasons, the anonymity of these SAAP services is protected in this paper. Interviewers asked SAAP managers about their thoughts on best practice for Women's IEA services responding to the needs of small children (0-5) who have been exposed to domestic violence. The interviews took the form of forty minute informal semi-structured discussions that used the following questions as a point of departure:

1. What are your thoughts about best practice ethos and principles (i.e. service culture and beliefs) for crisis accommodation services dealing with very young children 0-5 who have been exposed to domestic violence?
2. What do you see as best practice assessment of these children's needs? What specific assessment tools do you use/think services should use?
3. What advice can you give about best practice in making referrals/using the support of other agencies? How do these links and supports work for your agency?
4. What about best practice in intervention, including key activities and therapeutic play modules...what interventions, including key activities and therapeutic play modules does your service use? Why? What in your view works best for these young children?
5. What do you see as the key issues in developing best practice in recording and reporting data in this area of client need? What recording and reporting does your agency do in relation to such clients?
6. What staff (broad experience and qualifications) are needed for responding to the needs of children exposed to domestic violence? What are the issues of best practice in staffing crisis accommodation services so that the needs of these children are better met?
7. Looking at the big picture, what do you see as the key directions for developing Tasmanian crisis accommodation services so they better meet the needs of children 0-5 exposed to domestic violence?

Findings from the interviews were integrated into the consultant's report in sections dealing with Women's IEA SAAP practices. These sections were reviewed by Women's IEA SAAP managers and staff in a group meeting, in a manner consistent with hermeneutic approaches to interpretation of interview data, which emphasise successive iterations involving research subjects as part of the hermeneutic 'circle'. Hermeneutic approaches have been popular in some health service research contexts aimed at arriving at a holistic understanding of the client's service experience and 'life world' or total experience (4-10). They were particularly useful as a framework for developing an approach that was about participative styles of drafting interview analyses.

The project was able to identify elements of best practice and the tools either most commonly used and/or validated in the research literature. It was able to recommend steps that Women's IEA SAAP staff can take to develop their practices in line with the literature and the evidence of what is already occurring in Tasmanian Women's IEA SAAP services. However, in a project of this length, it was not possible to undertake a trial of sufficient size and technical robustness to support statements about the detail of what amendments need to be made to make particular tools more or less useful than other tools. To have confidence in such statements, given the nature and complexity of interventions for small children in this situation, a much larger study is required bringing careful validation and measurement techniques. The organisations currently producing such information would also need to give their consent for the use of their tools, including in amended form.

Accordingly, one of the findings of this study suggests that a large-scale empirical study be conducted to high academic standards. Ideally this would involve a national and international survey of the views of staff of crisis accommodation services about best practice in this area that builds upon the work in this study, and includes a well-developed empirical trial of specific resources used in interventions in different crisis accommodation settings.

THE FINDINGS

The study offers a suggested ethos statement and set of principles for guiding the work of Tasmanian IEA Women's SAAP services as it relates to the needs of children (0-5) exposed to domestic violence. The suggested ethos statement could include some elements from other models, though the advice given by IEA Women's SAAP agencies about their ethos matches and goes beyond many other statements, as follows.

- The child is a client in its own right and services should take a client-centred approach to meeting the child's needs: this approach should be individualised, culturally appropriate, non-judgmental, based on sound theoretical understandings of domestic violence, and delivered by qualified and well-equipped staff;
- The needs of the child are multi-faceted and therefore require a holistic approach involving networks with diverse community agencies and professionals;
- The safety and well-being of the child and mother is the first priority;
- The service should, where possible, support the authority of the mother and the positive development of the family unit, as part of family-based approaches;

- Children and their families should be treated with respect, dignity, and with a belief in their hopeful futures and their capacities to be empowered to build those futures;
- Effective interventions involve attention to both the child and the parent, separately and together;
- The service should create a supportive and safe environment with a non blaming ethos;
- The service has a role in educating not only the child and family, but also the wider community.

The study results also include a list of suggested assessment tools useful to SAAP services and related electronic links for practitioners. The researcher would suggest that practitioners in such services explore the value of the Child Behaviour Checklist (CBCL) for assessing children's emotional and behavioural functioning discussed in this report (11,12), as well as other tools listed in this section, particularly the Conflicts Tactics Scale, these two being the most commonly referred to tools in the literature scanned as part of this small project. On the basis of this research, it can be concluded that these tools appear more likely to work to develop broader staff capacities to recognise and respond to the needs of small clients. Clearly, however, it was beyond the scope of this small study to trial and evaluate the use of any such tools, however adapted, in the complex settings of crisis accommodation services—as noted, that should be the function of a second stage of research and must involve permission from the necessary organisations. As the information below will suggest, the development of these tools has been the result of very large investments of time and expertise (including expertise in the scientific validation of instruments) by particular individuals and organisations and naturally they are protected by copyright. However, the present study obtained sufficient evidence to support the value of practitioners examining such tools for professional development purposes (i.e. reading about the tools and discussing them in staff meetings to explore their implications for practices), pending further exploration of their usefulness in Australian SAAP services in a second stage of research.

Information about the child behaviour checklist: For ordering versions of the CBCL suitable for smaller children and related tools see this website http://www.aseba.org/products/cbcl1-5.html For information about the organisation (the Achenbach System of Empirically Based Assessment or ASEBA) that has developed and now sells these products see http://www.aseba. org/index. html and http://www.aseba.org/ ABOUTUS/aboutus_start. html For more detailed information on the empirical validation of the CBCL generally see http://vinst.umdnj.edu/VAID/TestReport.asp?Code=CBCA

•

Information about the conflicts tactics scale: For details of the instrument and information about who to contact to order it http://pubpages.unh.edu/~mas2/CTS15.pdf For information about its empirical validation http://pubpages.unh.edu/~mas2/CTS4.pdf

The study also provides directions for improving key support and links to other children's services relevant to Women's IEA SAAP agencies. The researcher's recommendations in this area, bearing in mind the literature on best practice and the issues raised by Women's IEA Tasmanian SAAP services, were as follows:

1. That agencies have regular community network meetings with other relevant agencies to develop improvements in co-ordinated responses to the needs of small children, such as timely referral responses, on site visits, development of programs tailor-made for small children, and professional training in the functions of collaborating agencies; that this collaboration place special emphasis on including education services to help design better access to pre-schools in particular
2. That a register of agencies be developed for referral of small children and their mothers exposed to domestic violence, including agencies offering on site visits
3. That the findings be referred to relevant Government offices, including the Department of Health and Human Services, for consideration of how to address the problem of the general overburdened nature of critical human services that are best positioned to meet the needs of small children exposed to domestic violence.

The study offered directions for interventions, including key activities and therapeutic play modules. These were as follows:

1. That a register of interventions suitable for children aged 0-4 years and the evidence for them be set up by a peak body in the field of domestic violence
2. That, in designing suites of activities for those children who need them, Women's IEA staff be informed by leaders in this field documented in this report such as the work of Leslie Givers (www.ggj.biz) and interventions listed by The Australian Domestic and Family Violence Clearinghouse (www.austdvclearinghouse.unsw.edu.au)
3. That Women's IEA staff explore the value of age-appropriate group approaches used with appropriate professional support such as those of Peled, particularly for children at the top end of the age range that is the focus of this study i.e. children 3-5 years.
4. That Women's IEA staff explore motivational interviewing techniques, implemented with appropriate professional support for its adult clients, particularly pregnant women exposed to domestic violence.
5. That specific funding arrangements be made for the development of play centres at Women's IEA, including their ongoing maintenance.
6. That the present study be used as a point of departure for a high quality empirical study of the effectiveness of commonly used tools for small children exposed to domestic violence, suitable for crisis accommodation service contexts; that this study utilise innovative social science methods that are able to deal with multi-dimensional client/service factors.

The task of describing the evidence for particular interventions for this age group is considerable. Researchers, including those focussing upon interventions specifically in crisis accommodation services, have commented on the dearth of evaluations of such programs (13), including inter-systemic programs aimed at addressing domestic violence (14). Even outside the sphere of crisis accommodation services, researchers have observed a lack of 'controlled outcome studies demonstrating the effects' of such interventions for children (15) as well as for pregnant women (16). Another study, referring to the evidence for interventions in domestic violence more generally, noted that despite almost twenty years of program evaluations, their effectiveness is still questionable (17). These authors were, however, able to conclude that effective treatment programs focus on the safety of victims, educate perpetrators and victims, emphasise the need for participants to be responsible, and are properly linked to, and educate participants about, the criminal justice system (17).

As noted in an Australian study, which was the first of its kind examining evidence from young people 12-20 about their exposure to domestic violence,

> ...we do not know whether the prevalence of these behaviours has been increasing, decreasing or remaining static. Without this information we cannot be sure which of our efforts to prevent domestic violence are effective. (18) (p. 3)

Of particular issue in the present study was the difficulty of accessing published academic research literature providing information about the post-intervention effectiveness of tools and kits commonly used by crisis accommodation services. The effectiveness of these resources, like many play activities and tools, and child-centered programs developed specifically for use in crisis accommodation settings (19), do not appear to be explored in the academic (peer reviewed literature).

This is not to say that research has not been used in the development of many resources—for example, St Luke's resources appear to involve partnerships with researchers and consideration of a great deal of research literature—or that research evaluations haven't been published outside the scholarly academic literature. It is to say that there is a need for high quality academic research that evaluates the effectiveness of tools currently in use by women's IEA services. This research might draw upon classical research designs (randomised control/experimental studies) but it would also need to utilise innovative quali-quantitative methods associated with such innovative social science researchers as Charles Ragin, in ways that examine the complex range of factors involved in intervention success in small populations (20-25).

Having said this, there are still significant learnings to be gained from the literature on intervention effectiveness, such as it is.

In the area of care for the in-utero child, there are indications of the value of peer mothering; advocacy and home visits have also been used with inconclusive evidence of success in the literature (16). Individual (as opposed to group) interventions that may have particular importance for very young children are even less well-researched in the literature (15). Specific interventions referred to in the literature include

- short-term group approaches for children in crisis accommodation situations such as those developed by Peled and others (26, 27); a major Australian report (28) outlining models of service for working with children describes the approaches developed by Peled as being most commonly used in women's refuges and counselling services; again though, the more commonly used group approaches referred to in the previous section have some evidence for their success though this relates to older children (3, 29)
- parenting skills training: one review refers to successful (leading to reducing externalising scores on the Child Behaviour Checklist) in-home sessions for 8 weeks conducted by a therapist-student team working with mothers and children (4-9 years) exiting domestic violence shelters, focusing on parent skills training relevant to

children's conduct problems, though it also includes family evaluation, tailoring services for each family, and working with extended family members (29); Carlson (2000) concludes that 'effective interventions with this population must be extensive and intensive' (p. 335); another leader in the field (3) notes that, in relation to behaviour issues 'parent management training' appears to be 'supported by a great deal of systematic clinical research' (p. 92)

- art therapy programs: for example, the literature refers to the work of the Center for Domestic Violence Prevention in San Mateo, California, which offers an on site art therapy program aimed at helping children in shelters who have been exposed to domestic violence which focuses upon giving children a safe medium for telling their stories (13)
- psychodynamic approaches to treating preschooler-mother pairs developed by the Child Trauma Research project at the San Francisco General Hospital, which focuses upon strengthening abilities in healthy family functioning, with some positive evaluation outcomes (15)
- counselling therapies: for example, the literature refers to the work of the Pro Bono Children's Mental Health project in Pittsburgh, Pennsylvania, which offers another approach to meeting the needs of children in shelters based on pro bono collaborations: therapists donate an hour of their counselling time every week to child residents, continuing to treat them pro bono after the child has left the shelter (13)
- motivatiional interviewing in interventions for pregnant women: at least one obstetrical study (30) points to the value of a 'stages of change' motivational interviewing approach that appears in the work of DiClemente (31) for use with pregnant women wanting to develop new attitudes and personal resources during this time
- clinical approaches to post-traumatic stress disorder in children, including an individual model for young children developed by the Boston Medical Center that is an outpatient and non-shelter-based program (15); as noted in the section on assessment, there are also clinical diagnostic and treatment guidelines developed by the American Medical Association (and Australian Medical Association) (32).

Some consideration was also given in this study to other issues to do with data collection, prevention, and staffing issues, as well as other key areas for development of these services, with findings as follows.

1. That data collection analysis of SAAP data include innovative quali-quantitative methods which have particular usefulness for service practitioners such as those developed by Charles Ragin
2. That the community agency network recommended by the study also target optimal data collection and data sharing procedures between agencies, subject to legal and ethical requirements.
3. That all staff in Women's IEA SAAP services who work with children exposed to domestic violence receive ongoing training through such bodies as the Partnerships Against Domestic Violence Program interstate, which can be contacted through the Office for Women. (http://ofw.facs.gov.au/womens_safety_agenda/index.htm)

4. That each Women's IEA SAAP service that deals with small children who may have been exposed to domestic violence receives dedicated funding for a child support worker.
5. That the community agency network recommended by the study also take a strong community education and prevention focus, expressed in a collaborative statewide plan, particularly through the involvement of pre-school and other early education specialists
6. That Women's IEA SAAP services receive dedicated funding for community education and prevention activities
7. That the limitation of six weeks be reviewed in a manner that is consistent with examining the issues of quality service delivery documented in this report.
8. That the community agency network recommended by the study develop strategies for ensuring that critical high priority needs of Women's IEA SAAP clients are met in a timely fashion, including as they relate to small children.
9. That the community agency network's plan for statewide collaborative training for all Tasmanian services, recommended by the study, include particular attention to training in legal issues and legal advocacy on behalf of community agencies to ensure their views are represented to government in the development of future legislation; that this work pay particular attention to the development of legislation that best positions services to respond to the needs of small children exposed to domestic violence.

Conclusions

The needs of children in emergency accommodation settings have often been neglected and are relatively poorly researched. This case study offers a number of directiions and supporting information that can be used in developing interventions for children exposed to domestic violence who present at immediate emergency accommodation services. In particular, it suggests that a whole-of-community approach is needed to ensure that government intentions are translated into real results for children at the grass roots level of service delivery.

References

[1] Bagshaw D, Chung D, Couch M, Lilburn S, Wadham B. Reshaping responses to domestic violence. Adelaide, Univ South Aust, 2000.

[2] Love L. Service provision in Tasmania for children who witness and/or experience domestic violence. Hobart, Tasmania, SHE (Support, Help and Empowerment), 2003.

[3] Jaffe PG, Wolfe DA, Wilson SK. Children of battered women. Thousand Oaks, CA, Sage, 1990.

[4] Allen D. Hermeneutics: philosophical traditions and nursing practice research. Nurs Sci Quart 1995;8:174-82.

[5] Angus J, Evans S, Lapum J, Rukholm E, St Onge R, Nolan R, et al. "Sneaky disease": the body and health knowledge for people at risk for coronary heart disease in Ontario. Can Soc Sci Med 2005;60: 2117-28.

[6] Clarke J. Hermeneutic analysis: a qualitative decision-trail. Int J Nurs Stud 1999;36:363-9.

[7] Daniel S. The patient as text: a model of clinical hermeneutics. Theoretical Med Bioethics 1986;7:195-210.
[8] Ekman I, Skott C. Developing Clinical Knowledge through a Narrative-Based Method of Interpretation. 2004 [online]. Available at: www.sciencedirect.com.ezproxy.library. uq.edu.au/ science?_ob.Accessed 2009 Apr 15.
[9] Hick C. The art of perception: from the life world to the medical gaze and back again. Medicine, Health Care Philosophy 1999;2: 129-40.
[10] Lowes L, Prowse M. Standing outside the interview process? The illusion of objectivity in phenomenological data generation. Int J Nurs Stud 2001;38:471-80.
[11] Koenen KC, Moffitt TE, Caspi A, Taylor A, Purcell S. Domestic violence is associated with environmental suppression of IQ in young children. Dev Psychopathol 2003;15:297-311.
[12] Levendosky AA, Huth-Bocks AC, Semel MA, Shapiro DL. Trauma symptoms in preschool-age children exposed to domestic violence. J Interpers Violence 2002;17(2):150-64.
[13] Saathoff AJ, Stoffel EA. Community-based domestic violence services. Future Child 1999;9(3):97-110.
[14] Edleson JL. Mothers and children: Understanding the links between woman battering and child abuse. 1995 [online]. 1-10. Minnesota Center Against Violence and Abuse. Available at: http://www. mincava.umn.edu/documents/ nij/nij.html. Accessed
[15] McAlister Groves B. Mental health services for children who witness domestic violence. Future Child 1999;9(3):122-32.
[16] Taft A. Violence against women in pregnancy and after childbirth: Current knowledge and issues in health care responses. Sydney: Aust Domestic Fam Violence Clearinghouse, Sydney, 2002.
[17] Romans SE, Poore MR, Martin JL. The perpetrators of domestic violence. Med J Aust 2000;173:484-8.
[18] Indermaur D. Young Australians and domestic violence. Canberra: Aust Inst Criminol, 2001.
[19] Becker P, Eden F. Children in Shelters: A training manual for working with women and children who have survived domestic violence. Adelaide: Southern Areas Women's Children's Shelter, 1994.
[20] Ragin C, Zaret D. Theory and method in comparative research: two strategies. Soc Forces 1983;61(3):731-54.
[21] Ragin C. The comparative method. Los Angeles, CA: Univ of Calif Press, 1987.
[22] Ragin CC. Introduction to qualitative comparative analysis. In: Janoski T, Hicks AM (eds). The Comparative Political Economy of the Welfare State. Cambridge: Cambridge University Press; 1994: pp.
[23] Ragin CC. Using qualitative comparative analysis to study configurations. In: Kelle U, ed. Computer-aided qualitative data analysis: Theory, methods and practice. London: Sage, 1995:177-89.
[24] Ragin CC. Turning the tables: How case-oriented research challenges variable-oriented research. In: Brady HE, Collier D, eds. Rethinking social inquiry: Diverse tools, shared standards. Lanham, MD: Rowman Littleford, 2004:123-38.
[25] Ragin CC. Using qualitative comparative analysis to study causal complexity. Health Serv Res 1999;34(5):1225-39.
[26] Peled E, Davis D. Groupwork with children of battered women: A practitioner's manual. Thousand Oaks, CA, Sage, 1995.
[27] Peled E, Edleson J. Process and outcome in small groups for children of battered women. In: Peled E, Jaffe P, Edleson J, eds. Ending the cycle of violence: community response to children of battered women. Thousand Oaks, CA: Sage, 1995:77-96.
[28] Gevers L. Models of service for working with children and young people who have lived with domestic violence. Canberra: Commonwealth Aust, 1999.
[29] Carlson BE. Children exposed to intimate partner violence: research findings and implications for intervention. Trauma Violence Abuse 2000;1(4):321-42.
[30] Mayer L, Liebschutz J. Domestic violence in the pregnant patient: obstetric and behavioral interventions. Obst Gynecol Survey 1998; 53(10):627-35.

[31] DiClemente C. Motivational interviewing and the stages of change. In: Miller W, Rollnick S, eds. Motivational interviewing: Preparing people to change addictive behavior. New York: Guilford, 1991:191-201.

[32] Flitcraft A. Physicians and domestic violence: challenges for prevention. Health Affairs 1993;12 (4): 154-61.

In: Rural child health: International aspects
Editors: Erica Bell and Joav Merrick ISBN: 978-1-60876-357-3

Chapter 6

A POLICY AND INTERVENTION FOR OVERWEIGHT CHILDREN AND ADOLESCENTS

Kimberly K McClanahan, PhD, Marlene B Huff, PhD and Hatim A Omar*, MD, FAAP
Division of Adolescent Medicine, Department of Pediatrics, Kentucky Children's Hospital, University of Kentucky, Lexington, United States of America

The global epidemic of childhood and adolescent overweight has become a major public health concern. Not only are these youth more likely to become obese as adults, and thus more prone to obesity-related diseases than their non overweight peers, they are also likely to suffer emotional and social effects associated with overweight. Overweight in youth has been linked to depression, low self-esteem, eating disorders, negative body image, and stigma. It appears to be bi-directional in nature, with overweight sometimes predicting certain psychological effects and psychosocial issues sometimes predicting overweight. Effective assessment and treatment of psychological and mental health issues in overweight youth will help overweight youth deal more effectively with their social and psychological milieus. Additionally, interventions for mental health concerns may have the added health benefit of increasing weight loss, thus decreasing obesity-related disease for which the overweight adolescent is prone.

INTRODUCTION

Adolescence is defined most simply by the word 'change'--physical, cognitive, emotional, and social. As physical and cognitive changes occur, so do changes in the domains of emotional/psychological development and social interaction/relationships. Psychological health and social adequacy are important components of mental health, but adolescence brings with it unique challenges, and interruption of development within any domain may

* Correspondence: Hatim Omar, MD, FAAP, Professor of Pediatrics and Obstetrics/Gynecology, Chief, Adolescent Medicine and Young Parent programs, J422, Kentucky Clinic, University of Kentucky, Lexington, KY 40536 United States. Tel: 859-323-6426 ext. 311; Fax: 859-257-7706; E-mail: haomar2@uky.edu

occur. Disruptions in emotional and social development can be influenced by many things, including physical and/or medical problems (1).

Obesity has become one of the most common diseases and disease-associated conditions in the United States (US) and other countries. In the year 2000, it was estimated that obesity would soon surpass tobacco smoking as the leading cause of preventable death in the United States (2) and it has also been suggested that today's young people may, on average, live less healthy and ultimately shorter lives than their parents due to overweight and obesity; in fact, this epidemic may reverse the modern era's steady increase in life expectancy (3,4). Further, it has been estimated that as this century progresses, more people will die from the complications of overnutrition than of starvation (5). Pinhas-Hamiel (6) noted that "life-style-related diseases are no longer the exclusive domain of adult medicine." Furthermore, overweight has a bi-directional relationship with mental and psychological health in that psychosocial factors have been shown to predict overweight, but overweight also impacts psychosocial factors such as psychological development and social functioning (7,8).

Overweight in children and adolescents is usually defined as a body mass index (BMI) equal to or greater than the 95th percentile, compared to pediatric population reference data when plotted on the appropriate age and gender chart; children and adolescents with a BMI between the 85th and 95th percentile are considered to be at risk for overweight, according to the Centers for Disease Control and Prevention (CDC); the CDC does not use the term obesity for children and adolescents. Most overweight preadolescent children and at least 70% of overweight adolescents will remain obese into adulthood (9), significantly increasing the chances of obesity-related disease as well as psychological complications associated with overweight (7,8).

Between 1980 and 2002, overweight prevalence tripled in children and adolescents ages 6 to 19 years (10-12). Comparing results obtained from the 1999-2000 National Health and Nutrition Examination Survey (NHANES) to results from the NHANES survey in 2003-2004, 13.9% vs. 17.1%, respectively, of US children and adolescents were overweight. For female children and adolescents, the percentage overweight increased from 13.8% in 1999-2000 to 16.0% in 2003-2004; for male children and adolescents, the increase went from 14.0% to 18.2% during the same time period (11). More than 10% of school age children are overweight worldwide with the Americas reporting rates as high as 32% (9). According to the 2005 Youth Risk Behavior Survey, a national probability sample of 9th – 12th graders which assesses risk behaviors and risk factors (13), approximately 16% of students in the US were at risk for overweight, and 13% were already overweight.

Childhood and adolescent overweight has some endogenous causes, but when those causes are ruled out, then behavioral and psychological factors, rather than biological ones, are primarily responsible for the upward trend in adolescent overweight.14 Behavioral factors such as lack of physical exercise, sedentary behavior, and poor dietary choices have been cited as common risk factors for weight gain, although psychological and mental health factors also factor into the equation (14,15).

PSYCHOSOCIAL RISKS

In the realm of psychological and social development, today's youth often face challenges in mental health and wellness as they progress from childhood to adolescence to adulthood. Over the past 20 years, the proportion of pediatric patient visits in general pediatric practices with psychosocial problems has increased from 7% to 19% (16). According to the 1999 US Surgeon General's report on children's mental health, 13% of children and adolescents have anxiety disorders, 6.2% have mood disorders, 10.3% have disruptive disorders, and 2% have substance use disorders, for a total of 20.9% having one or more mental health or substance abuse disorders (1). Of those needing active mental health interventions, 11% were found to have significant functional impairment and 5% were found to have extreme functional impairment (1). Other research has found that 27% of children ages 9, 11, and 13 years of age have mental impairment, and 20% have a diagnosable mental health condition (17). Further, suicide is the third leading cause of death in the US for children ages 15-24 years and suicide attempts reach a peak during the midadolescent years (1,18,19) highlighting the psychological vulnerability adolescents experience.

Many children and adolescents have both physical and mental disorders, and it has been found that the majority of children and adolescents with medical problems have higher levels of mental disorders (20), suggesting that having a chronic health condition, such as overweight, may increase the likelihood of mental health issues and concerns. In fact, one recent study found serious adverse consequences of overweight on health-related quality of life (HRQOL) in a clinical sample of severely overweight (BMI: 34.7) children and adolescents 5 to 15 years of age (21).

PSYCHO-SOCIAL RISKS FOR OVERWEIGHT ADOLESCENTS

Depression

Several studies have documented a clear correlation between depression and overweight in adolescents (22-24). Goodman et al (25) have shown in a nationally representative, longitudinal study of over 9,000 adolescents that depressed mood in non overweight individuals is associated with the development of overweight at one year and worsening overweight in baseline overweight participants, suggesting that depression may precede overweight. Other studies using community samples of overweight versus non overweight adolescents have found no differences in depressive symptoms between the two groups (26). Swallen et al (27) found a statistically significant relationship between BMI and general physical health in adolescents from age 12 to 20 years, but only young adolescents (12-14 years) evidenced a deleterious impact on emotional health as reported by depression and/or low self esteem. Several studies, including a recent one by Daniels (22), failed to confirm a relationship between overweight and symptoms of depression in adolescents. Thus, the relationship between depressive symptoms and overweight in children and adolescents is not completely clear, although depression appears to play a role in the mental health of a certain subpopulation of overweight adolescents.

Self-Esteem

Studies on self-esteem in overweight children and adolescents also report inconsistent results. Some studies have shown moderately lower self-esteem in overweight children and adolescents than their non overweight peers (28, 29), while others have shown no difference between population-based groups of overweight children and their non overweight peers (30,31). Studies also show that overweight females are at greater risk for self-esteem problems because body image is so important to self-image (28), perhaps because girls are expected to be thin, beautiful, flawless, sexy, cookie-cutter images of the super models and actresses they attempt to emulate. In clinical populations, there is a clear relationship between overweight and self-esteem in children and adolescents, with more heavily overweight children having lower self-esteem (31). One hypothesis is that clinically referred children represent a subgroup of overweight children associated with especially low self-esteem (15).

Eating disorders

The age of onset for 85% of all eating disorders is between 11 and 20 years (32) and eating disorders have been found to be associated with overweight in adolescents (33). Overweight youth are stigmatized (34), predisposing them to unhealthy dieting practices and attempts to lose weight. Britz et al (35) reported that the rate of eating disorders was six times higher in an overweight patient group than a population-based control group. The disorders included bulimia nervosa, eating disorders not otherwise specified, and anorexia nervosa. Sixty percent of females and 35.5% of males reported binge eating episodes.

Body image

Overweight in adolescents has been associated with negative body image (7). Overweight children as young as age five can develop a negative body image (36). A consistently replicated finding is that overweight children and adolescents have a more negative body image than their peers (37). A 1994 study by Grilo et al (38) demonstrated that "the greater the frequency of being teased about weight and shape while growing up, the more negative one's appearance is regarded, and the greater the degree of body dissatisfaction in adulthood" (p. 448). Studies have shown that overweight girls appear to have a more negative body image than overweight boys (29).

Stigmatization

Stigmatization of overweight children and adolescents is significant and has long been a part of western culture (39). Studies have shown that children as young as three years of age begin to have negative attitudes toward overweight and obesity. When given different methods for assessing stigmatizing attitudes, these children ascribe negative characteristics to overweight targets, including mean, ugly, stupid, and sloppy, compared to non overweight targets (40). These trends tend to worsen as children get older (41). Such stereotypes are born out in real-life when studies show that US women who were overweight adolescents become adults with lower educational attainment, lower paying jobs, higher rates of poverty, and less likelihood of marriage in comparison to thinner women (42,43). Stigma associated with overweight thought to be greater for girls than for boys (27).

Overweight impacts adolescents' relationships due to increased vulnerability to weight-related teasing and social isolation. Overweight adolescents may be socially marginalized among their peers and experience more weight-related stigmatization by peers and family members (7,44). Overweight youth have greater difficulty in gaining admission to college, although there is no indication that they are less apt to be able to complete the course work (39).

Evaluation of Mental Health

Overweight adolescents should be thoroughly evaluated to identify any psychological conditions that may affect the course of medical treatment for weight loss or other medical co-morbidities (15). However, most pediatric health care providers are not trained to assess mental health issues and may have limited experience in daily practice in addressing mental health related problems. Other factors, including limited visit time and lack of established office strategies (24), may also contribute to the lack of detection of the psychological and psychosocial factors leading to overweight or originating from it. Additionally, pediatricians may directly or indirectly express "fatism," which may contaminate the relationship with their young patients, and is particularly true with younger, overweight patients where parent-bashing or blaming is common (15).

Jonides et al (45) reporting results of a questionnaire to pediatricians asking about the routine evaluation of various psychological and emotional factors including self-esteem, eating disorders, concern about weight, family dynamics and history of abuse, showed that by far not every provider asks and elaborates on all of those important factors. Friedman (46) suggested that pediatricians are in an ideal position to detect psychological issues in young people, and they should be better trained to probe for and recognize signs of major mental illnesses. Weitzman and Leventhal (47) concluded that the pediatric practice setting is an optimal environment for behavioral health screening if the currently available tools are used effectively. However, training is lacking in these areas.

Given that most providers specializing in adolescent overweight are not trained in mental and behavioral health evaluations, having a team of providers, including mental health providers familiar with evaluation of and treatment options for various mental and behavioral health conditions in adolescents, would add significant value to the team caring for this particular patient subset. Evaluation and treatment of underlying psychological and behavioral problems by a health care provider trained in adolescent mental health will aid in the reduction of obesity-related psychological co-morbidity in adolescents.

SUGGESTIONS FOR MENTAL HEALTH EVALUATION

There is no consensus recommendation for the evaluation of mental health in overweight adolescents, and there are no studies comparing different methods for psychiatric assessment of affected children (15). An expert committee recommendation on overweight evaluation and treatment by Barlow and Dietz (48) suggested that asking the right questions in "objective, non accusatory language" would help establish a basis of trust between family and provider, which is key to long-term, successful management. Additionally, the use of well-validated instruments for evaluation is important.

A thorough psychiatric, psychological and family history regarding the patient needs to be taken. As rapport is established, questions regarding the patient's weight, concerns about weight, weight gain or loss, eating issues, and psychosocial issues associated with being overweight (e.g., friendships, teasing, depression, low self-esteem) need to be broached. It is also important to assess readiness for change. When dealing with an adolescent, the family context is important, and the entire family must have some readiness for change for any to occur.

Paper and pencil assessment instruments can be useful in the initial assessment of psychological variables associated with overweight. As noted earlier, no specific guidelines have been established, but the following instruments are suggested as a potential assessment packet which assesses depressive symptoms, behaviors across a variety of domains, eating issues, and acute and characterological psychological concerns. A summary of the suggested instruments may be seen in table 1.

Table 1. Psychological assessment instruments for overweight adolescents

Instrument	Age Group (yrs)	Measures	Method of report
Children's Depression Inventory (CDI)	6-17	Symptoms of depression	Self-report
Child Behavior Checklist (CBCL)	6-18	Child's activities, social relations, and school performance	Parent report
Children's Eating Attitude Test (chEAT)	7-14	Diet behaviors, food preoccupation, anorexia, bulimia, concerns about overweight	Self-report
Millon Pre-adolescent Clinical Inventory (M-PACI)	9-12	Emerging personality patterns and acute psychological symptoms	Self-report
Millon Adolescent Clinical Inventory (MACI)	13-19	Emerging personality patterns and acute psychological symptoms	Self-report

In order to assess level of depression, the Children's Depression Inventory (CDI), a 27-item, symptom-oriented scale for children ages 6 -17 years (49) may be utilized. The CDI is a highly reliable and valid measure (50) and has been used effectively in several studies with overweight children (51,52). Since the CDI is a self-report measure, it can be supplemented by a parent-completed Child Behavior Checklist (53) in order to obtain corroborating or conflicting data from parents. Issues regarding eating can be measured through completion of a version of the Eating Attitude Test (54,55). This is a 6-point, forced choice, self-report inventory that measures dieting behaviors, food preoccupation, anorexia, bulimia, and concerns about being overweight. Versions for teenagers and younger children (chEAT), have demonstrated concurrent and predictive validity as well as reliability (55). Finally, for overall symptom assessment, younger children (9-12 years) can complete the Millon Pre-adolescent Clinical Inventory (M-PACI), and adolescents (13-19 years) can complete the Millon Adolescent Clinical Inventory (MACI). Both instruments are designed to quickly and accurately identify psychological problems and determine both emerging personality patterns and acute psychological symptoms.

Addressing mental health by correct and timely assessment and intervention can be of significant importance in improving the outcome of obesity-related problems in adolescents. Also, the correct diagnosis and therapy of mental health problems, if associated with overweight, can improve weight management and decrease medical complications.

Conclusions

Overweight, obesity, and obesity-related diseases have become major problems in the developed and developing world in recent years. Adolescents are a high risk group for developing overweight, and most overweight teenagers will be unsuccessful in their attempts, should they make any, to lose weight; they move on to become an overweight or obese adult with the concomitant risk for medical disease. Along with obesity-related disease states, overweight adolescents are also likely to suffer from some psychosocial effects of overweight, such as depression, low self-esteem, eating disorders, negative body image, and stigmatization from peers, thus increasing the probability of obesity-related mental health co-morbidities.

The public health agenda with regard to overweight and obesity has shifted the focus toward primary prevention of overweight. Primary prevention is certainly the strategy for which to strive, but secondary and tertiary prevention are more reasonable strategies at this time since overweight and its potential complications are more prevalent than ever and need to be addressed aggressively and comprehensively.

To improve obesity-related morbidity and mortality in this age group, providers involved in their care need to develop a better understanding and increased focus on mental health in addition to physical health. One strategy is a comprehensive team approach, including a mental health specialist who not only addresses those issues in the patient and family but also teaches the pediatric provider better strategies for initial screening.

References

[1] Surgeon general. Mental health: A report of the surgeon general. Washington, DC: US Dept Health Hum Serv, 1999.

[2] Mokdad AH, Marks JS, Stroup DF, Gerberding JL. Actual causes of death in the United States, 2000. JAMA 2004;291(10):1238-45.

[3] Daniels SR. The consequences of childhood overweight and obesity. Future Child 2006;16(1):47-67.

[4] Olshansky SJ, Passaro DJ, Hershow RC, et al. A potential decline in life expectancy in the United States in the 21st century. New Engl J Med 2005;352:1135-7.
[5] Rossner S. Obesity: The disease of the twenty-first century. Int J Obes 2002;26(Suppl 4):S2-S4.
[6] Pinhas-Hamiel O, Zeitler P. "Who is the wise man?--The one who foresees consequences:". Childhood obesity, new associated comorbidity and prevention. Prev Med 2000;31(6):702-5.
[7] Jelalian E, Wember YM, Bungeroth H, Birmaher V. Practitioner review: Bridging the gap between research and clinical practic inpediatric obesity. J Child Psychol Psychiatry 2007;48(2):115-27.
[8] Hassink S. A clinical guide to pediatric weight management and obesity. Philadelphia, PA: Lippincott Williams Wilkins, 2007.
[9] Reilly JJ. Obesity in childhood and adolescence: evidence based clinical and public health perspectives. Postgrad Med J 2006;82(969):429-37.
[10] Hedley AA, Ogden CL, Johnson CL, Carroll MD, Curtin LR, Flegal KM. Prevalence of overweight and obesity among US children, adolescents, and adults, 1999-2002. JAMA 2004;291(23):2847-50.
[11] Ogden CL, Carroll MD, Curtin LR, McDowell MA, Tabak CJ, Flegal KM. Prevalence of overweight and obesity in the United States, 1999-2004. JAMA 2006;295(13):1549-55.
[12] Ogden CL, Flegal KM, Carroll MD, Johnson CL. Prevalence and trends in overweight among US children and adolescents, 1999-2000. JAMA 2002;288(14):1728-32.
[13] Danice Eaton DK, Kann L, Kinchen S,Ross J, Hawkins J, et al. Youth risk behavior surveillance--United States, 2005. MMWR 2006;55(SS05):1-108.
[14] Stice E, Presnell K, Shaw H. Psychological and behavioral risk factors for obesity onset in adolescent girls: A prospective study. J Consult Clin Psychol 2005;73(2):195-202.
[15] Zametkin AJ, Zoon CK, Klein HW, Munson S. Psychiatric aspects of child and adolescent obesity: a review of the past 10 years. J Am Acad Child Adolesc Psychiatry 2004;43(2):134-50.
[16] Kelleher KJ, McIrney TK, Gardner WP, Childs GE, Wasserman RC. Increasing identification of psychosocial problems: 1979-1996. Pediatrics 2000;105:1313-21.
[17] Burns BJ, Costello EJ, Angold A, et al. Children's mental health services use across service sectors. Health Affairs 1995;14(3):147-59.
[18] Lubell KM, Kegler SR, Crosby AE, Karch D. Suicide tends among youths and young adults aged 10-24 years, United States, 1990-2004. MMWR 2007;56(35):905-8.
[19] Hoyert DL, kochanek KD, Murphy SL. Deaths: Final data for 1997. Nat Vital Stat Report 1999;47(9).
[20] Spady DW, Schopflocher DP, Svenson Lw, Thompson AH. Medical and psychiatric comorbidity and health care use among children 6 to 17 years old. Arch Pediatr Adolesc Med 2005;159:231-7.
[21] Schwimmer JB, Burwinkle TM, Varni Jw. Health-related quality of life of severely obese children and adolescents. JAMA 2003;289:1813-9.
[22] Daniels J. Weight and weight concerns: are they associated with reported depressive symptoms in adolescents? J Pediatr Health Care 2005;19(1):33-41.
[23] Heo M, Pietrobelli A, Fontaine KR, Sirey JA, Faith MS. Depressive mood and obesity in US adults: comparison and moderation by sex, age, and race. Int J Obes (Lond) 2006;30(3):513-9.
[24] Kabir AA, Whelton PK, Khan MM, Gustat J, Chen W. Association of symptoms of depression and obesity with hypertension: the Bogalusa Heart Study. Am J Hypertens 2006;19(6):639-45.
[25] Goodman E, Whitaker RC. A prospective study of the role of depression in the development and persistence of adolescent obesity. Pediatrics 2002;110(3):497-504.
[26] Wardle J, Williamson S, Johnson F, Edwards C. Depression in adolescent obesity: Cultural moderators of the association between obesity and depressive symptoms. Int J Obes 2006;30:634-43.
[27] Swallen KC, Reither EN, Haas SA, Meier AM. Overweight, obesity, and health-related quality of life among adolescents: the National Longitudinal Study of Adolescent Health. Pediatrics 2005;115(2):340-7.
[28] Pesa JA, Syre TS, Jones E. Psychosocial differences associated with body weight among female adolescents: The importance of body image. J Adolesc Health 2000;26:330-7.
[29] Strauss RS. Childhood obesity and self-esteem. Pediatrics 2000;105:1-5.
[30] Renman C, Engstrom I, Silfverdal SA, Aman J. Mental health and psychosocial characteristics in adolescent obesity: A poulation-based case-control study. Acta Paediatr 1999;88:998-1003.

[31] Rumpel C, Harris TB. The influence of weight on adolescent self-esteem. J Psychosomat Res 1994;38:547-56.
[32] Yager J, Andersen A, Devin M, Mitchell J, Powers P, Yates A. American Psychiatric Association proactice guidelines for eating disorders. Am J Psychiatry 1993;150:207-28.
[33] Neumark-Sztainer D, Story M, French SA, Falkner NH, Beuhring T, Resnick MD. Sociodemographic and personal characteristics of adolescents engaged in weight loss and weight/muscle gain behaviors: Who is doing what? Prev Med 1999;28:40-50.
[34] Pipher M. Reviving Ophelia. New York: Ballantine, 1994.
[35] Britz B, Siegfried W, Ziegler A, et al. Rates of psychiatric disorders in a clinical study group of adolescents with extreme obesity and in obese adolescents ascertained via a population based study. Int J Obes 2000;24:1707-14.36. Ebbeling CB, Pawlak DB, Ludwig DS. Childhood obesity: public health crisis, common sense cure. Lancet 2002;360:473-82.
[36] Buddeburg-Fisher b, Klaghofer R, Reed V. Associations between body weight, psychiatric disorders and body image in female adolescents. Psychother Psychosomat Med 1999;68:325-32.
[37] Grilo CM, Wilfley DE, Brownell KD, Rodin J. Teasing, body image, and self-esteem in a clinical sample of obese women. Addict Behav 1994;19:443-50.
[38] Puhl RM, Latner JD. Stigma, obesity, and the health of the nation's children. Psychol Bull 2007;133(4):557-80.
[39] Cramer P, Steinwert T. Thin is good, fat is bad: how early does it begin? J Appl Dev Psychol 1998;19:429-51.
[40] Wardle J, Volz C, Golding C. Social variation in attitudes to obesity in children. Int J Obes 1995;19:562-9.
[41] Dietz WH. Periods of risk in childhood for the development of adult obesity--what do we need to learn? J Nutr 1997;127(Suppl):1884S-6.
[42] Maffies C, Tato L. Long-term effects of childhood obesity on morbidity and mortality. Horm Res 2001;55SS(suppl 1):42-5.
[43] Neumark-Sztainer D, Falkner NH, Story M, Perry C, Hannan PJ, Mulert S. Weight-teasing among adolescents: correlations with weight status and disordered eating behaviors. Int J Obes 2002;26:123-31.
[44] Jonides L, Buschbacher V, Barlow SE. Management of child and adolescent obesity: psychological, emotional, and behavioral assessment. Pediatrics 2002;110(1 Pt 2):215-21.
[45] Friedman RA. Uncovering an epidemic - screening for mental illness in teens. N Engl J Med 2006;355(26):2717-9.
[46] Weitzman CC, Leventhal JM. Screening for behavioral health problems in primary care. Curr Opin Pediatr 2006;18(6):641-8.
[47] Barlow SE, Dietz WH. Obesity evaluation and treatment: Expert committee recommendations. The Maternal and Child Health Bureau, Health Resources and Services Administration and the Department of Health and Human Services. Pediatrics 1998;102(3):E29.
[48] Kovacs M. The Children's Depression Inventory (CDI). Psychopharmacol Bull 1985;21:995-8.
[49] Knight D, Hensley VR, Waters B. Validation of the Children's Depression Scale and the Children's Depression Inventory in a prepubertal sample. J Child Psychol Psychiatry 1988;29:853-63.
[50] Sheslow D, Hassink S, et al. The relationship between self-esteem and depression in obese children. Ann NY Acad Sci 1993;699:289-91.
[51] Wallace WJ, Sheslow D, Hassink S. Obesity in children: A risk for depression. Ann NY Acad Sci 1993;699:301-3.
[52] Achenbach TM, Ruffle TM. The Child Behavior Checklist and related forms for assessing behavioral/emotional problems and competencies. Pediatr Rev 2000;21:265-71.
[53] Garner DM, Garfinkle PE. The eating attitudes test: An index of the symptoms of anorexia nervosa. Psychol Med 1979;9:273-9.
[54] Maloney MJ, McGuire JB, Daniels SR. Reliability testing of a children's version of the Eating Attitude Test. J Am Acad Child Adolesc Psychiatry 1988;27:541-3.

SECTION THREE: KNOWLEDGE, PERCEPTION AND CULTURE IN RURAL CHILD HEALTH

In: Rural child health: International aspects
Editors: Erica Bell and Joav Merrick

ISBN: 978-1-60876-357-3

Chapter 7

PARENTS' PERCEPTION ABOUT UNINTENTIONAL CHILDHOOD INJURIES AND ITS PREVENTION IN RURAL BANGLADESH LOCAL COMMUNITY

Salim Mahmud Chowdhury*, MBBS, MPH[1,2], Md, A Halim, BSS, MSS, MPhil[2], Leif Svanström, MD, PhD[1], Lars-Gunnar Hörte, PM, BSc, PhD[1], Ross Cox, BA[3] and Fazlur Rahman, MBBS, MPhil, PhD[1,2]

[1]Division of Social Medicine, Department of Public Health Science, Karolinska Institutet, Stockholm, Sweden

[2]Centre for Injury Prevention and Research, Bangladesh (CIPRB) and Alliance for Safe Children (TASC), Bangkok, Thailand

Injury is the leading killer of children aged 1 to 17 years in low and middle-income countries. In Bangladesh, like other low and middle-income countries, children exposed much higher levels of environmental hazards during their developmental stages that they do not have knowledge of safety and risk avoidance. But very little is known about parental knowledge regarding common childhood injuries which is very important for developing any intervention. Our study was conducted to ascertain parental knowledge regarding common childhood injuries and their prevention practices in rural Bangladesh. Participants were selected purposely from rural Bangladesh. Four focus group discussions (FGDs), ten in-depth interviews and five focused observations were conducted during November and December 2006 for this study. Results: Respondents stated that younger children appeared to be the victims of injury and the majority of these injuries occurred in and around the household. From the focused observations, different injury prevention measures seem to be practiced in a few households albeit unknowingly. Supervision and putting physical barriers (e.g. door barrier, fencing ponds etc.) were suggested as preventive measures. Participants also recommended government's involvement in raising mass awareness using different communication channels.

* Correspondence: Salim Mahmud Chowdhury, Epidemiologist, Centre for Injury Prevention and Research Banglades, Flat B-2, House 46, Road 12, Sector 4, Uttara Model Town, Dhaka 1230, Bangladesh. Tel: +880-2-8911404 (Res); Fax: ++880-2-9569234; E-mail: Salim.Chowdhury@ki.se, smchow_dhaka@yahoo.com, chowdhury@ciprb.org

Conclusions: The results of this study may be considered when designing childhood injury prevention programs for rural Bangladesh and also for similar socio-cultural settings in other low-income countries.

INTRODUCTION

Injury is the biggest killer of children between 1 and 17 years in low and middle-income countries (1). In Bangladesh, communicable and selected non-communicable diseases are still considered as the major concerns for children, especially for infants. However, child injury as a newly identified threat is significantly challenging the placement of this concern. In Bangladesh, there are over 30,000 children fatally being injured each year and almost two in every 100 children are being injured significantly enough to require medical care, or lose three days of school or work every year (2).

In Bangladesh, like other low and middle-income countries, children grow up exposed to much higher levels of environmental hazards in cultures that do not have an awareness of safety and risk avoidance, and where social situations make close adult supervision difficult. Prevention of childhood injuries is of great importance to both individuals and society, but unfortunately, it has largely been either excluded from attention or treated in an inappropriate manner. It is well established that identification of the context and mechanisms of injury, including injury risks and hazards, are the essential part of the injury prevention knowledge base (3,4). In recent years, qualitative studies have examined the antecedents of unintentional injuries (5) including both the social and physical environments in which injuries occur, as well as the behaviors that may contribute to injury occurrence (3,6). These studies have complemented the injury knowledge base. This study was an attempt to ascertain parental knowledge regarding common childhood injuries in rural settings of Bangladesh by exploring parents understanding about the causes of childhood injuries and their enculturation process with those events (coping mechanisms and as well as their preventative approaches).

OUR STUDY

This study was a qualitative investigation of the parents' perceptions of the risk factors that may contribute to the occurrence of childhood unintentional injury along with their prevention practices. Participants were selected purposely from the rural Bangladesh who had participated in focus group discussions (FGDs) and individual interviews. Different qualitative tools e.g. semi-structured interviews, FGD etc. guided both discussions and interviews.

Site information

This ethnographic study was conducted in a village of Raigonj sub-district of Sirajgonj district. Raigonj sub-district was chosen because of high injury risk status (2), presence of poor child health indicators, and the fact that the area can be characterized as typically representative of rural Bangladesh. After consultation with the different stakeholders, the village was selected for the study considering the size and the population density of the village, and the heterogeneity of the inhabitants regarding their occupations and religion.

Interview tools development and content

The interview tools were developed based on literature search and expert opinions on prevalent childhood injury risk factors. Experts reviewed the tools before pre-testing concerning the scope and coverage of the study. This range of tools allowed for the triangulation of findings, thus enhancing the interpretation of the data and facilitating our ability to validate information as the study evolved.

Extensive training was conducted for the junior research fellows on the use of the final tools after necessary correction following pre-testing. Free flow of opinions and conversation was encouraged. Box 1 shows the different tools used for this study along with participants' characteristics.

Box 1. Tools and characteristics of informants employed for data collection

Tools applied	Sex/characteristics of informants/target group	Number
Transect walk	Observed, taking notes and talked with villagers throughout the village	
Focus Observation (From 8 AM to 4 PM in the household level)	Mother (Having under five children)	5
Focus Group Discussion (FGD)	Mothers: 2 Fathers: 2	4
Key Informant Interviews	Fathers: 4 Mothers: 6	10

Four focus groups were included in the study: two groups of mothers and two groups of fathers. In addition, ten other parents (either mother or father) of different professions and religious groups were interviewed, which are illustrated in box 2.

Box 2. Introduction to key informants

Male Key Informants	Female Key Informants
Health Inspector, BA	Grand mother, 65 yrs and Hindu
Community Leader	Grand mother, 55 yrs and Muslim
School teacher	Mother, wealthier household and Muslim
A shopkeeper	Mother, poor household and Hindu
	BRAC school teacher
	Family Planning Volunteer

Procedure

The group discussions with the mothers and fathers were conducted on resident premises with 8 to 12 respondents in each group. In selecting respondents preference was given to those who had heard of or seen any unintentional childhood injury event. Two trained teams consisting of one facilitator, two note-takers and one organizer were deployed to conduct the

FGDs. After welcoming participants in each session during FGD, the facilitator gradually introduced a series of prompts to explore the desired information. A semi- structured check list was used for the in-depth interviews. Before the interview or discussion, the aims of the study were explained to the participants, confidentiality guaranteed, and permission asked to record the interview, thus obtaining informed verbal consent. Structured observation was conducted in the families having children under five years of age for 8 hours, from 8 am to 4 pm, with the prior permission of the residents.

The study was carried out during November and December, 2006. Facilitators conducted the interviews and the focus group discussions in the preferred language of the respondents. Major themes were identified, coded and categorized from content analysis.

RESULTS

Participants' views about unintentional childhood injury

Communicable diseases, e.g. fever, catching colds, diarrhea and dysentery etc. and poverty related to socioeconomic issues during the growing stages of the children were the most common responses to the question "What are the problems of your children". Surprisingly, when respondents were asked about the injuries, most of them said that they used to say 'bipod apod' a Bengali word, which means 'some unpredictable events' to understand injuries. A few of them said that they used to say 'accident' to understand injury events though they also agreed that generally the word 'accident' referred to road accident. Respondents classified their children in to four categories to describe age-sex specific priority issues for their children (Box 3). However, there was no consensus in this regard.

Box 3. Age-sex specific priority issues for the children perceived by parents

Distribution of age	**Local terminology of children**	**Priority issues for children**	
		Male	**Female**
0-12 months	'*Gheda*' (Very young)	a. Non injuries: 1. Fever, 2.Catch-cold, 3.diarrhoeal disease, 4.measles, 5. '*Khesa utha*' (A like measles), 6. '*dena utha*' (A kind of pain at the upper arms) b. Injuries: nothing	
13 months-36 months	'*Sishu*'(Child)	a. Non injuries: 1. Fever 2. Catch-cold 3.Cough. 4. Poxes. 5.Measles b. Injuries: 1.Limb fracture during playing 2. Cut by sharpen object. 3. Cut by fallen objects 4. Burn. 5. Drowning c. Others: 1. water/foreign body in the ear 2. Unwillingness to take food	
4-10 years	a. 4-6= *Nabalok* b. 7-10= *Saishob* (Childhood)	a. Non injuries: 1. Diarrhoea b. Injuries: 1. Injury during play 2. Burn 3. Drowning, 4. Injury following quarrel during play 5. Fall from tree 6. Cut by sharp objects 7. Electrocution 8. Snake bite c. Others: 1. Reluctant to attend at school 2. Inattentive in the class	a. Non Injury: 1. Diarrhoea b. Injuries: 1. Injury during play 2. Burn. 3. Cut by sharpen object.
> 10 years	10-14 years = Adolescent/ *Layek* >14 years = Adult	a. Non Injuries: nothing b. Injuries: 1.Burn 2. Cut 3. Attacked by terrorist/ Snatcher 4. Road traffic injury c. Others: 1. Reluctant to obey parent's advice 2. Drug addiction	a. Non injuries: nothing b. Injuries: 1.Burn 2. Cut c. Others: 1. Marriage

Who gets injured?

They majority of the respondents affirmed that most of the injuries occurred when the children are very young, between 3 to 5 years. They stated that children 7 to 8 years old have less chance to be injured, as in that age group they become capable of perceiving differences between risky items such as water, fire and even 'bish' (poison) and honey. A 35 year old mother from a Hindu family expressed:

> "........... Very young children are most vulnerable as they just learned how to walk. It is a matter of scaring, as they may drown in the water or they may disappear during this age........"

Only one respondent who was a schoolteacher at a non-formal primary school pointed out:

> "........Childhood (6 years and above) is more risky as there are none to look after them, but when they are below five years, then at least their parents can give attention to them."

When does a child get injured?

Most of the respondents stated that during noon children mainly get injured. But one respondent mentioned that during school holidays older children get injured. He stated:

> "......Older children (more than 7 years) jump into the water, and climb the tree to catch baby birds from their nests, when their school remains close. And then they get injured......"

Where do childhood injuries take place?

Regarding the place of injury occurrence, the majority of the respondents affirmed that most of the unintentional childhood injuries take place in and around the home, and only road traffic injuries take place far away from the home. One participant (Saleha Khatoon, a grand mother) stated that her grandson fell into the backyard 'pagar' (ditch). According to the respondents it was evident that most of the injuries occur in the backyard ditch/pond, and around the 'chula' a locally made earthen burner in the courtyard and inside the houses.

Why do childhood injuries happen?

The most common response to the question "Why do unintentional childhood injuries happen?" was that unintentional injury is simply an inevitable part of early age for the children. Only a few respondents indicated that injuries occurred because of insufficient parental supervision. A male respondent mentioned:

"………Everything is decided, and there is nothing to do for its change. That will happen what is supposed to happen ………"

In our observation we found that sharpen objects like 'da boti' (a kind of traditional iron-made sharp object used in the kitchen or in agricultural fields for cutting purposes) were not stored carefully. We have also found that children 4 to 5 years old play with these objects. We also found girls were playing 'jola bati' (a kind of pretend cooking). They collected fire by 'kupi' (a kind of open kerosene lamp which is very risky for burns), and assembled a knife for cutting vegetables, dry straw as firewood, and small dishes for cooking. They even prepared an earthen 'chula' (burner). Children could be injured while playing with these objects.

Existing preventative practices

Although in the study it was evident that the community people were not significantly concerned either individually or collectively about preventing their children from various injury opportunities, we still observed scattered approaches to injury prevention at the societal and individual level. We have seen that in a few households, parents tie waist belts with bells called 'gungur' on their children's waist. By hearing the sound of the 'gungur' parents usually follow their children's movement. To prevent children from drowning they believe in super natural things. They forbid their children going to the pond, river, or big paddy fields alone at noon. They believe that the devil may attack children in these places at noon. In a poor family we found an earthen 'chula' walled by mud. Although, they made this wall to protect the flame from wind, the height of the wall was acceptable to keep the children safe from burns.

Parent's suggestions for preventing injuries

Most of the participants felt that it is the parents' responsibility to keep their children safe and to make them aware of injury risks and hazards. Preventive measures suggested included: 1) parental supervision; 2) keeping children under supervision of other elder relatives during working time; 3) putting up physical barriers, e.g door barrier, fencing ponds etc.; 4) swimming teaching at an early age to prevent drowning; 5) employing different communication channels, e.g. courtyard meetings, door to door campaigns and mass media etc. to inform the community about injury; and 6) government policy planners should be involved in the process from the beginning. All were of the opinion that, without government's direct assistance, it is not possible to motivate community people to prevent injuries with local resources. Participants strongly recommended that there should be collaboration between government authorities and local social development organizations in this respect.

Discussion

The study results showed that injury prevention was not identified as a high priority in parenting; mothers were mostly concerned about other health problems of their children.

Most of the respondents did not believe that injuries could be prevented. This belief is not unusual. Several studies on mothers' attitudes towards injury prevention established injury as an unpreventable event (7,8). It is perceived that their attitudes consider these events as a normal process of a child becoming an adult. Even in their mosque base ('samaj' – the informal community organization), the injury issue has never been talked about. An awareness program through education (9,10) and advocacy in this regard can be important in changing their beliefs.

The study also revealed that mostly younger children were the victims of injury, though only a few mentioned that older children were more vulnerable. Similar findings have been observed in many quantitative studies (2,11,12). But when we analyzed box 3, we observed injuries appeared as an alarming events in the older age with different patterns. Thus, there was no consensus in this regard among the participants. From this study it was evident that parents believe injuries predominantly happen without any cause, but insufficient parental supervision was also identified as another important contributing factor for child injuries. In our study we also found that most of the child injuries occur in and around the home and its premises. In some quantitative studies similar findings have been observed (13,14). Thus, assisting parents in identifying the risks to their children in their specific environments could be one of the most effective interventions (15,16).

For a childhood injury prevention initiative participants identified several approaches, other than mentioning common safety devices and barriers. Most of the respondents commonly gave indistinct and impossible responses for child injury prevention, such as, "never take your eyes off of him." Although supervision is important in preventing injuries (17), watching alone does not prevent injuries. There has been no consistent research support for either supervision or parental competence in preventing injury (18). Rural mothers, especially when at work or busy with household chores, are not in a position to supervise their children constantly (19). Furthermore, in cases such as in a large family, constant supervision of each child is not possible. Hence, a feasible intervention for the supervision of the children needs to be identified.

While most of the participants were reluctant to consider child injuries as preventable, amazingly we observed different injury prevention measures unknowingly in practice in a few households. Some of these measures have already been proven as effective interventions (20). Promoting these indigenous good practices in a systemic way could also be an important strategy for the prevention of childhood injuries.

It was obvious from the study that supervision is very important issue for childhood injury prevention, while at the same time different communication channels could be utilized for raising community awareness involving the government authority. From the study it is also evident that a comprehensive effort is needed to address child injury by education, engineering including environmental modification (21,22) and enforcement of safety laws and procedures (23,24).

Before drawing conclusion, we must explain its limitations as well as strengths of the study. Since, the study was conducted in one rural area of Bangladesh; result of this study may not reflect the perception of parents' of other parts of the country due to socio-cultural variation to certain extent. However, this open-ended process provided participant-generated, rather than researcher generated information, which is an important knowledge base for the development of appropriate intervention. Thus, we feel the information on parents' perception on child injuries reported in this study is acceptable, though there were some limitations.

Conclusions

The qualitative data obtained in this study have provided important insights into the community's knowledge and perceptions regarding unintentional childhood injuries and their suggestions for effective prevention. The findings of this study will help the injury prevention experts to detail their cultural model of etiology of different injuries from the rural community's perspective. The information could be considered when designing childhood injuries prevention programs for rural communities of Bangladesh as well as for similar socio-cultural settings of other low-income countries. In practice, safety promotion at community level is the essence of a safe child friendly community, and this must be based on an understanding of local cultural beliefs.

References

[1] Krug E, ed. Injury: a leading cause of global burden of disease, Geneva, World Health Organization, 1999.

[2] Rahman A, Rahman F, Shafinaz S, Linnan M. Bangladesh Health and Injury Survey. Dhaka: DGHS, ICMH, UNICEF, TASC, 2005

[3] Galal S. Working with families to reduce the risk of home accidents in children. Mediterranean Health J 1999;5:572–83.

[4] Welander G, Svanström L, Ekman R. Safety promotion: An introduction. Kristianstad, Sweden: Kristianstad Boktyckeri, 2000.

[5] Butchart A, Kruger J, Lekoba R. Perceptions of injury causes and solutions in a Johannesburg township: implications for prevention. Soc Sci Med 2000;50:331–44.

[6] Saluja G, Brenner R, Morrongiello BA, Haynie D, Rivera M, Cheng TL. The role of supervision in child injury risk: definition, conceptual and measurement issues. Inj Contr Saf Promot 2004; 11:17–22.

[7] McCormick LK, Bartholomew LK, Lewis MJ, Brown MW, Hanson IC. Parental perceptions of barriers to childhood immunization: results of focus groups conducted in an urban population. Health Educ Res Theory Pract 1997;12:355-62

[8] Langley J, Silva P. Childhood accidents: Parents' attitudes to prevention. Aust Paediatr J 1982;18:247-9.

[9] Murphy LMB. Adolescent mother's belief about parenting and injury prevention: Results of a focus group. J Pediatr Health Care 2001;15:194-9.

[10] Skinner AM, Brown TL, Peat BG, Muller MJ. Reduced hospitalisation of burns patients following a multi-media campaign that increased adequacy of first aid treatment. Burns 2004;30:82–5.

[11] Tarim A. Nursal TZ. Yildirim S. Noyan T. Moray G. Haberal M. Epidemiology of pediatric burn injuries in southern Turkey. J Burn Care Rehabil 2005;26:327-30.

[12] Ahmed MK, Rahman M, Ginneken JV. Epidemiology of child deaths due to drowning in Matlab, Bangladesh. Int J Epidemiol 1999;28:306-11.

[13] Ong ME, Ooi SB, Manning PG. A review of 2,517 child injuries seen in a Singapore emergency department in 199 – mechanisms and injury prevention suggestions. Singapore Med J 2003;44(1):12-9.

[14] Engeland A. Kopjar B. Injuries among children treated at emergency medical centers and hospitals 1990-97, Tidsskr Nor Laegeforen 1999;119(6):784-7. [English abstract]

[15] Babul S, Olsen L, Janssen P, McIntee P, Raina P.A. Randomized trial to assess the effectiveness of an infant home safety program. Int J Inj Contr Saf Promot 2007;14(2):109-17.

[16] King WJ, Klassen TP, LeBlanc J, Bernard-Bonnin AC, Robitaille Y, Pham B, Coyle D, Tenenbein M, Pless IB. The effectiveness of a home visit to prevent childhood injury. Pediatrics 2001;108(2):382-8.

[17] Munro SA. Niekerk AV. Seedat M. Childhood unintentional injuries: the perceived impact of the environment, lack of supervision and child characteristics. Child Care Health Dev 2006; 32:269-79.
[18] Matheny AP. Accidental injuries. In: Routh DK, ed. Handbook of pediatric psychology. New York: Guilford, 1988:108-34.
[19] Issac R, Helan J, Minz S, Bose A. Community perception of childhood drowning in South India: a qualitative study. Ann Trop Pediatr 2007;27:225-9.
[20] Niekerk AV, Seedat M, Menckel E, Laflamme L. Caregiver experiences, contextualizations and understandings of the burn injury to their child. Accounts from low-income settings in South Africa. Child Care Health Dev 2007;33:236-45.
[21] Wilson C, Willis C, Hendrikz JK, Bellamy N. Speed enforcement detection devices for preventing road traffic injuries. Cochrane Database Syst Rev 2006;19(2):CD004607.
[22] The University of North Carolina. Highway Safety Research Center. Highway Saf Direction 1997;5:1-23.
[23] Davis JW, Bennink LD, Pepper DR, Parks SN, Lemaster DM, Townsend RN. Aggressive traffic enforcement: a simple and effective injury prevention program. J Trauma 2006;60(5):972-7.
[24] Thompson DC, Rivara FP, Thompson R. Helmets for preventing head and facial injuries in bicyclists. Cochrane Database Syst Rev 2000;2:CD001855.

In: Rural child health: International aspects
Editors: Erica Bell and Joav Merrick

ISBN: 978-1-60876-357-3

Chapter 8

ETHNICITY AND ETHNIC IDENTITY AMONG BEDOUIN ADOLESCENTS IN ISRAEL

***Salman Elbedour, PhD**[*1]*,
***Anthony J Onwuegbuzie, PhD, PGCE, FSS**[2]*,
***Qun G Jiao, MEd**[3]**, Aref Abu-Rabia, PhD**[4]*,
***Mohammed Morad, MD**[5,6]*
***and Joav Merrick, MD, MMedSci, DMSc**[6-10]*

[1]Department of Human Development and Psychoeducational Studies, School of Education, Howard University, Washington, DC, United States
[2]Department of Educational Leadership and Counseling, Sam Houston State University, Huntsvill, Texas, United States
[3]Newman Library, Baruch College, City University of New York, New York, United States
[4]Department of Middle East Studies, Ben-Gurion University of the Negev, Beer-Sheva, Israe
[5]Department of Family Medicine, Faculty of Health Sciences, Ben Gurion University of the Negev, Beer-Sheva, Israel
[6]National Institute of Child Health and Human Development
[7]Office of the Medical Director, Division for Mental Retardation, Ministry of Social Affairs, Jerusalem, Israel
[8]Zusman Child Development Center, Soroka University Medical Center, Beer-Sheva, Israel
[9]Interuniversity College for Health and Development, Castle of Seggau, Graz, Austria
[10]Kentucky Children's Hospital, University of Kentucky, Lexington, United States

* Correspondence: Professor Salman Elbedour, Department of Human Development and Psychoeducational Studies, School of Education, Howard University, 2441 Fourth Street, NW, Washington, DC 20059, USA. E-Mail: (selbedour@howard.edu).

While the focus on ethnic identity in the Middle East conflict has tended to be on Israeli Jews and Palestinian Arabs, there has been a paucity of research on the effects of this social construct on the marginal groups that are directly or indirectly affected by this political dispute. Methods: A sample of high-school students from five Bedouin schools in the south of Israel (n = 351). Results: Sample members (46.9%) ranked religion as the most important factor in forming their identity. Although they were Israeli citizens, 73% of the participants stated that the term "Israeli" was not an appropriate definition of their identity, and 44.9% stated that the term "Palestinian" was. Moreover, when given a list of six ways of characterizing themselves (i.e., Arab, Israeli Arab, Israeli, Palestinian Arab, Israeli Palestinian, Palestinian), "Palestinian Arab" received the highest endorsement (33.5%), followed respectively by "Israeli Arab" (29.7%), "Arab" (18.7%), Israeli Palestinian (11.7%), and Palestinian (3.5%); only 2.9% characterized themselves as Israelis. Conclusions: This indicates that their Arab/Palestinian ethnic identity is predominant and that an acceptance of their Israeli identity, while secondary, also is widespread. More than two-thirds (68.6%) of the respondents were in favor of establishing a Palestinian state alongside Israel. The implications of these and other findings are discussed.

INTRODUCTION

Much that has been written about the Arab Bedouins of the Negev has focused on the significant impact of the state of Israel and its attempts to settle this semi-nomadic group (1-3). Not surprisingly, the Negev Bedouins have occupied the attention of many Israeli social scientists (4-6). One evident exception, however, is that they have rarely addressed the ethnic identity of these Bedouin Israeli citizens.

The present study goes further by focusing on the formation of ethnic consciousness and ethnic identity among Bedouin adolescents. Studies have established the association between ethnic identity and self-esteem (7), ethnic identity and psychological functioning (8), as well as ethnic identity and experiences of racism and discrimination (9). According to Phinney et al (9), "when one's group faces rejection and discrimination, a common strategy, in order to preserve one's self-respect, is to reaffirm and strengthen group identity, through movements, which stress ethnic pride" (p. 179). In a similar vein, Smith (10) found that ethnic identity is formed by a person's majority or minority group membership and the quality and nature of interaction with out-groups members. As outside forces challenge identity, it is actually further reinforced as the group attempts to regain its collective sense of security and empowerment.

The primary objective of this paper is to examine how sociopolitical and historical factors are shaping the ethnic identity of the Bedouin Arab citizens of Israel. This group has a dual identity that is both Palestinian Arab and Israeli, although they hold a marginal status with respect to both groups. Thus, the process of ethnic identity formation is becoming more challenging and complex for this group. First, as Arab Bedouin, they are an oppressed minority within Israel, although they are Israeli citizens (11). Second, by virtue of their Israeli citizenship, they are outsiders within the Palestinian community, although they are part of that community by racial origin (11,12). Through no choice of their own (13), the Israeli Bedouin belong to both warring factions, and their joint membership in both groups may have the potential to impose psychological conflict as well as cognitive dissonance and incongruence, cognitive processes that elicit self and ethnic searching.

Generally speaking, most of the Israeli Jewish population perceives the Bedouin Arab community as a marginal and neutral group that is not allied with either the Israeli Jews or the Palestinian Arabs. Based on the assumption that marginal individuals are psychologically unbiased and ideologically uncommitted, they do not expect the Bedouin to show any loyalty or favoritism toward either group. This offers the Bedouin the potential of emerging as social critics (13), who use their marginality to play the role of bridging the warring Israeli and Palestinian Arab parties. Thus, they have the potential to respond creatively to a polarized political situation, combining their knowledge and experience as insiders with the critical attitude of outsiders, to the advantage of both the Israelis and the Palestinians. But, as the minimal group paradigm (14) suggests, an arbitrary single factor alone is capable of eliciting emotional bias among participants randomly assigned to two groups: ingroup "us" and outgroup "them." Israelis and Palestinian Arabs have a long history of antagonism, conflict over land and power, which exacerbates group categorization and differentiations, thereby accelerating their ethnic pride and ethnic self-identification (15).

RECENT RESEARCH

Over the last decade, research on the development of ethnic identity has garnered increased attention among social scientists (10,16-18). Ethnic identity refers to a set of ideals, values, behaviors, and attitudes that pertain to one's membership in an ethnic group (19,20). Feagin (21) defined an ethnic group as a "socially distinguished" entity formed by those who embrace a specific culture or nationality. Ethnic identity also is viewed as a selected social domain in which the shared values of the in-group merge with its interactions with the out-group (18,22,23). However, Thompson (24) argued that groups engage in behaviors within a social context, based on relevant cultural or physical criteria.

Theoretically speaking, an individual's ethnic identity provides information about the degree to which the individual has reflected on and examined the meaning of his or her ethnicity, thereby developing and nurturing a sense of obligation to a particular ethnic background and lineage (25,26). According to Garcia and Hurtado (17), racial ethnic identity and awareness has been reported among children as young as five years old. It has also been established that identification with an ethnic group is associated with positive self-esteem and self-concept, as well as resiliency (27). According to Tajfel (28), ethnic identity relates to some extent to social identity, and is defined as "that part of an individual's self-concept which derives from his knowledge of his membership in a social group (or groups) together with the value and emotional significance attached to that membership" (19).

Phinney (20) attempted to expand on this premise by defining ethnic identity as a dynamic process that entails one's identity and cultural practices, along with other ethnic involvements, such as a common ancestry, culture, race, religion, language, kinship, or place of origin. According to Phinney (29), some researchers stress that self-identification is the key component of ethnic identity; others believe that feelings of belonging and commitment are the essential elements of ethnic identity. Ethnic identity is chosen, and, in some cases, may be invisible to those who are not members of the relevant group. However, in other cases, a racial identity founded upon outwardly discernable features may be imposed on a group (30).

When evaluating the worth and adaptation of individuals, Euro-American cultural values place considerable emphasis on individualism, materialism, physical attributes, and social status. Marginalized groups, such as African Americans, are compelled to adapt to this monocultural Western worldview (31), which are often quite different from their own cultural value systems (32,33). When minority groups fail to abide by the attitudes and worldviews held by the dominant group, they become subject to discrimination, stereotyping, and prejudice (34). As result of these experiences, minority groups "carve up" their ethnic identities and group categorization and differentiation become inevitable. Ethnic identity is a direct function of these values and worldview frameworks, and is mediated by other social and historical forces such as distribution of power, quality of contact with dominant group, ethnic worry, ethnic discrimination, and racism (25,34,35).

The Bedouin Arab community in Israel is a minority group. It consists of nearly 1,400,000 people from 27 different tribes. Since the aftermath of the 1948 war, the community's traditional social structure has collapsed, and they have been forced to abandon their traditional semi-nomadic lifestyles and move into urban settlements (36,37). From 1948 until the present, the successive governments of Israel have followed a policy of urbanization of the Bedouin population, ostensibly in order to a) more efficiently provide government services such as education, health, and welfare; and b) use the large tracts of land traditionally used by the nomadic Bedouin to establish cities, towns, and villages for the ever-increasing Israeli Jewish population (11,36). However, the Bedouin community has resisted this forced urbanization policy and over time, their resistance has grown more active (12). The Bedouin are currently being forced out of and restricted from using open lands, and the Israeli government appears to be indifferent to their needs (4,38). Israeli scholars have supported this policy, on the grounds that the "people of the desert" lack a sense of ownership, and in the Western worldview, ownership is the primary means of valuing property. This fundamental conflict over land has shaped the contacts that the Bedouin have had with the Israelis, and has led to negative attitudes towards Israeli Jews (12,38).

The Bedouin Arabs themselves have been unable to express their connection to the land in a way that is understandable to sedentary Westernized people. However, their attachment to the land is poignantly reflected in their actions since the displacement of more than half of their population in 1948. To this day, most of them have refused to take any compensation for their land, despite the Israeli government's attempts to encourage them to do so. After more than 50 years, they are still prohibited from using their traditional lands (38,39) and they believe that in this respect they are being targeted and discriminated against because of their ethnicity.

Before the establishment of the Israeli state, the Bedouin represented the majority of the population in the Negev. However, since the creation of Israel, they have been reduced to the status of a minority in what they see as their homeland. This change has occurred for many reasons, including the fact that a) many Bedouin Arabs were forced to leave the Negev region by the Israeli authorities; b) some Bedouin voluntarily left the region to go to an Arab country (e.g., Jordan) in search of a more secure environment; and c) there has been an influx of Jewish immigration into the area (40). Another external force that significantly altered the condition of the Bedouin was the social change that occurred after the occupation of the West Bank (Judea and Samaria) and Gaza Strip in 1967. Historically, Negev Bedouin Arabs have been isolated from other Arab communities, because they have been subject to restrictions on their movements. In fact, any Bedouin who wished to travel across Israel required special authorization from the Israeli army (3). However, after 1967, Bedouin Arabs were no longer isolated from other Arabs in these areas (12,41). Some of them reconnected with relatives, while others married Palestinian Arabs and formed families in the Negev. Because of the relatively higher education levels of Palestinian Arab women compared to Bedouin women, some well-educated Bedouin men chose to marry Palestinians from Jordan. Some of the Bedouin (although a relatively small proportion) resettled in the West Bank and Gaza Strip. After the peace accord between Israel and Jordan, many Bedouin were able to reconnect with relatives who had been expelled to Jordan (40,42). In recent years, many Bedouin college students have attended educational institutions outside Israel, in the Gaza Strip, West Bank, or Jordan, and many Bedouin schoolchildren have been taught by Palestinian Arab teachers (43).

The development of ethnic identity is not only influenced by in-group membership, but also shaped by the quality of interactions with members of out-groups (10). The ongoing dispute between the Israelis and the Palestinian Arabs has deeply affected the course and direction of Bedouin ethnic awareness, self-identification, preferences, and attitudes. Previous studies have established an inverse relationship between the self-identification of ethnic, national, and social groups and their attitudes towards out-groups (16,44-46). Consistent with this finding, group identification has been found to induce individuals to prefer in-group members over out-group members (47), to view themselves as being a representative in-group member, and to exhibit high levels of cooperation with in-group members, often sacrificing personal interests in an attempt to preserve the interests of the in-group (48,49).

The Israeli and Palestinian groups have deep-seated, persistent attitudes not only about the conflict per se, but also about their in-group and the members of the out-group. According to Kelman (15), each side in the conflict "holds the view that only one can be a nation: "Either we are a nation or they are. They can acquire national identity and rights only at the expense of our identity and rights" (p. 354, emphasis in original). In the course of this conflict, both sides believe that they are competing for the same resources (e.g., land), using a "winner-takes-all" approach. According to Heraclides (50), this ethnic-based conflict "is based on a vertical psychological boundary—an 'intermediary' between ingroup and outgroup, which has the potential to give rise to group mobilization and politicization" (p. 197). As such, the conflict has served neither group; rather, it has politicized interpersonal relationships among ordinary people from both groups, including the Bedouin community. Moreover, the ongoing conflict has exacerbated each person's sense of belonging to the in-group, to the point where the thoughts and feelings of the in-group are taken on as the individual's own (51, 52). The result of this prolonged and intense conflict is that significant pressure has been placed on the individual to differentiate his or her in-group from that of the out-group, and each group has dehumanized and even demonized the other.

While the focus on ethnic identity in the Middle East conflict has tended to be on Israeli Jews and Palestinian Arabs, there has been a paucity of research on the effects of this social construct on the marginal groups that are directly or indirectly affected by this political dispute. However, dual identification with both two groups is becoming problematic. As a result of the regional conflict, the Bedouin community has become more politically active, and has been increasingly forced to choose between their Palestinian Arab ethnicity and their bicultural ethnic identity, which has become difficult to maintain in this political context.

The threats to their cultural and traditional ways of life, their socioeconomic disadvantages and their position on the fringes of Israeli society (5,12) all make it challenging for the Bedouins to develop a positive association with the Jewish majority in Israel. The

Israeli government anticipated that establishing towns for the Bedouin would increase their opportunities for employment and access to welfare services, which in turn would build their levels of self-confidence, self-worth, and sense of control over their destinies. However, the urbanized Bedouin, who are no longer employed in their traditional occupations, such as sheep or camel herding and agrarian activities, are still suffering from a grossly inadequate economic infrastructure and a paucity of employment opportunities (53). Many of their dwellings resemble those found in shantytowns in the world's poorest urban environments. The result is that, for the average Bedouin, life has gone from bad to worse. The seven towns into which the Bedouin have been relocated are desolate settlements; paved roads are scarce, and there is a lack of basic, essential services, including healthcare facilities, public libraries, playgrounds, and cultural centers (53,54). In towns such as Tel Sheva, Kessifa, Ar Ara, and Lakya (with populations ranging from 5,000 to 9,500 people), most of the roads are in poor condition—incomplete, unpaved, or nonexistent altogether. These settlements also are characterized by extremely high rates of poverty and unemployment. In the 1999 Haaretz report, the unemployment rates were 17.7% in Rahat, 12.2% in Tel Sheva, and 10.4% in Ar Ara. Using survey research, Abu-Saad and Lithwick (54) also noted that out of the seven Bedouin towns, six were ranked last in Israel for employment opportunities. In addition, the Bedouin towns have not been classified as national development areas, which would make them eligible for tax incentives for industry, educational development, and housing. These factors heighten the sense of vulnerability and distinctiveness within the Bedouin community, and increases their sense of alienation from Israeli society.

Formal education has the potential to help this minority group adjust successfully to the new Western way of life in Israel and expedite its full integration into mainstream society. However, the Bedouin education system has not received the needed attention and funding from the Israeli government (36,43,55).

It comes as no surprise, therefore, that the school achievement levels of Bedouin children are substantially lower than that of Jewish children (56). The Bedouin schools are poorly built and maintained, overcrowded, understaffed, and staffed by unqualified teachers (36,43,55). School dropout rates have reached 40% in Rahat, 45% in Tel Sheava, and 50% in Kessifa. Furthermore, the percentage of high school students who have passed the matriculation exams is among the lowest in the country. Because of the poor quality of the Bedouin educational system, there is little incentive for Bedouin students to remain in the school. During the 1991–92 school year, only 16% of Arab 17-year-olds earned their matriculation certificates, compared to 38% of Jewish seventeen-year-olds (56). And the proportion of Negev Bedouin graduates was even lower, due to not having access to the programs intended to increase their participation in higher education. The gap in educational outcomes and resources allocated to the Bedouin schools compared to the schools in the Jewish areas of Israel reflects discriminatory practices and reinforces the Bedouin Arabs' attitudes that their ethnicity and minority status are negatively impacting their lives and the quality of their education.

Unfortunately, there is a lack of empirical data on the ethnic identity of the Bedouin in Israel. While the focus of ethnic identity in the Middle East conflict has tended to be on Israeli Jews and Palestinians, there has been little research on the effects of this conflict on the marginal communities with allegiances to both groups. The present study investigates how sociopolitical factors (e.g., minority status, the Israeli-Arab conflict, the lack of power and resources) have influenced the development of ethnic identity in the Bedouin. For the first time, this study allows Bedouin youth to define themselves and demonstrate their self-identities, as well as express their ethnic self-consciousness (consciousness of self within a particular group) (57). Therefore, the primary purpose of the present study was to investigate the development of the ethnic identity of Bedouin-Arab adolescents in the context of their life experiences. Bachay (58) stated that the formation of ethnic identity is "a function of adolescence, but it neither begins nor ends in adolescence" (p. 107). Our objective in this study is to examine the ethnic identity of this cohort and provide empirical evidence about four possible ethnic orientations:

- Integration or biculturalism: The Bedouin group identifies strongly with both the Palestinian Arab and the Israeli groups.
- Marginality: The Bedouin group identifies with neither group.
- Assimilation: The Bedouin group identifies exclusively with the majority Israeli group and culture.
- Separation: The Bedouin group identifies only with the ethnic Palestinian Arabgroup and culture.

Our prediction is that the Bedouin Arab adolescents in this study will embrace their Palestinian Arab ethnicity as the central component of their identity, will perceive Palestinian Arabs as their primary reference group, and will relegate their identity as Israeli citizens to a secondary status. Despite research findings that minorities who are discriminated against tend to identify with the majority culture rather than their own cultural groups, we still predict that the Bedouin minority will embrace its Palestinian ethnic identity more prominently and assert a greater sense of belonging to its racial group. These expected results will raise the question whether it is still possible, in the face of the Middle East conflict, for the Bedouin to maintain a unique ethnic identity that involves marginalization or dual identification with both Israelis and Palestinian Arabs.

Because the Bedouin-Arab community is characterized by distinct gender differences and a patriarchal social structure, and because boys enjoy higher levels of social interaction than do girls (6,51,59), we also predict that there will be gender differences among Bedouin adolescents with respect to the thoughts, values, ideals, attitudes, feelings, and behavior that they hold about their identity as a member of the in-group. Thus, the second purpose of this investigation was to compare male and female adolescents with respect to their ethnic identity. Also because approximately 40% of the Bedouin in the Negev live in towns and villages, and 60% live semi-nomadically in unrecognized villages that are devoid of infrastructure or services (12), it is probable that level of urbanicity also will be related to ethnic identity among the sample group. Because Bedouin children experience severe disadvantages in the Israeli education system, including high attrition rates, low high school graduation rates, and low enrollment and completion rates in colleges and universities (60), it is likely that the ethnic identity of Bedouin-Arab adolescents will vary as a function of education level. Thus, the final purpose of the study was to determine whether the fathers' level of education is associated with the ethnic identity of Bedouin adolescents. It should be noted that because the majority of Bedouin women are homemakers and have limited access to education and contact with Israelis (43), we decided not to disaggregate the data by the mothers' level of education.

The present study is unique is several ways. First, it represents the initial empirical investigation of ethnic identity among the Bedouin Israeli population. Second, this inquiry is one of a few that has examined the ethnic identity of a group that has been forced to change its citizenship. Third, it is one of the first investigations to disaggregate ethnic identity within a population. Finally, previous studies (51) mostly have investigated the mental health of Palestinian and Israeli children and adolescents. Other investigations have examined various attitudes of these group members. The current inquiry expands on these studies associated with the Israeli-Palestinian conflict by examining, for the first time, a group that is not a direct combatant in the dispute. As such, it was hoped that findings from this study would increase our understanding of the social and ethnic dynamics of the Middle-East conflict.

OUR STUDY

The sample involved students from five Bedouin-Arab urban high schools located in Israel: Rahat School, Arur School, Segev-Shalom School, Tel-Sheva School and Lakiya School. These schools were located in the areas that have been formally recognized by the Israeli authorities for the settlement of the Bedouin. Efforts were made for the participants to be divided as evenly as possible among each school, so that the sample represented all the schools in the area. All the sample members were residents of the Negev in the southern part of Israel, and all the participants and their parents were born in the Negev. The Israeli government has established high schools in these six Bedouin-Arab settlements, despite the fact that 60% of the Bedouin continue to live in the unrecognized villages, all Bedouin children have to attend one of these six high schools (54). The Israeli authorities have deemed these villages as unrecognized and unplanned (11,52).

This study received authorization from the Israeli Ministry of Education, and the permission for each student to participate was obtained through their parents' signed permission. The participants and their parents were promised full anonymity and the right to pull out of the study at any time, if so desired. The participants received no material or other payment; however, they were informed that their participation would help the researchers add to the body of knowledge.

A total of 351 students participated in the study. Males represented 48% of the sample. The ages of the participants ranged from 14 to 20 years (M = 16.35, SD = 1.17). Approximately one-fifth (i.e., 21.6%) of the sample resided in the city, with 48.8% living in a village, 17.5% living as part of a tribe, and the remainder (i.e., 12.1%) residing in an unrecognized village. In addition, 44.2% of participants lived in houses that they classified as modern, 33.5% lived in single wood houses, 19.8% lived in huts, and 2.4% lived in tents. The number of members in each household ranged from 1 to 27 (M = 9.46, SD = 3.96). In line with this, the number of rooms in each dwelling ranged from 1 to 20 (M = 5.42, SD = 2.59). Only slightly more of the participants (54.5%) lived in places that had separate bedrooms than lived in abodes with no separate bedrooms.

Although the majority (68.1%) of sample had telephones in their homes, relatively few of them (14.7%) lived in dwellings that had hot water. With respect to the father's level of education, the adolescents reported that approximately one-third (33.7%) of the fathers had no formal education at all, with another third (37.6%) having only an elementary school education. A complete high school education was the highest level of attainment earned by 15.5% of fathers. Only 13.3% of fathers had a college or university education. With regard to the mothers, the majority (61.1%) had no formal education, with an additional 19.1% experiencing only an elementary school education. A further 14.2% had attained a high school education, with the remaining 4.7% attaining a college or university education. These distributions pertaining to parental education were similar to those reported by Elbedour, Onwuegbuzie, Caridine and Abu-Saad (61), who studied the effect of polygamy on Bedouin third graders.

INSTRUMENTS

All participants were administered the Ethnic Identity Questionnaire (EIQ), an instrument designed by Smooha (62) to be administered within 90 minutes. The EIQ consists of three sections. The first section, entitled, "Lifestyle," extracts demographic information (e.g., gender, age). The second section, entitled, "Ethnic Identity," contains items that attempt to assess the ethnic identity of each respondent, as well as her/his attitudes toward Arab-Jewish relations. Some of the items on the questionnaire represent categories (e.g., "daily," "quite often," "sometimes," "almost never"); whereas some of the items involve rating scales (e.g., "not good at all," "not good," "good," "very good"), with the remaining items representing Likert-format scales (e.g., "definitely willing," "willing," "uncertain," "unwilling," "definitely unwilling"). In order to maximize validity (i.e., content-related validity and construct-related validity), all items were read aloud by the first author and a research assistant to participants, and sufficient time was given to respond to each questions. Unfortunately, because of the mixed item format, score reliability pertaining to the instrument could not be computed.

PROCEDURES

In order to maximize the internal validity of the findings by minimizing threats via differential selection of participants and instrumentation (63), the study was carried out within the school framework according to the following criteria. First, the sample members participated in small groups of 10 adolescents only. Second, all participants were residents of the Negev area and from Bedouin backgrounds, from whom the researchers received their permission and that of their parents to participate in the study. Third, questionnaire instructions and explanations were delivered to the participants on a pre-prepared audio tape. Fourth, in an attempt to collect independent observations, the study did not include siblings from the same family. Fifth, the researchers and their assistant—Arabic speakers who were familiar with the culture—were present during the administration of the instrument to clarify and answer any student questions, as well as to emphasize the importance of the study and stress that anonymity would be maintained. Finally, the study was undertaken consecutively, without breaks.

OUR FINDINGS

In line with the purposes of the study, the results are presented in four major sections. The first section contains descriptive statistics pertaining to ethnic identity and attitudes towards Arab-Jewish relations of the full sample. The remaining three sections involve the presentation of inferential statistics, using a series of chi-square analyses to examine ethnic identity as a function of gender, urbanicity, and parental education level, respectively. It should be noted that because of the length of the EIQ, only items considered to yield the most notable responses were reported.

ETHNIC IDENTITY AND ATTITUDES TOWARDS ARAB-JEWISH RELATIONS OF FULL SAMPLE

Dwellings. The Bedouin-Arab adolescent participants were asked to indicate the degree to which they were satisfied with their dwellings. Encouragingly, only 9.7% of the respondents deemed their homes to be either "not good" (2.9%) or "not good at all" (6.9%). The remaining 91.3% rated their abodes as being either "good" (54.2%) or "very good" (36.1%). However, the picture was not as positive with respect to the adolescents' attitudes towards the cultural and educational services (e.g., schools, extra-curricular education, libraries, and entertainment opportunities) in their places of residence. Indeed, only 36.0% were either "satisfied" (18.6%) or "definitely satisfied" (17.4%) with these services, with 28.3% "not too satisfied", 22.6% "not satisfied", and 13.1% "definitely not satisfied".

Social relationships. Somewhat surprisingly, nearly one-half of the sample members (44.4%) almost never had contact with Jews, with a further 37.2% having only occasional contact with Jews. Only 12.9% and 5.4% had frequent and daily contact, respectively. Moreover, half of the participants (50.1%) reported having no Jewish acquaintances or friends. Also, an additional 23.1% of adolescents who had Jewish friends had never visited them at their homes in the last two years. Only 13.5% and 13.3% had visited Jewish friends once/twice and on three or more occasions, respectively. With respect to having Jewish people as one of two immediate neighbors, one-fourth (25.7%) were either willing (15.0%) or definitely willing (10.7%) for this to occur. A further 38.4% were willing to have a Jewish person as an immediate neighbor, although they would prefer Arab neighbors. Finally, 35.8% of the teenagers wanted to have exclusively Arab people as immediate neighbors.

All research participants were asked whether they believed that their relations with Jewish people were on an equal footing. Responses were very mixed. Whereas 15.1%, 24.9%, and 7.8% indicated that they believed this to be always the case, mostly the case, or often the case, respectively, slightly more than half (52.2%) of the adolescents reported either that they believed that this was almost never the case (27.8%), or that they had no contacts with Jewish people for them to hold this belief (24.3%). Another interesting split occurred when the teenagers were asked whether they believed that there should be separate schools for Arabs and for Jews. Slightly less than one-half (42.9%) agreed with this idea, with 36.0% uncertain, and 20.5% against this plan. A very similar distribution occurred when the question was raised as to whether there should be separate residential quarters for Arabs and Jews. Here, 46% agreed, with 31.9% uncertain, and 22.1% disagreeing. Finally, an extremely large proportion (97.1%) of the teenagers indicated that their thinking and behavior were affected by their Arabic origin either to a great extent (60.6%) or to some extent (36.5%).

Political representation. When asked whether they thought that political parties should be separate for Arabs and Jews, responses were very evenly split. Specifically, 34.1% agreed, 34.4% were uncertain, and 31.5% disagreed. Approximately two-thirds (66.4%) of adolescents reported that they did not favor the imposition of compulsory military service on Arabs in Israel, with only 16.2% in favor of this and the remainder (17.4%) uncertain.

The following issues led to approximately two-thirds of sample members deeming them to be important, with less than one-fifth regarding these issues as not important: Arabs controlling their own educational system (68.6% vs. 9.1%); Arabs controlling their own local governments (62.3% vs. 13.5%); Arabs controlling separate Arab departments (55.3% vs. 15.6%); establishing an independent Arab university (62.7% vs. 19.1%); establishing a new, independent Arab-language newspaper, radio, or television station (66.6% vs.15.0%); establishing an independent Arab trade union (68.9% vs.13.1%); establishing an independent Arab industry (64.5% vs. 15.8%); and establishing a new, independent Arab national political party (63.0% vs. 12.5%).

Of the types of political organizations presented as being the most desirable for Arabs in Israel at the current time, independent Arab national political parties received the greatest endorsement (43.0%), followed, respectively, by non–Zionist parties composed of Arabs and Jews (27.9%), no political parties at all (19.3%), Arab parties affiliated with Zionist parties (6.5%), and the existing Zionist parties but joining as individuals with equal status (3.3%).

Ethnic identity. The adolescents were asked to rank which identities they found to be the most important. Interestingly, religion was rated as being by far the most important component of identity (46.9%), followed, a long way behind, by nationality (15.8%), socioeconomic status (15.5%), extended family (11.1%), and citizenship (10.6%), respectively. Not only did citizenship receive the lowest endorsement, but when asked whether they were satisfied with being an Israeli citizen, only 44.5% reported that they were either definitely satisfied (24.9%) or satisfied (19.7%), with the remaining 55.5% expressing dissatisfaction. Further, nearly three-fourths of the adolescents (73.0%) believed that the term "Israeli" was not appropriate in describing their identity. Also, a relatively large, albeit smaller, proportion of sample members (44.9%) believed that the term "Palestinian" was appropriate in describing their identity. Moreover, when given a list of six ways of characterizing themselves (i.e., Arab, Israeli Arab, Israeli, Palestinian Arab, Israeli Palestinian, Palestinian), "Palestinian Arab" received the highest endorsement (33.5%), followed respectively by "Israeli Arab" (29.7%), "Arab" (18.7%),"Israeli Palestinian" (11.7%), and "Palestinian" (3.5%); only 2.9% characterized themselves as Israelis.

Approximately one-third of the adolescents (36.5%) revealed that they felt closer to Oriental Jews than to Ashkenazic Jews. The reverse was true for only 12.8%. Half of the sample (50.4%) stated that it made no difference. A similar proportion of study participants (47.9%) indicated that they felt closer to Arabs in the West Bank and Gaza Strip than they did to Jews in Israel. Disturbingly, nearly one-half of the sample (48.2%) did not recognize Israeli's right to exist, with a further 33.8% recognizing this right with reservations. Only 17.9% of the adolescents unequivocally recognized Israeli's right to exist.

More than two-thirds (69.2%) indicated that Israel should recognize the Palestinians as a nation, with an additional 17.7% supporting this under certain circumstances. Only 13.1% were against the creation of a Palestinian nation. Similarly, 68.6% of sample members were in favor of establishing a Palestinian state alongside Israel, 18.2% supported this under certain circumstances, and only 13.2% opposed this scenario. Also, 65.1% of study participants reported that they would definitely (27.9%) or would consider (37.2%) moving to a Palestinian state if one were established alongside Israel.

Finally, when asked where they felt most at home, 45.4% revealed that they felt most at home in Israel, 21.8% felt most at home in an Arab country, and 13.6% felt more at home in the West Bank and Gaza Strip, with 19.2% reporting that it made no difference.

GENDER COMPARISONS

A series of chi-square analyses was conducted to compare the male and female adolescent participants with respect to the items presented in the previous section. The items falling under each of the four sub-sections above (i.e., Dwellings, Social Relationships, Political Representation, and Ethnic Identity) were treated as a family, and the Bonferroni adjustment was used to maintain a 5% familywise error rate. Due to space constraints, only differences that were statistically significant after this adjustment are discussed. In all cases, Cramer's V statistic was used as an index of effect size (i.e., practical significance), using Cohen's (1988) criteria to determine whether the statistically significant differences represented small (V = .10 to .29), medium (V = .30 to .49), or large (V > .49) effects.

After applying the Bonferroni adjustment, six gender comparisons emerged as statistically significant. With respect to the four sub-sections, these six statistically significant differences were distributed as follows: dwellings (no gender differences), social relationships (one gender difference), political representation (two gender differences), and ethnic identity (three gender differences).

Social relationships. A statistically significant difference emerged between the male and female adolescents with regard to the number of times they visited their Jewish friends (p2[3] = 10.91, p < .01), with a small-to-moderate effect size (Cramer's V = .19). Interestingly, females (57.5%) were more likely to declare that they had no Jewish friends/acquaintances than were males (41.7%). On the other hand, females (19.0%) were less likely than were males (35.2%) to have visited a Jewish friend/acquaintance at least once.

Political representation. A statistically significant gender difference was found among the adolescents in terms of whether they supported that an independent Arab national political party be established (p2[2] = 12.33, p < .001). Here, males (74.1%) were more likely to endorse the establishment of this political party than were females (58.9%). The converse also was true. That is, males (5.2%) were less likely than were females (17.9%) to support this formation. The effect size (Cramer's V = .21) was small-to-moderate. Further, the male and female participants differed with respect to the types of political organizations they believed were the most desirable for Arabs in Israel at the current time. In particular, females (25.9%) were statistically significantly (p2[2] = 12.60, p < .01) more likely than were males (11.6%) to endorse no political parties at all. The effect size (Cramer's V = .21) again was small-to-moderate.

Ethnic identity. A statistically significant gender difference was found among the adolescents in terms of whether they felt closer to Oriental Jews or to Ashkenazic Jews (p2[3] = 10.65, p < .01). Specifically, a greater proportion of males (16.5%) than did females (6.7%)

revealed that they felt closer to Ashkenazic Jews than to Oriental Jews. At the same time, a higher percentage of females (58.7%) than did males (43.9%) stated that it made no difference. The effect size (Cramer's V = .19) again was small-to-moderate.

Interestingly, a statistically significantly (p2[2] = 8.29, p < .01) greater proportion of males (58.4%) than did females (41.4%) did not recognize Israeli's right to exist. At the same time, females (39.5%) were more likely than were males (28.5%) to recognize this right with reservations. The effect size (Cramer's V = .17), once again, was small-to-moderate.

Finally, a statistically significant gender difference was observed with respect to what the adolescents believed should be the borders of the state of Israel (p2[2] = 16.01, p < .001). The effect size (Cramer's V = .24) associated with this difference was small-to-moderate. Although a similar proportion of males (30.9%) and females (31.7%) believed that Israel should return to the 1947 United Nations Partition Resolution borders, a higher percentage of males (39.0%) than did females (19.0%) supported the pre-1967 borders. At the same time, a smaller proportion of males (30.1%) than did females (49.3%) endorsed the present borders with certain modifications.

URBANICITY COMPARISONS

After applying the Bonferroni adjustment, three urbanicity comparisons emerged as statistically significant. With respect to the four sub-sections, these three statistically significant differences were distributed as follows: dwellings (one difference), social relationships (no difference), political representation (two differences), and ethnic identity (no difference).

Dwellings. A statistically significant relationship was found between urbanicity (i.e., city/village vs. unrecognized village) and whether adolescents liked their dwellings (p2[3] = 20.42, p < .0001). The effect size (Cramer's V = .27) associated with this relationship was moderate. Specifically, adolescents who lived in unrecognized villages (26.8%) were the most likely to deem their homes as being either "not good" or "not good at all." In contrast, only 5.9% of those living in either cities or villages were dissatisfied with their dwellings.

Political representation. A statistically significant relationship was found between urbanicity and how important the adolescents believed it was for Arabs to control separate Arab departments (p2[2] = 7.02, p < .05). The effect size associated with this relationship was small-to-moderate (Cramer's V = .15). In particular, adolescents living in villages and cities (51.9%) were less likely than were those living in unrecognized villages (63.4%) to endorse Arabs controlling separate Arab departments.

Further, a statistically significant relationship was found between urbanicity and whether the adolescents believed that there should be separate political parties for Arabs and Jews (p2[2] = 8.17, p < .01), with a small-to-moderate effect size (Cramer's V = .17). Specifically, adolescents living in cities and villages (31.2%) were less likely than were those living in unrecognized villages (45.0%) to endorse separate political parties for Arabs and Jews.

PARENTAL EDUCATION LEVEL

After applying the Bonferroni adjustment, four parental education level comparisons emerged as statistically significant. With respect to the four sub-sections, these four statistically significant differences were distributed as follows: dwellings (one difference), social relationships (one difference), political representation (two differences), and ethnic identity (no differences).

Dwellings. A statistically significant relationship was found between parental education level and whether adolescents liked their dwellings (p2[9] = 20.11, $p < .01$). The effect size (Cramer's V = .25) associated with this relationship was small-to-moderate. Specifically, adolescents whose fathers had received no formal education at all (14.3%) were the most likely to deem their homes as being either "not good" or "not good at all." This was followed, respectively, by teenagers whose fathers had received elementary school education (11.1%), those whose fathers had received college/university education (4.5%), and those whose fathers had received high school education (4.0%).

Social relationships. A statistically significant relationship was found between parental education level and whether adolescents believed that their relations with Jewish people were on an equal footing (p2[12] = 31.65, $p < .001$). The effect size (Cramer's V = .31) associated with this relationship was moderate. Most notably, adolescents whose fathers had received high school education (26.9%) and college/university education (25.6%) were more likely than were those whose fathers had received elementary school education (10.3%) and no formal education (11.0%) to believe that their relations with Jewish was on an equal footing.

Political representation. A statistically significant relationship was found between parental education level and whether adolescents believed in the imposition of compulsory military service on Arabs in Israel (p2[6] = 15.69, $p < .01$). The effect size (Cramer's V = .22) associated with this relationship was small-to-moderate. Interestingly, adolescents whose fathers had received college/university education (20.5%) and no formal education (20.9%) were more likely than were those whose fathers had received high school education (9.6%) or elementary school education (11.3%) to support the imposition of compulsory military service on Arabs in Israel.

Finally, a statistically significant relationship was found between parental education level and whether adolescents supported the establishment of an independent Arab university (p2[6] = 14.36, $p < .025$). The effect size (Cramer's V = .21) associated with this relationship was small-to-moderate. Interestingly, adolescents whose fathers had received college/university education (54.5%) were less likely than were those whose fathers had received high school education (73.1%), elementary school education (61.3%%), and no formal education (63.4%) to be in favor of the establishment of an independent Arab university.

DISCUSSION

Identity formation in adolescence is remarkably significant (64). More than four decades ago, Strauss (65) pointed out that if you "wish to understand persons—their development and their relations with significant others—you must be prepared to view them as embedded in historical context" (p. 164). And with this in mind, "we must recognize that all ethnic groups and units can change genes, while yet remaining whole and retaining their identity" (66). As the present authors assert, the historical and political events experienced by contemporary Bedouin adolescents are likely to strengthen their identity as a separate group from the Israeli Jewish population and reinforce their emotional and symbolic ties to the Palestinian Arabs. Because this is the first comprehensive study to document the ethnic identity of Bedouin adolescents, it is difficult to determine whether a sense of Palestinian ethnic membership has been growing among this population. However, it also appears that this group is now displaying a much stronger sense of its Palestinian Arab identity, becoming more attached to its Palestinian heritage, pride, and nationalist philosophy. In response to the profound sociopolitical events that they have experienced in recent years. Although they are Israeli citizens, 73% of the participants stated that the term "Israeli" was not an appropriate definition of their identity, and 44.9% stated that the term "Palestinian" was. Moreover, when presented with various ways of characterizing themselves (Arab, Israeli, Israeli Arab, Palestinian Arab, Israeli Palestinian, Palestinian), the term "Palestinian Arab" received the highest endorsement (33.5%), followed by "Israeli Arab" (29.7%), "Arab" (18.7%), "Israeli Palestinian" (11.7%), and "Palestinian" (3.5%); only 2.9% of the sample characterized themselves as Israelis. As these results indicate, the participants showed a strong preference for an Arab or Palestinian identity, while a significant minority also acknowledged their status as Israeli citizens. This indicates that their Arab/Palestinian ethnic identity is predominant and that an acceptance of their Israeli identity, while secondary, also is widespread. Although this dichotomy is viewed as a fundamental conflict by Jewish Israelis, it is not seen that way by Israeli Arabs (11).

Interestingly, the results show that religion plays a significant role in the ethnic identity in this group; they ranked it as by far the most important factor in forming their identity (46.9%). Religion is a learned frame of reference—a set of beliefs, values, and attitudes that, once adopted, serve to shape and guide a person's behavior and identity (37). The participants (11.1%) identified religion as a more potent aspect of their ethnic identity than their tribal heritage or their extended family--the parameters by which they traditionally defined themselves (67). It appears that as social change has transformed their traditional culture, the Bedouin have coped by revising their collective identity to fit into the culture of politicized Islam that has enveloped the region. Consistent with this observation, the psychological literature shows that religious identification tends to increase when an individual's control over his or her environment is weakened (68,69).

THE EFFECTS OF ISRAELI STATE POLICIES ON ETHNIC IDENTITY

Since the establishment of the state of Israel in 1948, the Bedouin community of the Negev has suffered the cumulative effects of neglect, which have continually intensified their sense of alienation (70,71). Their traditional culture and way of life has been threatened with extinction by the Israeli state policy of forced settlement. As they witness continuing pressure, the Bedouin continue to resist assimilation into the larger Israeli culture (12,72). This is reflected in our study. When asked whether they were satisfied with being an Israeli citizen, only 44.5% of the sample members reported that they were either definitely satisfied

(24.9%) or satisfied (19.7%). As the identity theorist Erikson (73) pointed out, when an oppressed minority group becomes "aware of the dominant cultural ideals but prevented from emulating them, [they] are apt to fuse [their identify with] the negative images held up to them" by the majority dominant group (p. 237). Experiences of rejection and discrimination pose a threat to a person's sense of self, motivating a reevaluation of the old identity and the creation of a new identity to reinvent the self (34).

The political point of reference of our participants shows that their ethnic identity also encompasses a salient political foundation. Disturbingly, nearly half of the sample (48.2%) does not recognize Israeli's right to exist (58.4% for males and 41.4% for females) and a further 33.8% recognize it only with reservations. Only 17.9% of the adolescents unequivocally recognize Israeli's right to exist. These results reflect a widespread sense of socioeconomic and political marginalization among Israeli Arabs. The dominant Jewish group has implemented a variety of policies to control other groups and maintain a psychological distance from them. One such policy is the principle that Israel was established as a Jewish state to serve the Jewish people and another policy, based on security considerations, fundamentally regards all non-Jewish Israelis as a security threat or potential danger to the existence of the state (70,71).

Over the years, Bedouin-Arabs have been either ignored or viewed with suspicion by the Israeli authorities. For example, the state imposed restrictions on the movements of Bedouin-Arabs, so that those who wished to travel within Israel had to seek special authorization from the army (74). The Israeli state and its institutions are based on the values and culture of its dominant Jewish group; the Bedouin (and other non-Jewish groups) are excluded and viewed with suspicion. Therefore, it should be no surprise to find that the Bedouin Arabs are completely alienated from the majority Jewish community. It can be argued that the "disloyalty" of the Bedouin youth in our study is a natural response to the fact that they have been treated as a separate racial group that is subordinate to the Jewish Israelis and a threat to their security.

The literature suggests that the cohesion of two groups and the ethnic and racial separation between them is most evident when the groups interact less frequently and posses unequal power status (75). When the participants in this study were asked whether they believed that their relations with Jewish people were conducted on an equal footing, the responses were very mixed. While 15.1%, 24.9%, and 7.8% of the respondents indicated that they believed this to be always, mostly, or often the case, more than half (52.2%) of them reported either that this was almost never the case (27.8%), or that they never had any interaction with Jewish people (24.3%). These results clearly demonstrate the polarizing negativity of the interethnic contacts between the two groups and the view that Israeli Arabs should be assimilated and treated as equals has failed to gain significant support.

Almost a century ago, Sumner (76) theorized that there is a strong relationship between identification within an ethnic group and the group's experiences of maltreatment or hostility from outside groups. Branscombe and Wann (77) made a distinction between symbolic and material threats to identity. However, the threats that the Bedouin community of Israel are facing have been both symbolic (threats to their social and cultural continuity) and material (hostility and neglect). A succession of Israeli governments largely has ignored the social and economic needs of the Bedouin community, and the minimal attention that they have received has been random rather than far-reaching or sustained. Israeli Bedouins have responded to their highly threatening environment by increasingly defining themselves in contrast to Israeli

Jews. It is worth noting that this attitude is a significant change from their traditional self-definition in contrast to the fellahin, the sedentary Arab farmers.

This continuous neglect has deepened the frustration of the Bedouin community and disrupted its trust of the Israeli government. The lack of trust in the Israeli government is especially strong among the 70,000 Bedouin (approximately half of the Israeli Bedouin population) who live in 45 villages that have not been authorized by the Israeli government—the so-called "unrecognized" villages. These are illegal settlements, and the Bedouin who live there are not allowed to build houses. These communities suffer from a lack of essential services, including medical services, schools, power, water, and paved roads. These abysmal conditions are reflected in the current study; 26.8% of the respondents living in unrecognized villages described their home as "not good," as opposed to only 5.9% of those living in recognized villages and towns. The members of the unrecognized villages also lack political representation in local government (11). Although under Prime Minister Itzhak Rabin the Israeli government did recognize many of these communities and provide funding to develop their services and infrastructure, in subsequent years, these budget allocations have not been spent (11). Also, despite the fact that these communities suffer from the highest unemployment rates in the country (11,53,54), none of the Bedouin villages have been designated as "national priority" economic zones, a designation that brings additional funding and tax exemptions for economic development (11). Because of the political neglect and lack of government services in the unrecognized villages, as the findings demonstrate, the sample members who live there are more inclined to endorse political autonomy for Israeli Arabs and separate political parties for Arabs and Jews. In our results, this is reflected in higher levels of ethnocentrism and pro-Palestinian sentiment in the respondents from the unrecognized villages.

THE BEDOUIN SCHOOL SYSTEM

In Bedouin communities, the only law-abiding ways to make a living are teaching and taking low-paying jobs such as construction work and truck driving. However, any Israeli Arab who wishes to become a teacher must first pass strict tests of security and loyalty and be approved by the Israeli authorities (12). Once working, a teacher's subsequent promotions are based on his or her connections with the authorities, rather than credentials and experience. Any teacher who is believed to favor the Palestinian cause or otherwise to lack loyalty to the state may be dismissed or pressured to leave (70). School principals are appointed based not on their qualifications but on their political loyalty and influence within a political party (either the party that is in power, or the party favored by their chief superintendent). Because of the rampant political corruption and state control in the schools, there are many Bedouin with excellent educational credentials (PhDs) and experience who are unemployed and unable to find positions in the school system.

In 1998 the Israeli government formed a committee to report on the Bedouin school system. It found that the "schools in the unrecognized villages were poorly equipped, with low budgets, inadequate facilities, poor buildings and furniture, and few teaching materials . . . they were not supplied with running water and electricity, although some are [located] next to water pipes and electric lines. Schools in the planned settlements, although they are housed in modern buildings and have electricity and water, do not have sufficient laboratories, libraries or other teaching materials".

The poor state of the Bedouin schools is especially alarming, because it further perpetuates the divide between Arab and Jewish Israelis. For example, in our study the adolescents whose fathers had a high school (26.9%) or college (25.6%) education were more likely than those whose fathers had an elementary school (10.3%) or no formal (11.0%) education to believe that their relations with Jewish Israelis were on an equal footing. By treating the Bedouin educational system as if it were a threat to the state, rather than a potential uniting force, the Israeli authorities further alienate their Bedouin citizens.

THE POLITICAL IMPLICATIONS OF SEGREGATION AND ETHNIC COHESION

Our results indicate that Bedouin adolescents experience a strong awareness of their racial and ethnic identity. The Jewish character of the state of Israel (12), the Arab-Israeli conflict, the state-sanctioned discrimination in jobs, funding, and services (74,78), the lack of political equality, participation, and representation (12), and the negative portrayal of Arabs in the media have all influenced the development of identity in our respondents and made them more likely to identify themselves from a racial/ethnic perspective.

Overall, the Bedouin culture in Israel has been marginalized and (at best) tolerated, instead of being integrated into the larger society. Israeli Arabs have been segregated, forced by official government policy into a few overcrowded cities (Rahat, Tel Sheva, Laquia), in order to ensure their separation from the surrounding Jewish population. Their traditional ways of life have been destroyed; their land and other cultural and economic resources have been appropriated by the state and transferred to other uses (11,12).

The result of these segregationist policies is that the Bedouin community now perceives itself as a distinct group, socially and ethnically separate from the Jewish population of Israel (35) and marginalized into social isolation. Almost half of the respondents in our study (44.4%) almost never had contact with Jews, and a further 37.2% had only occasional contact with Jews. An additional 23.1% of those who did have Jewish friends had never visited them in their homes in the last two years. Interestingly, although females (57.5%) were more likely to have no Jewish friends or acquaintances than males (41.7%), females (19.0%) were less likely than males (35.2%) to have visited a Jewish friend or acquaintance at least once.

The state policies also have conveyed the message that the rights associated with being a member of the state of Israel are awarded not on the basis of citizenship, but based on Jewish racial heritage. So it is not surprising that the respondents also evidence the ideology of an oppressed minority—they emphasize the similarities between themselves and other oppressed groups in Israel. Specifically, almost one-third of the respondents (36.5%) stressed that they felt closer to the Oriental Jews than to Ashkenazic Jews. Deprived minority groups compare themselves with other disadvantaged groups. As the social, psychological, and cultural barriers between Israeli Jews and Bedouin grow larger, the individual's need to align, identify with, and rely on his or her own ethnic group is reinforced. Among the adolescents in our study, Arab ethnicity has become integral to their self concept. Most of them are no longer able to relate to or identify with the symbols and values of the Jewish state that has failed to respect either their group identity or their rights as citizens, and that has actively pursued discrimination in religion, education, politics, security, and employment (12).

However, the findings also demonstrate that although the participants identify with their Palestinian heritage, they demonstrate no hatred for the Jewish people of Israel. In the words of Siham Fahoum, a local political leader and member of the Nazareth local council, "Our objection is not to the state, but to the state's discriminatory policy" (11). One-fourth of the respondents were either definitely willing (10.7%) or willing (15.0%) to have a Jewish neighbor. An additional 38.4% also were willing to have a Jewish neighbor, although they would prefer an Arab neighbor. These responses are surprisingly positive, considering that the relationship between these two groups has been characterized in recent generations by racial discrimination, political inequality, and a bitter competition for land and resources. In addition, the two groups live in segregated villages and neighborhoods, attend separate educational systems, speak different languages, and observe different religious and cultural traditions.

More than two-thirds (68.6%) of the respondents were in favor of establishing a Palestinian state alongside Israel. A similar number (69.2%) believed that Israel should recognize a Palestinian state, and an additional 17.7% expressed conditional support for this recognition. The Israeli-Palestinian conflict has contributed to the self-perception and attitudes of our respondents and their relationships with Israeli Jews and the larger world. However, the results also appear to show that our sample group perceives surprisingly little contradiction between their identification with Palestinian Arab causes and their connection to Israel as citizens of that country. When participants were asked where they felt most at home, 45.4% revealed that they felt most at home in Israel. Although the Israeli part of their self-perception is subordinate to their ethnic self-identification as Palestinians, our findings suggest that it is also a critical characteristic of their self-description.

The respondents in the current study were asked to respond to a list of specific suggestions for furthering equality and coexistence within the Jewish state. Their responses (pro and con) were as follows, in order of positive responses:

- establishing an independent Arab trade union (68.9% vs.13.1%)
- Arabs controlling their own educational system (68.6% vs. 9.1%)
- establishing a new, independent Arab-language newspaper, radio, or television station (66.6% vs.15.0%)
- establishing an independent Arab industry (64.5% vs. 15.8%)
- establishing a new, independent Arab national political party (63.0% vs. 12.5%)
- establishing an independent Arab university (62.7% vs. 19.1%)
- Arabs controlling their own local governments (62.3% vs. 13.5%)
- Arabs controlling separate Arab departments (i.e., political divisions within the state) (55.3% vs. 15.6%). The respondents from unrecognized villages endorsed this by a wide majority (63.4%), whereas those from recognized villages were more evenly split (51.9%).

These results raise a fundamental challenge for the Israeli state—is it willing and able to confront the undemocratic attitudes of its Israeli citizens and take steps to provide the equity and fairness that it has so far failed to deliver to its Arab citizens, who constitute a major (and growing) proportion of its population? If the current policies of discrimination and marginalization are allowed to continue, it will only increase the volatility of the regional conflict and further polarize the Israeli Arabs who are caught in the middle. In the words of Elie Rekhess of the Moshe Dayan Centre, "a concrete, integrated plan of action, showing observable achievements, will offer a palpable alternative to many Arab citizens who seek their place in the state of Israel without confrontation" (11).

CONCLUSIONS

As with all studies, the present investigation has limitations. In particular, population validity and temporal validity threaten the external validity of the findings (63). Thus, replications of this study are needed. However, by collective empirical data from a relatively large sample, the current inquiry has taken an important first step towards identifying the ethnic identity of Bedouin-Arab adolescents in the context of the Middle East conflict.

REFERENCES

[1] Lavie S. The poetics of military occupation: Mzeina allegories of Bedouin identity under Israeli and Egyptian rule. Berkeley, CA: Univ California Press, 1990.
[2] Marx E. Bedouin of the Negev. Manchester: Manchester Univ Press, 1967.
[3] Meir A. Nomads and the state: The spatial dynamics of centrifugal and centripetal forces among the Israeli Negev Bedouin. Political Geography 1988;17: 251-270. [Hebrew]
[4] Ben-David Y. The Negev Bedouin: From nomadism to agriculture. In: Kark R, ed. The land that became Israel: Studies in historical geography. Jerusalem, Israel: The Magness Press, 1989:181-95.
[5] Fenster T. Spaces of citizenship for the Bedouin in the Israeli Negev. Prog Plann 1997;47(4):291-306.
[6] Ginat J. Blood revenge: Family honor, mediation, and outcasting. Portland, Oregon: Sussex Acad Press, 1997.
[7] Goodstein R, Ponterotto JG. Racial and ethnic identity: The relationship and their contribution to self-esteem. J Black Psychol 1997;23(3):275-92.
[8] Phinney JS, Kohatsu EL. Ethnic and racial identity and mental health. In: Schulenberg J, Maggs J, Hurrelmann K, eds. Health risks and developmental transitions during adolescence. New York: Cambridge Univ Press, 1997:420-43.
[9] Phinney JS, DuPont S, Espinosa C, Revil J, Sanders K. Ethnic identity and American identification among ethnic minority youths. In: Bouvy A, van de Vijver FJR, eds. Journeys into cross cultural psychology: Selected papers from the eleventh international conference of the International Association for Cross-Cultural Psychology held in Liege, Belgium. Lisse, Netherlands: Swets Seitlinger, 1994:167-83.
[10] Smith EJ. Ethnic identity development. Toward the development of a theory within the context of majority/minority status. J Couns Dev 1991;70(1):181-88.
[11] International Crisis Group. Identity crisis: Israel and its Arab citizens. Amman/Brussels: ICG Middle East Report No. 25. Retrieved February 18, 2009, from http://www.crisisweb.org//library/documents/middle_east___north_africa/arab_israeli_conflict
[12] Ghanem A. The Palestinian-Arab minority in Israel. 1948-2000: A political study. Albany: State Univ New York Press, 2001.
[13] Stonequist EV.The marginal man: A study in personality and culture conflict. New York: Russell Russell, 1961.
[14] Hogg MA, Abrams D. Social identifications: A social psychology of intergroup relations and group processes. London: Routledge, 1988.

[15] Kelman HC. The political psychology of the Israeli-Palestinian conflict: How can we overcome the barrier to a negotiated solution? Political Psychol 1987;8(3):347-63.
[16] Chang E, Ritter E. Ethnocentrism in Black college students. J Soc Psychol 1976;100(1):89-98.
[17] Garcia EE, Hurtado A. Becoming American: A review of current research on development of racial and ethnic identity in children. In: Hawley WD, Jackson AW, eds. Toward a common destiny: Improving race and ethnic relations in America. San Francisco, CA: Jossey-Bass, 1995;164-83.
[18] Waters MC. Ethnic options: Choosing identities in America. Berkeley, CA: Univ California Press, 1990.
[19] Phinney JS. Ethnic identity in adolescents and adults: Review research. Psychol Bull1990;108(3):499-514.
[20] Phinney JS. Ethnic identity. In: Kazdin AE, ed. Encyclopedia of psychology. New York: Oxford Univ Press, 2000:254-9..
[21] Feagin JR. Racial and ethnic relations. Englewood Cliffs, NJ: Prentice Hall, 1978.
[22] Sherif M, Sherif CW. Groups in harmony and tension. An integration of studies on intergroup relations. New York: Harper, 1953.
[23] Shibutani T. Reference group and social control. In: Rose AM, ed. Human behavior and social processes: An interactionist approach. Boston, MA: Houghton Mifflin, 1962:128-47.
[24] Thompson RH. Theories of ethnicity: A critical appraisal. New York: Greenwood Press, 1989.
[25] Fischer AR, Moradi B. Racial and ethnic identity: Recent developments and needed directions. In: Ponterotto JG, Casas JM, Suzuki LA, Alexander CM, eds. Handbook of multicultural counseling, 2nd ed.). Thousand Oaks, CA: Sage, 2001:341-70.
[26] Phinney JS. The multi-group ethnic identity measure: A new scale for use with diverse groups. J Adolesc Res 1992;7(2):156-76.
[27] Avery ME. The relationship between child variables, parent and family functioning variables, and aspects of African American children's ethnic identification. Unpublished master's thesis. Atlanta, GA: Georgia State Univ, 1995.
[28] Tajfel H. Social psychology of intergroup relations. Ann Rev Psychol 1982;33:1-39.
[29] Phinney JS. Stages of ethnic identity development in minority group adolescents. J Early Adolesc 1989;9:34-49.
[30] Helm JE, Talleyrand RM. Race is not ethnicity. Am Psychol 1997;52(11):1246-7.
[31] Katz J. The sociopolitical nature of counseling. Couns Psychol 1985;13(4):615-24.
[32] Myers LJ. Understanding an Afrocentric world view: Introduction to an optional psychology. Dubuque, IA: Kendall/Hunt, 1988.
[33] Seidman E, Rappaport J. Framing the issues. In: Seidman E, Rappaport J, eds. Redefining social problems. New York: Plenum, 1986:1-8.
[34] Breakwell GM, ed. Threatened identities. New York: Wiley, 1983.
[35] Benziman U, Mansour A. Subtenants: Israeli Arabs, their status and
[36] state policy towards them. Jerusalem: Keter, 1992. [Hebrew]
[37] Abu-Saad I. Bedouin Arab education in the context of radical social Change: What is the future? Compare Journal Comp Educ 1995;25(2):149-60.
[38] Elbedour S, Van Slyck M, Stern M. Psychosocial adjustment in Middle Eastern adolescents: The relative impact of violent versus non-violent social disorganization. Community Ment Health J 1998;34(2):191-205.
[39] Ben-David Y. The land conflict between the Bedouin and the state of Israel. Historical, legal, and actual perspectives. Karka 1995;40:61-91. [Hebrew]
[40] Porat C. The land policy of the Jewish National fund, 1940-1956. Jerusalem: Res Inst History Jewish Natl Fund, 1998. [Hebrew]
[41] Dinero S. Planning for an ethnic minority: The Bedouin Arabs of Israel. In: Burayidi MA, ed. Urban planning in a multicultural society. Westport, CT: Praeger, 2000:169-91.
[42] al-Haj M. The impact of the Intifada on Arabs in Israel: The case of double periphery. In: Cohen AA, Wolfsfeld G, eds. Framing the intifada: People and media. Norwood, NJ: Ablex, 1993:64-75.

[43] Elbedour S, Bastien D, Center BA. Identity formation in the shadow of conflict: Projective drawings by Palestinian and Israeli Arab children from the West Bank and Gaza. J Peace Res 1997;34(2):217-31.
[44] Abu-Rabia S, Elbedour S, Al-Atawana F. Profile of the status of education within the Bedouin school system. Shevaion [J Equality Justice] 1996;5:1-32. [Hebrew]
[45] Adorno TW, Frenkel-Brunswick E, Levinson DJ, Sanford RN. The authoritarian personality. New York: Harper Row, 1950.
[46] Morse NC, Allport FH. The causation of anti-Semitism: An investigation of seven hypotheses. J Psychol 1952;34:197-233.
[47] Ruttenberg J, Zea MC, Sigelman CK. Collective identity and Intergroup prejudice among Jewish and Arab students in the United States. J Soc Psychol 1996;136(2):209-220.
[48] Mullen B, Brown R, Smith C. Ingroup bias as a function of salience, relevance, and status: An integration. Eur J Soc Psychol 1992;22(2):103-22.
[49] Karau SJ, Williams KD. The effects of group cohesiveness on social loafing and social compensation. Group Dynamics 1997;1(2):156-68.
[50] Turner JC, Hogg MA, Oakes PJ, Reicher SD, Wetherell MS. Rediscovering the social group: A self-categorization theory. Oxford: Blackwell, 1987.
[51] Heraclides A. Conflict resolution, ethnonationalism and the Middle East impasse. J Peace Res 1989;26(2):197-213.
[52] Elbedour S, Bouchard TJ Jr, Hur Y. Similarity in general mental ability in Bedouin full and half siblings. Intelligence 1997;25(2):71-82.
[53] Mahjoub A, Leyens J, Yzerbt V, Di Giacomo J. War stress and coping modes: Representations of self-identity and time perspective among Palestinian children. Int J Ment Health 1989;18(2):44-62.
[54] Bailey C. The condition of the Bedouin towns in the Negev: Interim Report. Jerusalem: Truman Res Inst Adv Peace, Hebrew Univ, 2002.
[55] Abu-Saad I, Lithwick H. A way ahead: A development plan for the Bedouin Towns in the Negev. Beer-Sheva, IL: Center Bedouin Stud Dev, Negev Center Regional Dev, Ben-Gurion Univ Negev, 2000.
[56] Abu-Saad I. Towards an understanding of minority education in Israel: The case of the Bedouin Arabs of the Negev. Comp Educ 1991;27(2):235-42.
[57] Ministry of Education, Culture and Sports. The education system in numbers, 1995. Jerusalem: Econ Stat Div, Econ Budgets Adm, 1995. [Hebrew]
[58] Spencer MB, Markstrom-Adams C. Identity processes among racial and ethnic minority children in America. Child Dev 1990;61(2):290-310.
[59] Bachay J. Ethnic identity development and urban Haitian adolescents. J Multicultural Couns Dev 1998;26(2):96-109.
[60] Elbedour S, Shulman S, Kedem P. Adolescent intimacy: A cross-cultural study. J Cross Cultural Psychol 1996;28(1):5-22.
[61] Fishkoff S. Shifting sands. Jerusalem Post Magazine 1997;45:11-12 (16 May 1997).
[62] Elbedour S, Onwuegbuzie AJ, Caridine C, Abu-Saad H. The effect of polygamous marital structure on behavioral, emotional, and academic adjustment in children: A comprehensive review of the literature. Clin Child Fam Psychol Rev 2002;5(4):255-71.
[63] Smooha S. The orientation and politicization of the Arab minority in Israel. Haifa, IL: Univ Haifa, Jewish-Arab Center, Inst Middle Eastern Stud, 1984.
[64] Onwuegbuzie AJ. Expanding the framework of internal and external validity in quantitative research. Res Schools 2003;10(1):71-90.
[65] Phinney JS, Traver S. Ethnic identity search and commitment in Black and White eighth graders. J Early Adolesc 1988;8(3):265-77.
[66] Strauss A. Mirrors and masks: The search for identity. Glencoe, IL: Free Press, 1959.
[67] Forbes JD. The manipulation of race, caste and identity: Classifying Afro Americans, Native Americans and Red-Black people. J Ethnic Stud 1990;17(4):1-51.
[68] Haider A. The different levels of Palestinian ethnicity. In: Esman J, Rabinovich I, eds. Ethnicity: Pluralism and the state in the Middle East. Ithaca, NY: Cornell Univ Press, 1988:95-120.

[69] Bornman E. Etnisiteit ub 'n oorgangsperiode: 'N Sisuaak-sielkundige Studie [Ethnicity in a transitional period: A social psychological study]. Dissertation, Pretoria: Univ South Africa, 1995.
[70] Korf L, Malan J. Threat to ethnic identity: The experience of White Afrikaans-speaking participants in postapartheid South Africa. J Soc Psychol2002;142(2):149-69.
[71] Lustick I. Arabs in the Jewish state: Israel's control of a national minority. Austin, TX: Univ Texas Press, 1980.
[72] Smooha S. Control of minorities in Israel and Northern Ireland. Comp Stud Soc History 1980;22(2):256-80.
[73] Rouhana N. The civic and national subidentities of the Arabs in Israel: A psycho-political approach. In: Hoffman JE, ed. Arab-Jewish relations in Israel: A quest of human understanding. Bristol: Wyndham Hall Press,1988:123-54.
[74] Erikson EH. The concept of identity in race relations: Notes and queries. In: Parsons T, Clark KB, eds. The Negro American. Boston: Beacon Press, 1966:227-53.
[75] Sikkuy (Assoc Adv Equal Opportunity). The socioeconomic level of Jewish and Arab communities in Israel: Comparative data. Jerusalem: Sikkuy, 1996. [Hebrew]
[76] Katz PA. Towards the elimination of racism. New York: Pergamon Press, 1976.
[77] Sumner WG, Keller AG. Folkways: A study of the sociological importance of usages, manners, customs, mores, and morals. Boston: Ginn, 1906.
[78] Branscombe NR, Wann DL. Collective self-esteem consequences of out-group derogation when a valued social identity is on trial. Eur J Soc Psychol 1994;24(6):641-57.
[79] Zureik E. The Palestinians in Israel: A study in internal colonialism. London: Routledge Kegan Paul, 1979.

In: Rural Child Health: International Aspects
Editors: Erica Bell and Joav Merrick

ISBN: 978-1-60876-357-3

Chapter 9

FEMALE GENITAL CUTTING IN IGBO-ORA COMMUNITY, NIGERIA

Daniel Adedayo Adeyinka, MBBS*[*1], Olanrewaju Oladimeji, MBBS[1] and Chris Aimakhu, MBBS, FWACS, FMCOG, Cert. ARSH[2]

[1]College of Medicine, University of Ibadan, Nigeria
[2]Department of Obstetrics and Gynecology,
College of Ibadan, University of Ibadan, Nigeria

Female genital cutting (FGC) or female circumcision is a human rights violation that prevents girls from enjoying optimal health and maturation. Despite international agreements, it is still common worldwide and affects millions especially in the developing countries. Objective. To assess the knowledge, prevalence, practice and attitudes to FGC and its health implication in Igbo-Ora Community. Methods. A survey was conducted among 280 people above the age 18 years in Igbo-Ora town using a multi-staged sampling technique with an appropriate interviewer administered semi-structured questionnaire. Results. More than 78.7% girls and women in Igbo-Ora had undergone FGC. Despite high awareness (97.5%), only a few (30.7%) knew about the health consequences. It was practiced by people from all social classes and women with more education were less likely to practice FGC. There was strong adherence to tradition and beliefs and the patriarchal nature of the society as many disapproved its abolition especially people of younger age group (58.1%) with more men than women. More practiced among Muslims, 63.8%. The traditional doctors did not have health training, use anesthesia or sterilize the circumcision instruments. A majority (84.8%) had no knowledge about the enacted legislation regarding FGC in Nigeria. Conclusion. This suggests that the younger generations may have lesser access to FGC information and are more influenced by tradition. Hence, efforts to end it require understanding and changing their beliefs. Focusing largely on gathering information and speaking out about FGC at international, regional and national levels is critical in encouraging its abandonment.

* Correspondence: Daniel Adeyinka, MBBS, POBox 27058, Agodi Post Office, Ibadan, Oyo State, Nigeria. E-mail: greatguymedic@yahoo.com

Introduction

Several traditional practices have been termed bad and harmful. Among these is female genital cutting, which is gender specific. Female Genital Cutting (FGC) or female circumcision involves the removal of part or the whole of a female's external genitalia for non-medical reasons (1). The traditional practice is conducted in many cultures and in many countries. The extent of genital cutting and stitching varies considerably from country to country. Female circumcision is mainly carried out in western and southern Asia, the Middle East and large areas of Africa. It is also known to take place among immigrant communities in the USA, Canada, France, Australia and Britain.

The health consequences of FGC are both immediate and lifelong depending on the type of FGC performed and the proficiency of the circumciser (2). The procedure is fraught with a lot of physical consequences, which in the short term include pain, hemorrhage, shock, fractures, acute urinary retention, while the long term consequences include difficulty with passing urine, recurrent urinary tract infections which could also become ascending, abscesses and keloids may develop as may clitoral neuromas, prolonged labour, gynaetresia, vesicovaginal fistula, rectovaginal fistula and infertility. Sexual consequences include sexual dysfunction, dyspareunia and lack of fulfillment of sexual desire in both the man and the woman. Mentally, she copes with pain and the disabilities imposed on her without being able to voice her opinions and feelings. The risk of HIV infection through this practice is a strong possibility through the use of unsterilized instruments (3).

The reasons given for circumcision include dampening of sexual desire, easier childbirth; preserve their virginity, hydrocephalus prevention and reduction of vaginal secretion (4).

Considering the heath importance, the Nigerian government declared on the 9th of February, 2007 to observe the International Day for Zero Tolerance to FGC, which is the 6th of February. The date had earlier been declared by the World Health Assembly and approved by the Federal Executive Council. Estimates suggest that more than 130 million girls and women have been subjected to various forms of FGC worldwide (5,6). Another two million females are estimated to undergo the procedure every year. Africans are believed to comprise 24% of this number. It is common in a band that stretches from Senegal in West Africa to Somalia on the East coast, as well as from Egypt in the north to Tanzania in the south. In this region, an estimated 95% of all women have undergone the operation. In Nigeria FGC is widespread, cutting across regional, ethnic and religious lines. The prevalence in Nigeria ranged from 34% to about 70% of women (4).

It is not a problem of developing countries alone and the basis of this can be traced to immigration, as a result of which the prevalence has increased in countries such as Australia, the United States and Europe. FGC has become recognized not only as a health hazard and a form of violence against girls and women, but also as a human rights issue under international law. Efforts at the international level particularly United Nations agencies have placed FGC on women's health and human rights agenda.

Legally, there are no Federal laws banning Female Genital Cutting in Nigeria. Opponents of the practice rely on Section 34(1) (a) of the 1999 Constitution of the Federal Republic of Nigeria that states, “No person shall be subjected to torture or inhuman or degrading treatment”, as the basis for banning the practice nationwide. Ogun, Cross river, Osun, Rivers, Bayelsa, and Edo States have banned the practice since 1999.

In United Kingdom (UK), it was found out that even though the practice had been legally prohibited since 1985(7), it has continued among ethnic groups that migrated to the UK. The main groups are from Ethiopia, Eritrea, Somalia and the Yemen, countries in which over 85% of the female population have been circumcised (8). In 1993, a medical practitioner was brought before the General Medical Council on charge of performing female circumcision and struck off the council's register. Although data on prevalence is scarce, it is thought that about 4,000 new cases of FGC are seen in developed countries per annum (9)

About 27,000 women form countries with high prevalence of FGC are living in Sweden and about 30,000 in Italy (9)

The United States 1995 federal prohibition of FGC Act passed in 1996 stipulates up to five years or more for anyone involved in female genital cutting (FGC) or on anyone less than 18 years of age. It also requires that United States representatives and foreign agencies oppose financial loans to countries in which FGC is prevalent. In the Netherlands, discussions on FGC in the early 1990s following the arrival of Somali immigrants among whom it is traditional performed on girls between 6 and 12 years of age as part of an initiation ceremony. The type done is infibulation. Recent research from Amsterdam's free university found that the practice is also common among the Egyptians, Sudanese and Eritrean immigrants even though the parents know it is forbidden under the Dutch law (10)

It has been supported in the past by some African leaders such as Jomo Kenyatta, who saw it as a traditional heritage and a ritual which must continue (4,11). However, considering the grave health consequences, it has been banned in some countries such as Sudan, Burkina Faso, Guinea, Cote d'Ivoire (12)

We conducted this study to assess the knowledge, prevalence, practice and attitudes to FGC and its health implication in the Igbo-Ora community in Nigeria.

OUR STUDY

Igbo-Ora town, the study area is in the rain forest region in the outskirts of Oyo State in the Southwestern part of Nigeria. It is a semi-urban community. The town is divided into six blocks, which are further divided into 62 enumeration areas each containing varying number of family compounds. There is also a Primary Health Care system.

This was a cross-sectional study carried out between February-March 2007 in the community. With the use of a multi-staged sampling technique, an appropriate interviewer administered semi-structured questionnaire was developed. The questions were translated into Yoruba language then back translated into English language to ensure that the meanings of questions were retained. A pretest was done after which all ambiguous questions were removed. A minimum sample size of 226 was obtained which was oversampled to 280 and was used for the study to allow for greater precision. Hence, 280 males and females above age 18 years in Igbo-Ora town constituted the study population. The statistical analysis was done with Statistical Package for Social Sciences (SPSS) version 12 software. Tables and charts were used for the descriptive variables and Chi-square test was used to determine the associations between independent variables.

The Yoruba culture does not consider matters like circumcision to be discussed openly thereby some of the respondents did not want to respond favourably but we ensured privacy when administering the questionnaires and confidentiality of information.

Our Findings

A total of 280 people aged between 18 to 80 years (mean age of 36.53 years (S.D 14.40) were interviewed. The majority of the respondents; 263 (94.9%) were Yoruba; 155 (56%) of the respondents were female; 191(69%) were married; 153(55%) had at least Secondary school education; 103 (37.2%) were traders and 162 (58.5%) were Muslims (see table 1).

More than 78.7% girls and women in Igbo-Ora had undergone FGC. Despite high awareness (97.5%), only a few (30.7%) knew about the health consequences. It was practiced by people from all social classes and women with more education were less likely to practice FGC as majority (57.1%) of respondents with post secondary education knew about complications that may arise from this practice and 81.5% of respondents with no formal education (19.9%) knew no complication, while only 42.9% of those with post secondary education did not know any complication.

There was strong adherence to tradition and beliefs (62.2% of the 55% of those who supported FGC) and the patriarchal nature of society was seen as many disapproved its abolition especially (58.1%) of younger age group with more men than women (75.6% of men and 58.7% of women supported its continuation). The major reason given for this practice is that it prevents promiscuity (36.8%) and other reason given were that it assists delivery, it is a taboo if it is not done, enhances fertility while 30% said they did not know why it is done (see table 4). Majority of those with post secondary education did not support the practice (54.4% of respondents with post secondary education). 55.1% of respondents that have been circumcised and 67.4% with no knowledge of complication supported FGC. More practiced among Muslims, 63.8% compared to 42.5% of the Christian respondents. The traditional doctors did not have health training, use anesthesia or sterilize the circumcision instruments. Majority (84.8%) had no knowledge about the enacted legislation regarding FGC in Nigeria.

Discussion

The results of this study revealed that the awareness of female genital cutting (female circumcision) was very high as 97.5% of the respondents knew about this practice. The awareness of female genital cutting had no significant association with level of education, tribe or occupation. This is similar to the results of similar studies in Bere(1) and Kano (2) with 91.4% and 100% respectively. However, only 30.7% of those who knew about female genital cutting knew any complication or health consequences. Also a statistically significant association exists between the knowledge of complications and level of education as majority of respondents with post secondary education (57.1%) knew about complications that may arise from this practice and 81.5% of respondents with no formal education knew no complication while only 42.9% of those with post secondary education did not know any complication.

Only 15.2% of the respondents knew about a law against female genital cutting in Oyo state and this was significantly influenced by their level of education. The major reason for given for this practice is that it prevents promiscuity (36.8%) , others were; it assists delivery, it is a taboo if it is not done, enhances fertility while 30% said they didn't know why it is done. This study also revealed that female genital cutting is still widely practiced and favoured by quite a large proportion of the populace of Igbo-Ora as in other communities in Nigeria. 78.7% of the female respondents admitted to have been circumcised while 55.9% of the respondent supported the practice similar to what was found in a similar study conducted in Ibadan(3) which also revealed 71.3% prevalence of the practice and 72.6% supported the practice and contrary to the 34% prevalence in Zaria. This difference might be as a result of this study being community based and the other hospital based.

The majority of respondents who supported it said they did because it is an integral part of their tradition, while those who did not support said it was harmful and others said they had been advised against it.

It is noteworthy that majority of those with post secondary education did not support the practice (54.4%), while a staggering 28.6% supported it. The possible reason for this may be the fact that female genital cutting is deeply rooted in culture. There was also a statistically significant association between religion and support of the practice as 63.8% of Muslims respondents supported the practice compared to 42.5% of the Christian respondents, this was also evident in a similar study by Onadeko et al (4) with 70.3% of Muslim respondents and 29.7% of Christian respondents supported the practice. The possible reason for this is that the majority of the respondents were Muslims. Another reason might be the fact that some Muslims "erroneously" believe that the Quran supports female genital cutting.

Also worthy of note is that most of those who supported the practice do not know any complication that may arise from this practice, as 59% of those who knew any complication did not support the practice compared to 22.5% of those ,who knew no complication and yet supported it. The knowledge of a law against female genital cutting in Oyo State also had a statistically significant association with support of the practice as only 26.8% of those who knew the law supported this practice, while 61.1% of those who did not know any law supported it.

In this study, sex had an influence on the attitude of the respondents to female genital cutting, as 24.4% of the males and 41.3% of the females did not support this practice unlike the 64.3% of the male respondents in the study by Onadeko et al (4) who did not support the practice.

Furthermore, a comparison of the attitude of the age groups to this practice revealed that a higher percentage of the younger age group supported the practice (58.1% to 53.7%) in keeping with the findings of a similar study in Ibadan (3), which revealed that majority of the younger age group do support the practice.

The fact that "misery loves company" is clearly demonstrated from this study as a majority of females, who were circumcised supported this practice and had their daughters circumcised, a fact also seen in the study form Ibadan (3).

CONCLUSIONS

There is no doubt that this practice is still prevalent among the natives of Igbo-Ora, due to the fact that it is an integral part of their tradition, which is difficult to change rapidly. The knowledge about complications or health consequences was poor and hence continuous support of the practice. Surprisingly, younger members of this community still wanted the practice to continue. It was also noticed that some people question the importance of female genital cutting and hence its continuity. This is attributed to the health talks at various primary health care centers. It is therefore important that:

- Continuous and adequate health education on the dangers of female genital cutting and other harmful traditional practices is carried out at health centers, primary and secondary schools so that the younger generation will be aware of it before they become parents
- The right of a female child to physical integrity, education speech and freedom must be protected as this will increase her knowledge and bargaining power when it comes to issues that will affect her
- Health workers who perform female genital cutting should be discouraged from doing it and educated on its health consequences
- Mass campaigns on female genital cutting and its consequences should be carried out at market places or schools, which should include health workers, elders of the town and the local circumcisers
- Female genital cutting and its consequences should be inculcated into primary and secondary school curriculum
- Alternative job opportunities should be provided for the local circumcisers by the government
- A specific law prohibiting female genital cutting should be passed as a national law and enforced with severe punishment for anyone who is found guilty of this offence.

ACKNOWLEDGMENT

The authors thank professor MO Onadeko and Dr. Adewole for their invaluable comments and suggestions.

REFERENCES

[1] Inter-African committee on traditional practices affecting the health of women and children (IAC). Addis Abeba, Etiopia, 1997.

[2] Kiragu K. Female genital mutilation. A reproductive health concern. Population report supplement. Baltimore, MD: John Hopkins Popul Inform Prog, 1995.

[3] World Health Organization. A systemic review of health complications of female genital mutilation including sequelae in childbirth. Geneva: WHO, 2000.

[4] Onadeko MO, Adekunle LV. Female circumcision in Nigeria: A fact or a farce? J Tropical Pediatrics 1985;31(4);180-4.

[5] PATH/WHO. Female genital mutilation programs to date. What works and what does not?. Geneva: WHO, 1999.
[6] Population Reference Bureau. Abandoning female genital cutting. Prevalence, attitude, and efforts to end the practice. Washington, DC: PRB, 2001.
[7] Prohibition of female genital mutilation (Scotland) Bill. Norwich: HMSO, 2004.
[8] Healey T. Historical aspect of female circumcision and sexual sacrifice. Br J Sex Med 1979;8:23-6.
[9] Bosch X. Female genital mutilation in developed countries. Lancet 2001;358:1177-9.
[10] van Kolfschooten F. Dutch government cracks down on female circumcision. Lancet 2004;363:1531.
[11] Kenyatta J. Initiation of boys and girls: facing mount. New York: Vintage Books, 1965;6:125-49.
[12] Marion D, Dreyfus S.Female genital mutilation and African AIDS. Religious Tolerance, 2005. URL: www.religioustolerance.com
[13] Onuh SO, Igberase GO, Umeora JO, Okogbenin SA, Otoide VO, Gharoro EP. Female genital mutilation: Knowledge, attitude and practice among nurses. J Natl Med Assoc 2006;9813:409-14.
[14] Female genital cutting. Available at www.wikkipedia.com
[15] Herieka E, Dhar J. Female genital mutilation in the Sudan: Survey of the attitude of Khartoum University students towards this practice. BMJ 2003;79(3):220-3.
[16] Chugulu J, Dixey R. Female genital mutilation in Moshi rural district. Tanzania. Int Quart Community Health Educ 2000;19(2):103-18.
[17] Abubakar I, Iliyasa Z, Kabir M, Uzoho CC, Abdulkadir MB. Knowledge, attitude and practice of female genital cutting among antenatal patients in Aminu Kano Teaching Hospital, Kano. Nigerian J Med 2004;13(3):254-8.
[18] Mandara MU. Female genital mutilation in Nigeria. Int J Gynaecol Obstet 2004;84(3):291-8.
[19] Ehigiegba AE, Selo-Ojeme DO, Omorogbe FI. Female circumcision and determinants in southern Nigeria. East Afr Med J 1998;75(6):374-6.
[20] Adeneye AK, Oke EA, Adeneye AA. Knowledge of the health consequences of female genital mutilation in Bere community of Oyo State, Nigeria. World Health Popul 2006;8(4):1-7.
[21] Briggs LA. Male and female view points on female circumcision in Ekpeye, Rivers State. Afr J Reprod Health 2002;6(3):44-52.
[22] Sangowawa AO, Onadeko MO, Ekanem SE, Faserub. Knowledge and Attitudes of staff of health facilities in Igbo-Ora , Nigeria about female genital cutting. Int Conf AIDS, Bangkok, Thailand, 2004.

SECTION FOUR: DEVELOPING HEALTH SERVICES FOR CHILDREN IN RURAL COMMUNITIES

In: Rural child health: International aspects
Editors: Erica Bell and Joav Merrick

ISBN: 978-1-60876-357-3

Chapter 10

CHILD SELF TREATMENT AND USE OF HEALTH SERVICES IN A RURAL DISTRICT IN VIETNAM

Le Thi Hoan*, MD, MSc, Nguyen Thi Thu, MD, PhD and Peter Allebeck, MD, PhD

Faculty of Public Health, Hanoi Medical University, Vietnam and Department of Public Health Science, Karolinska Institute, Stockholm, Sweden

The aim was to analyze patterns of use of health services among children under 5 years of age with respiratory symptoms and/or diarrhoea. Specific aims were to: 1) describe use of health services among children with respiratory symptoms and/or diarrhoea and 2) examine determinants of use of health services in relation to socio-economic groups in a rural district in Vietnam. Methods: A population-based survey of 4087 children under five was conducted in Bavi district, a Demographic Surveillance Site in rural Vietnam and a structured questionnaire was used. Logistic regression was applied to assess determinants for use of different type of health services as well as self-treatment. Results: We identified 1,415 children with an episode of respiratory symptoms and/or diarrhoea. Measures reported were 54.5% self-treatment, 31.4 % use of private practitioners, 8.8 % use of community health centre, and 5.3 % use hospital. There were no significant differences by socio-economic groups in use of health services. Conclusions: Self-treatment was the most common measure taken in cases of respiratory symptoms and/or diarrhoea, followed by private health services, and community health centre. There were no significant differences in use of health services by socio-economic groups.

INTRODUCTION

Studies from several countries indicated that the decision to seek treatment for sick children was influenced by several factors: disease severity, household economic status, education of mothers/caregivers and gender of the child (1-3).

* Correspondence: Le Thi Hoan, Faculty of Public Health, Hanoi Medical University, No. 1 Ton That Tung St., Dong Da district, Hanoi, Vietnam. Tel: 84-4-8524141; Fax 84-4-8523032; E-mail: hoan.lethi@gmail.com

This study focuses on children with respiratory symptoms and/or diarrhoea. These diseases remain the main causes of child morbidity and mortality in Vietnam (4). According to the National Health Survey, the proportion of children who had acute respiratory infections and diarrhoea during the past four weeks was 19 percent and 5.8 percent respectively (5).

Studies on health care utilization in Vietnam have shown that a significant proportion of illness is handled by self-treatment (6-9). However, there are few studies on determinants and pattern of use of health services among children in Vietnam.

Since 1989 a number of reforms in the health care sector have been implemented. User fees were introduced in public health facilities, drug dispensing was liberalized and private providers were allowed in health services. Concern has been raised about negative effect of these reforms on the poor (10). However the government has issued laws and policies on free health care services for children under 6 years at public health facilities. The Law on the Protection of Population Health in 1991 also pointed out the rights of children to receive immunization, treatment and other preventive, curative services. However, it has been difficult to implement this law in reality due to the lack of resources, especially in curative health services. To deal with this constraint the Prime Minister made a decision in 2004 to allocate government resources for providing free of charge health services for children under 6 years.

This study aims to analyze the pattern of use of health services among children under 5 years of age with acute respiratory symptoms and/or diarrhoea. Specific aims were to: (1) describe use of health services among children with respiratory symptoms and/or diarrhoea; and (2) examine determinants of use of health services in relation to socio-economic groups.

OUR STUDY

The study was carried out in the rural Bavi district in the north of Vietnam. The district covers an area of 410 km2, including lowland, highland and mountainous area. The total population of this district is 240000 people with domination of Kinh ethic group (91%). Agricultural production and livestock breeding are the main economic activities (81%) and the others such as forestry (8%), handicraft (6%), small trade (3%), fishing and transport (2%). In 1998, an Epidemiological Field Laboratory for demographic surveillance (FilaBavi) has been established in Bavi.

STUDY POPULATION

All children under 5 years of age in the households comprise in the FilaBavi sample were included in the study. There were 4087 children under 5 years in the study. The FilaBavi sample was selected randomly with probability proportional to the size of population in the area and covered all different geographical regions in the district. The sampling unit was based on village. There were 69 out of 352 clusters in the sample with about 51 000 inhabitants in 11 038 households. The study was carried out from October to December in 2004.

DATA COLLECTION

Longitudinal surveillance data of Filabavi are collected every three months by trained interviewers. On a regular basis, questions are asked about household information such as housing conditions, housing assets, expenditures and income from different sources, geographical access to health services, and household members' information such as demographic characteristics, education and occupation. For this study, a structured questionnaire was added to collect information on acute respiratory symptoms and diarrhoea in children under five years of age and use of health services during two weeks prior to the survey among these cases. Mothers/caregivers were asked about illness events, symptoms during illness episodes, and use of health services among ill children. Symptoms related to respiratory infection and diarrhoea were reported and evaluated by mothers/ caregivers.

Respiratory symptom case in this study was defined as a child with cough and fever symptoms. Diarrhoea was defined as a child with loose stool at least 3 times per day. This study has got ethical approval from Research Ethical Committee of Hanoi Medical University.

DATA ANALYSIS

Logistic regression was applied to calculate odds ratio for use of private services, commune health centre (CHC) and hospitals as well as self-treatment in each socioeconomic group. Independent variables were sex of the child, education and occupation of mothers and economic status. Other factors such as number of ill days, combination of illness, distance to health facilities, mother's marriage status, and household size, were also included in this model. The children who did not report any treatment (not even self treatment) were excluded in the model.

VARIABLES

Mother's education was categorized into three levels based on the highest level completed: primary, secondary and high school. Economic status was measured by the wealth index, which is based on a weighted sum of household assets and income source. Use of health services term in this study was mentioned about use of curative health services, and classified into self-treatment or informal care, seeking health care from private health facilities, visiting a communal health centre, and policlinic/ hospital. All cases in this analysis were not inpatient because number of inpatient in this study was small. Self-treatment was classified as buying and using modern or traditional medicine without medical professional consultation.

OUR FINDINGS

Out of 4,087 children under five years of age, 1,415 children had an episode of respiratory illness and/or diarrhoea during 2 two weeks prior to the survey. Thus 34.6 % of the children had any of these conditions during 2 weeks period. All most of mothers/caregivers reporting child illness did something in response to the episode.

Out of 1,414 measures reported by mothers or caregivers to these episodes, 54.5 percent were self-treatment (informal care) 31.4 per cent were use of private practitioners, 8.8 per cent were use of CHC, and 5.3 percent used hospital (see figure 1).

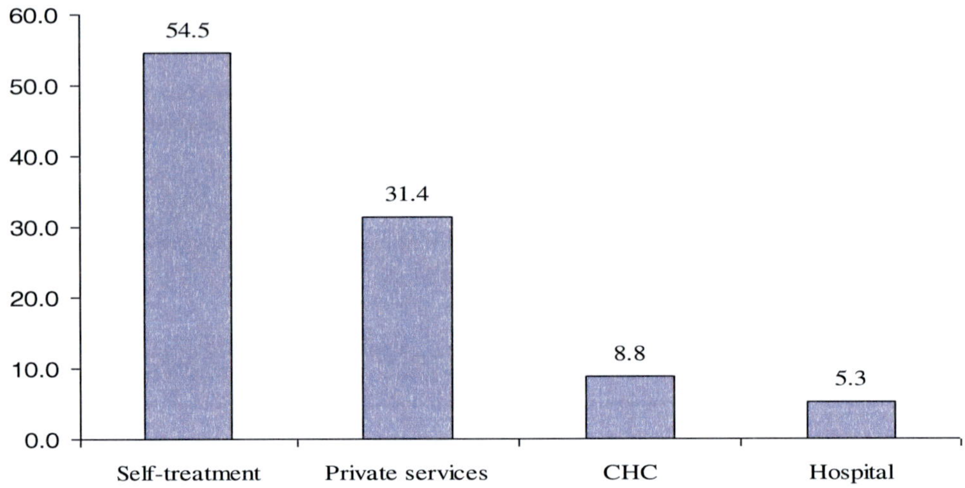

Figure 1. Proportion of use of health services among children with respitory systems and/or diarrhea.

DETERMINANTS OF USE OF HEALTH SERVICES

As shown in table 1 and figure 2, self-treatment was the most common measure taken regardless of socio-economic status. Private health services and CHC, respectively, was the next most common in all socio-economic groups. Use of hospital services, which in most of the cases are at district level, accounted for only a small proportion of use of health services, and this applied to all socio economic groups.

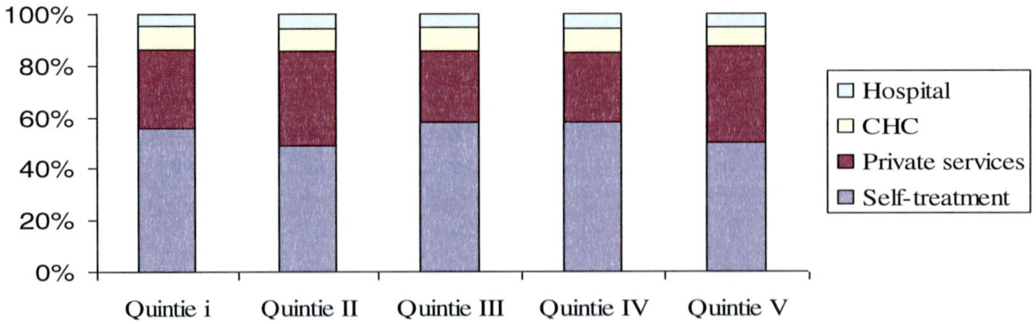

Figure 2. Proportion of use of health services among children with respitatory systems and/or diarrhea by household economic groups.

Table 1. Proportion of use of health services among children with respiratory symptoms and/or diarrhea by socio-economic characteristics

	Self-treatment	Private Practitioners	CHC	District Hospital
Sex				
Male	52.7	31.7	10.1	5.5
Female	56.6	31.1	7.2	5.1
Mother's education				
Primary School	51.9	33.5	10.8	3.8
Secondary School	55.8	30.2	8.5	5.5
High School and College	52.7	34.1	8.0	5.3
Household size				
<=4 people	54.1	31.2	8.9	5.8
> 4 people	54.8	31.5	8.7	5.0
Mother's occupational				
Farmer	54.7	31.7	8.5	5.1
Employers	55.6	36.1	2.8	5.6
Others	54.5	27.0	12.2	6.4
Economic status (wealth index)				
Poor	55.7	30.3	9.3	4.7
Moderate poor	49.1	36.8	8.6	5.5
Average	58.3	27.4	8.9	5.4
Better-off	58.3	26.6	9.2	6.0
Rich	50.3	37.3	7.3	5.1

Table 2. Estimated odds ratios for determinants of use of health services

	Self-treatment	Private services	CHC	District Hospital
Sex				
Male	1	1	1	1
Female	1.21(0.97,1.51)	0.94(0.74,1.19)	0.73(0.49,1.08)	0.9(0.55,1.49)
Mother's education				
Primary School	1	1	1	1
Secondary School	1.08(0.76,1.52)	0.91(0.63,1.31)	0.83(0.47,1.47)	1.4(0.58,3.41)
High School and above	0.85(0.53,1.36)	1.13(0.69,1.86)	0.91(0.41,2.02)	1.53(0.5,4.67)
Mother's occupation				
Farmer	1	1	1	1
Employees	1.17(0.6,2.28)	1.02(0.51,2.04)	0.26(0.03,2.19)	1.15(0.26,5.11)
Others	1.01(0.71,1.45)	0.73(0.49,1.08)	1.62(0.9,2.9)	1.49(0.7,3.19)
Illness conditions				
Respiratory symptoms or diarrhoea only	1	1	1	1
Respiratory symptoms and diarrhoea	0.91(0.7,1.17)	0.94(0.71,1.24)	1.38(0.85,2.24)	1.51(0.84,2.72)
Respiratory symptoms and difficult breath	0.61(0.4,0.94)	1.58(1.02,2.46)	1.28(0.59,2.75)	1.3(0.45,3.75)
Number with symptom days	0.99(0.95,1.04)	1.02(0.97,1.08)	1.04(0.96,1.12)	0.86(0.76,0.98)
Economic status				
Poor	1	1	1	1
Moderate poor	0.8(0.58,1.1)	1.28(0.91,1.81)	0.88(0.5,1.55)	1.23(0.58,2.61)
Average	1.16(0.83,1.6)	0.83(0.58,1.19)	0.92(0.52,1.63)	1.21(0.57,2.57)
Better-off	1.08(0.73,1.59)	0.82(0.53,1.25)	1.04(0.53,2.05)	1.57(0.65,3.76)
Rich	0.71(0.46,1.1)	1.4(0.88,2.23)	0.91(0.41,2.01)	1.68(0.62,4.53)

Note: Odds ratios with 95 per cent confidence interval in brackets.

Logistic regression analysis indicated that there were no significant differences by socio-economic groups in use of health services (table 2). However, children with respiratory symptoms and difficult breath used somewhat private health services (OR=1.58, 95 per cent CI 1.02-2.46) than children with one single illness.

The most common reasons given for use of health services were previous experience of dealing with a similar condition and convenience. Economic reasons played only a minor part in determining type of use of health services (see table 3).

Table 3. Reasons given for use of health services

Reasons given for use of health services	Self-treatment	Private services	CHC	Hospital	Total
Mild illness	93 (12.1)	53 (11.9)	16 (13.0)	11 (14.7)	173 (12.2)
Previous experiences	347 (45.1)	190 (42.5)	44 (35.8)	30 (40.0)	611 (43.2)
Conveniences	274 (35.6)	167 (37.4)	50 (40.7)	30 (40.0)	521 (36.9)
Economic reasons	60(0.8)	61 (0.3)	3 (2.4)	0 (0.0)	15 (1.1)
Others	49 (6.4)	31 (6.9)	10 (8.1)	4 (5.3)	94 (6.7)
Total	769 (100)	447 (100)	123 (100)	75 (100)	1,414 (100)

Note: frequency with column percentages in brackets

Discussion

In this study we found that for the majority of cases, self-treatment was the most common measure taken. A smaller proportion of the cases sought care at public health facilities, such as commune health centre and hospital. A high proportion sought care in private health services. However, we did not find any difference in use of health services by socio economic groups.

The high proportion of self-treatment is an agreement with other studies in Vietnam (6-10). According to sentinel surveillance in Vietnam, self-treatment is the most common for the sick in all economic groups. This situation is rather similar in other countries (11,12). Several studies have shown that pharmacy, which is part of the self-treatment category in our study, is the most common place where care was sought (13,14). Certain minor health problems may not require any special care and are appropriately cured by self-treatment. However, the capacity to provide self-treatment varies with educational background and knowledge of appropriate care as well as perception on illness seriousness. When self-treatment is not appropriate it may cause complications of the disease or irrational drug use. An important issue is the quality of private health services. While studies on quality of private health services in Vietnam are scarce, a recent study on quality of private and public health service in rural Vietnam showed that the quality of private health services is not controlled and is significantly poorer than public services (15).

We did not find that the sex of the child influenced use of health services, although this has been documented from other countries (2, 3, 16, 17). However, this is an agreement with other studies in Vietnam that did not find any significant difference in use of health services between men and women (7, 18). Neither did we find any association between maternal education, occupation and use of health services as indicated in studies in other setting (13, 19). This is opposite to the case among adults in Vietnam. It has been shown that people with higher education tend to use more public health services than those with lower education (5). Severity of illness and type of illness is according to many studies related to the likelihood of using health services, while this trend was only partially seen in our study (2,13, 20, 21). Children with respiratory illness and difficult breath were likely to seek health care at private health services (OR, 1.58; CI, 1.02- 2.46). This difference may be caused by the different measurement of illness severity. We measured number of days of illness instead of perceived severity of illness as in other studies. However the higher use of professional care for children having difficult breath symptom indicates that mothers may recognize serious signs and seek professional care.

The pattern of use of health services for children did not vary markedly between socio-economic groups. CHC and district hospital outpatient care were used as much by the poor as the better-off group. This is not in line with findings from previous studies in Vietnam, in which the non-poor made more use of CHC and hospital than the poor (10). The probability of use of hospital is strongly and positively related to household income and health insurance (8). The economic status of the family also has been found to be an important determinant of use of health services in many studies (2, 13, 17, 20-23). The reason for this difference may be that previous studies have concerned adults and that children are looked after and brought to care to a higher extent. A study from the Ministry of Health in Vietnam showed that the proportion of self-treatment among children under 5 years of age is lower than in other age groups (5). Some studies have not distinguished different levels of hospital care. The difference may occur in use of hospital at high level, which needs larger database and future study. There was evidences that a means of finance, which protect families against financial burden in health care, such as health insurance, improved access to health services among children (24-26). In this perspective, it may be that the policy on free health services for the children under six years in Vietnam have contributed at least partly to our findings. In addition the use of health services may mainly be influenced by previous experiences of dealing with the illness and the convenience.

CONCLUSIONS

Self-treatment was the most common use among children with respiratory and/or diarrhoea, followed by private services and CHC. The pattern of use of health services did not vary between socio-economic groups and economic reasons were only a minor reason given for use of health services among children with respiratory infections and/or diarrhoea.

ACKNOWLEDGMENTS

The author(s) declare that they have no competing interests. This research was conducted within the Epidemiological Field Laboratory for Health System Research (FilaBavi) Vietnam, which is supported by Sida/SAREC, Sweden. The authors thank all child mothers or caregivers, and all interviewers who participated in the study.

REFERENCES

[1] Hjortsberg C. Why do the sick not utilise health care? The case of Zambia. Health Econ 2003;12(9):755-70.

[2] Pillai RK, Williams SV, Glick HA, Polsky D, Berlin JA, Lowe RA. Factors affecting decisions to seek treatment for sick children in Kerala, India. Soc Sci Med 2003;57(5):783-90.

[3] Pokhrel S, Snow R, Dong H, Hidayat B, Flessa S, Sauerborn R. Gender role and child health care utilization in Nepal. Health Policy 2005;74(1):100-9.

[4] UNICEF. Vietnam children and women: A situation analysis. Vietnam: UNICEF, 1999.

[5] MoH. Report of Vietnam National Health Survey. Hanoi: Min Health, General Statistic Office, 2003.

[6] Dzung T, Doan NV, et al. Sentinel surveillance in health care utilization in 28 rural communes during 2000-2001. Hanoi: Health Policy Unit, Min Health, 2002.

[7] Khe ND, Toan NV, Xuan LT, Eriksson B, Hojer B, Diwan VK. Primary health concept revisited: where do people seek health care in a rural area of Vietnam? Health Policy 2002;61(1):95-109.

[8] Sepehri A, Chernomas R, Akram-Lodhi AH. If they get sick, they are in trouble: health care restructuring, user charges, and equity in Vietnam. Int J Health Serv 2003;33(1):137-61.

[9] Toan NV, Khe ND, Hojer B. Expenditure and payment sources for treating acute respiratory infections in rural Vietnam. Southeast Asian J Trop Med Public Health 2001;32(4):682-8.

[10] Segall M, Tipping G, Lucas H, Dung TV, Tam NT, Vinh DX, Huong DL. Economic transition should come with a health warning: the case of Vietnam. J Epidemiol Community Health 2002;56(7):497-505.

[11] Leyva-Flores R, Kageyama ML, Erviti-Erice J. How people respond to illness in Mexico: self-care or medical care? Health Policy 2001;57(1):15-26.

[12] Shankar PR, Partha P, Shenoy N. Self-medication and non-doctor prescription practices in Pokhara valley, Western Nepal: a questionnaire-based study. BMC Fam Pract 2002;3:17.

[13] Sreeramareddy CT, Shankar RP, Sreekumaran BV, Subba SH, Joshi HS, Ramachandran U. Care seeking behaviour for childhood illness--a questionnaire survey in western Nepal. BMC Int Health Hum Rights 2006;6:7.

[14] Heuveline P, Goldman N. A description of child illness and treatment behavior in Guatemala. Soc Sci Med 2000;50(3):345-64.

[15] Tuan T, Dung VT, Neu I, Dibley MJ. Comparative quality of private and public health services in rural Vietnam. Health Policy Plan 2005;20(5):319-27.

[16] Pandey A, Sengupta PG, Mondal SK, Gupta DN, Manna B, Ghosh S, et al. Gender differences in healthcare-seeking during common illnesses in a rural community of West Bengal, India. J Health Popul Nutr 2002;20(4):306-11.

[17] Thind A, Andersen R. Respiratory illness in the Dominican Republic: what are the predictors for health services utilization of young children? Soc Sci Med 2003;56(6):1173-82.

[18] Long NH, Johansson E, Lonnroth K, Eriksson B, Winkvist A, Diwan VK. Longer delays in tuberculosis diagnosis among women in Vietnam. Int J Tuberc Lung Dis 1999;3(5):388-93.

[19] Thind A, Cruz AM. Determinants of children's health services utilization in the Philippines. J Trop Pediatr 2003;49(5):269-73.

[20] Goldman N, Pebley AR, Gragnolati M. Choices about treatment for ARI and diarrhea in rural Guatemala. Soc Sci Med 2002;55(10):1693-712.

[21] Taffa N, Chepngeno G. Determinants of health care seeking for childhood illnesses in Nairobi slums. Trop Med Int Health 2005;10(3):240-5.

[22] Schellenberg JA, Victora CG, Mushi A, de Savigny D, Schellenberg D, Mshinda H. Inequities among the very poor: health care for children in rural southern Tanzania. Lancet 2003;361(9357):561-6.

[23] Levin A, Rahman MA, Quayyum Z, Routh S, Barkat e K. The demand for child curative care in two rural thanas of Bangladesh: effect of income and women's employment. Int J Health Plann Manage 2001;16(3):179-94.

[24] Heck KE, Parker JD. Family structure, socioeconomic status, and access to health care for children. Health Serv Res 2002;37(1):173-86.

[25] Newacheck PW, McManus M, Fox HB, Hung YY, Halfon N. Access to health care for children with special health care needs. Pediatrics 2000;105(4 Pt 1):760-6.

[26] Woods CR, Arcury TA, Powers JM, Preisser JS, Gesler WM. Determinants of health care use by children in rural western North Carolina: results from the Mountain Accessibility Project. Pediatrics 2003;112(2):143-52.

In: Rural child health: International Aspects
Editors: Erica Bell and Joav Merrick

ISBN: 978-1-60876-357-3

Chapter 11

MOBILE FAMILY RESOURCE SERVICE FOR PARENTS AND YOUNG CHILDREN

John Guenther*, BAppSc (App Chem), DipTh (Miss), PhD and Margaret Arvier, RN, BA, Grad Dip Management Arts
University of Tasmania, University Department of Rural Health, Ulverstone and Burnie City Council, Burnie, Tasmania, Australia

Programs typically produce activities that have an impact on service users or clients with measurable impacts in terms of service use outcomes. However health promotion activities and community information initiatives often do not have 'clients' in the same way. Impact evaluation of such programs can therefore be more problematic. This chapter reports on an outcomes evaluation of a health and community information program, described as a mobile family resource centre, to demonstrate how impact may be measured. The evaluation draws on program logic assumptions but uses these in a way that informs the development of an impact model. The evaluation has found that while some of the impact can be measured quantitatively in terms of increased uptake of information, the impact can also be measured qualitatively in terms changes in access to social networks and improvements in interagency networks. The chapter concludes that impact of health promotion and community information programs like the mobile family resource centre can be effectively measured using innovative approaches to data collection and analysis.

INTRODUCTION

Programs typically produce activities that have an impact on service users. For example a playgroup will have a direct, observable and measurable impact on those parents and children attending. A breastfeeding program will have immediate outcomes for mothers and babies. The tangible outcomes of these programs can be measured with any number of evaluation instruments including perception surveys, monitoring records that track changes in behaviour

* Correspondence: John Guenther, PhD, PO Box 469, Ulverstone, TAS 7315, Australia. Tel: 03 6425 9016; E-mail: john@catconatus.com.au

and other measures that assess impact in terms of health and early learning indicators. Such outcomes fit neatly with a standard program logic model that shows a clear progression from inputs and processes through to outputs and outcomes. However, many programs do not have outcomes that are easily measured in terms of service use or community impact. For example, how can the immediate impact of a poster campaign promoting healthy eating or exercise be measured? How can the outcomes of an information pack for new parents be determined? How can the impact of a health information DVD resource delivered in doctors' waiting rooms be assessed? While it is possible to easily measure aspects of these program in terms of how many posters/DVDs/advertisements have been distributed the key problem for impact assessment lies in the difficulty associated with tracking the users of the programs.

The subject of this paper is a program funded under an Australian Government initiative designed to build health, early learning and capacity outcomes for parents and their 0-5 year old children. The program, based in a regional Australian city with a relatively high degree of disadvantage, is described as a mobile family resource centre. It provides outreach information, referral and educational services to all families with children 0-5 years, with a focus on 'hard to engage' and isolated families within the local community. By 'hard to engage' we mean those who are socio-economically disadvantaged (in terms of education, income, housing, employment) and those who may be socially isolated (e.g. people who speak a language other than English). The centre operates from a van that is staffed and located strategically at community events, in busy places within the city's CBD and at specific activities organised by community groups. Ethically, the program is not able to collect names and contact details for those it engages with. As with the other examples mentioned above, it is not possible to evaluate the program's impact on individual service users.

The question posed in this paper—and related to the above scenario— is: Within a program logic framework, how can impact of a program where the service users are not known, be evaluated? To answer this question, the paper will first consider an evaluation of this kind within the context of a program logic framework. It will then outline the methodology used for the evaluation of the mobile family resource centre. Some results from the evaluation will be provided and the implications of the findings will be discussed. The lessons learned from this evaluation are directly applicable to other programs—particularly health promotion initiatives including media campaigns and other public health awareness raising initiatives.

OUR STUDY

The literature considered here will focus on the nature and purpose of program evaluations with a particular emphasis on those based on program logic assumptions. Examples from health and community development literature will be highlighted.

Evaluation approaches

Depending on the purpose and the nature of the activity to be evaluated, the approach used will differ. On the one hand evaluations can be simply categorised as either formative or summative. The former, is conducted during the life of a program to help shape the outcomes, while the latter is conducted at the end of a program's life to evaluate what the outcomes were. Within these two broad categorisations there are several approaches that can be used discretely or in combination. Stufflebeam and Shinkfield (1) for example, identify 26 approaches to evaluation, which they describe under headings of 'Pseudoevaluations', 'Quasi-evaluation studies', 'Improvement and accountability oriented evaluations', 'Social agenda and advocacy approaches' and 'Eclectic' or 'utilization focused evaluations'. Within these fields they identify case study evaluations, benefit-cost analyses, accreditations and certifications, objective based studies and empowerment evaluations. While acknowledging this diversity, evaluations that are commissioned by the program's funding body often have a focus on outcomes. Evaluations in this context are sometimes described as 'theory of change' and/or 'realistic' evaluations (2,3) where the focus is on causal linkages between programs and outcomes.

Program logic assumptions and evidence based practice

Program logic may be based on 'theories of change' assumptions—emphasising the theoretical foundations of a program; or an 'outcome approach' which emphasises the causal linkages between outputs and outcomes; or an 'activities approach' which emphasises intended work plans (4,5). One of the perceived benefits of a program logic approach is that it builds an 'evidence base' (6). An important use of a logic model is to assist with the identification of indicators that will measure the intended outcomes. The choice of indicators is critical for determining impact. There is a tendency in some program evaluations to incorrectly ascribe process and output statements to outcomes (7). There is also a risk that use of program logic may prescribe an outcomes framework that ultimately is not valid. Stufflebeam and Shinkfield (1) warn that evaluators using this approach may 'focus attention on theory developed early in the program and later discover that the program has evolved to be a quite different enterprise from what was theorised at the outset'.

Measuring outcomes of health promotion programs

Models of evaluating outcomes of public health initiatives have often in the past depended on experimental designs based on scientific approaches dependent on randomised control trials. The approach to this kind of research is largely deductive using a hypothesis testing approach. For example: Does a particular drug make a statistically significant difference to a trial group compared to a control group of patients? However there is a growing recognition that such approaches are inadequate for more complex initiatives (8, 9) particularly in the area of health promotion (10) and that theories of change approaches may offer a more thorough and adequate way of addressing the complexities of community health initiatives.

In the literature there are examples of different approaches used to evaluate health promotion. For example, recent work published by McKenzie et al (11) uses a largely qualitative framework with a broad range of indicators to assess a number of public health promotion programs across a matrix of areas described as reach, effectiveness, adoption, implementation and maintenance. Katz (12), discussing evaluations in the context of children and family interventions, notes the challenges of using secondary data sources—which he noted are generally qualitative—in evaluations but acknowledges the cost effectiveness and contribution that such methods can make to an impact evaluation structured around program logic assumptions.

Qualitative data can sometimes best be used as a part of a 'discovery process' where evaluators allow 'emergent questions to shape the collection and analysis' of information (1). This process could be described in terms of 'inductive strategies of theory development in contrast to theory generated by logical deduction from a priori assumptions' (5). In practice, theory generated by induction can be used to build hypotheses that can then be tested deductively to produce results that in turn can be used with further inductive strategies in a 'cyclical process' (13). Qualitative data also has an important role to play in building an understanding of the local context. Drawing on findings of several health program evaluations, Stevenson and Thomas (14) assert that 'external evaluators cannot design effective evaluations without incorporating "local knowledge"'.

METHODOLOGY

The methodology used for the evaluation of mobile family resource centre was built around an overarching program logic framework which prescribed outcomes under five high-level outcome areas: 1) early learning and care; 2) healthy young families; 3) supporting families and parents; 4) child-friendly communities; and 5) family and children's services working together effectively as a system. While the mobile family resource centre was identified as an activity under the 'supporting families and parents' outcome area it could equally fit under any of the areas because of the multiple foci of the program.

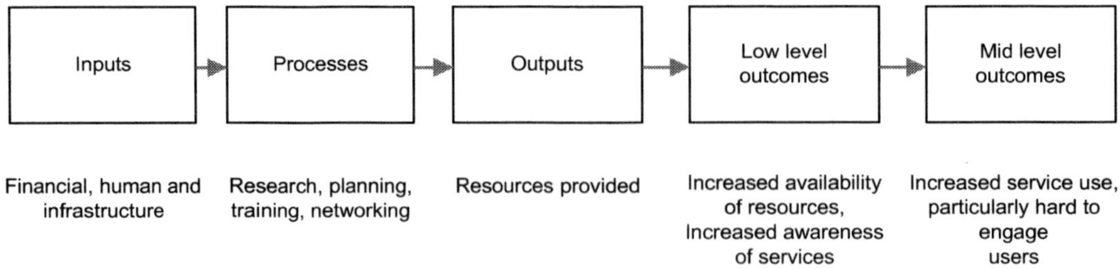

Figure 1. Mobile family resource centre logic model.

The assumptions underpinning the design of the program—reflected in the logic model shown at figure 1—included an expectation that in order for health and community service use to increase among the population and therefore increase overall community health and well-being, an initiative was required that would be flexible enough to reach into those parts of the community that have not taken advantage of available services. A mobile family resource centre would support this initiative because it is inherently flexible, non-threatening and mobile.

Having identified the expected outcomes, a set of evaluation tools was developed by the program manager with the support of a local evaluator that could serve to record aspects of service delivery and use. These tools used a combination of quantitative and qualitative measurement instruments. Quantitative measures included a) collection and collation of data about the numbers and types of resources taken at each event; and b) categorisation and summation of the number and type of conversations held with different people at each event. Qualitative data was collected using a journaling method which allowed for the description of the key learnings from each event together with a summary of the kinds of conversations the program manager engaged people in along with any outstanding observations. The quantitative data gives a clear picture of the outputs (resources provided) and to some extent the low level data (in terms of increased availability of resources). However the qualitative data provides a rich source of information about the outcomes in terms of increasing awareness and the nature of service use. The program manager has collected over 50 journal entries from activities she has attended and this in itself provides a valuable reference point and source of information about the program outcomes in terms of a) what people want to know about, b) where people come from (socio-economically, demographically and geographically) and c) who people are connecting with to gain information and access services in the community. The records do not include personal information such as names and contact details.

However, on reviewing the data with the local evaluator it became apparent that the information could be more important for understanding the dynamics of this kind of community health and well-being promotion initiative. It also became apparent from a review of the data that the expected outcomes of the program which related to the information and resources provided to people, were a relatively minor contributor to the program's effectiveness. As the data was analysed it became evident that the more significant aspect of the program was the way that it facilitated connections between individuals and organisations within the community. This understanding of the program's outcomes has then informed the evaluation of program impact in an unexpected way. At the time of writing, the evaluation was still continuing. The program and the accompanying evaluation is scheduled for completion in 18 months.

EVALUATION RESULTS

While the program manager collected quantitative data about the distribution of various resources and the number of contacts made at events within the community, the focus of the presentation here will be on the qualitative results of the evaluation. In particular, we will draw on an analysis of the nature of networks formed and the apparent role of the program manager in this.

Figure 2 represents a portion of the findings following an analysis of the qualitative data contained in the journal entries. It represents the low and mid-level outcomes in terms of the change in awareness and use of services. The diagram places the mobile family resource centre in the middle of a number of interactions between individuals and organisations. The mobile resource centre acts as a first point of contact for parents, some of who are otherwise disconnected from existing networks. While on the one hand the centre provides information, it also makes referrals informally to other organisations, such as the health clinic or a playgroup association. The data also shows that the program manager facilitates interagency networks. An example of this occurred when the program manager was talking to a nurse at the local health clinic, who was coordinating guest speakers for a new mothers group. Because of the program manager's relationship with the local playgroup association, a connection was made that in turn facilitated additional support for those mothers who wished to form a new playgroup. Similarly, because of the referrals the program manager made to the playgroup association there is the potential for that organisation to feed those referrals to new or existing playgroups.

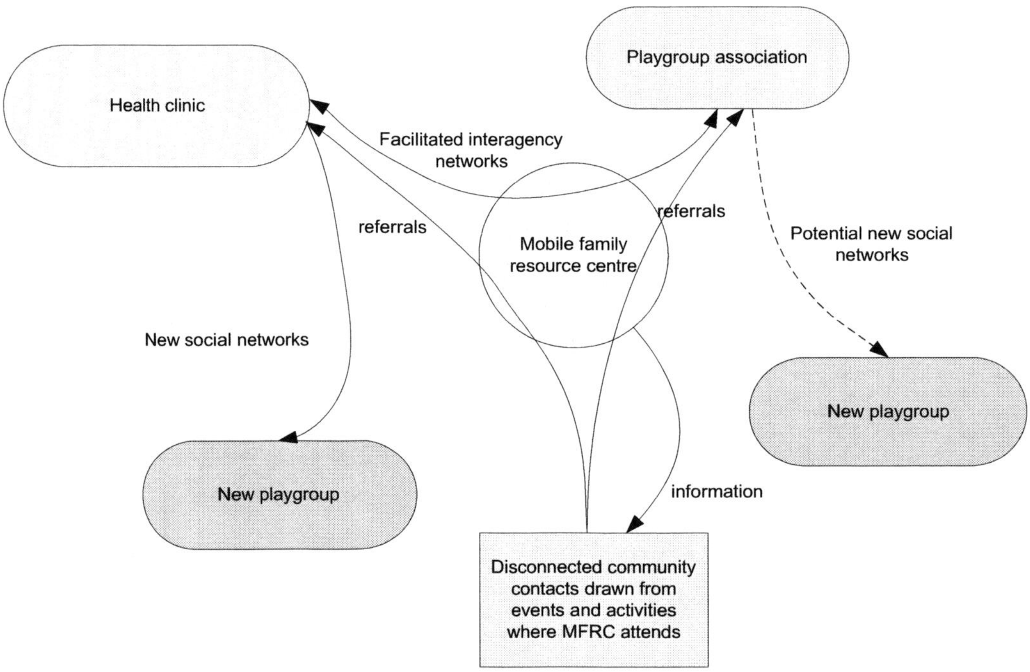

Figure 2. Representation of the Mobile Family Resource Centre as a catalyst for networking.

Another illustration of how these connections are made is given by the program manager who describes her observations below:

> There is one family that I see quite often now. I would consider them "hard to engage". Neither parent is employed and they live in a low-cost housing area. Initially, the young couple would push their three year old past me in the shopping mall. I would offer them a balloon for the boy or a list of useful phone numbers which they could display on their refrigerator. Sometimes they would walk by and just smile or wave. One day—probably the fifth time that I had seen them—they stopped and asked what the van was about. On this occasion, they took information on a playgroup and a fun day that was about to happen, and some parenting classes. They told me that they were concerned about their parenting and were concerned that their boy might find it difficult when he went to school. Later in the year I was a guest speaker at the parenting classes mentioned above and this couple was present. The next day I was out in the van in the shopping

> mall and they dropped by and talked about the parenting classes. I told them about a reading program that was available for a small cost and a regular time commitment. This was when they told me that neither could read very well themselves. I asked if I could get the reading program coordinator to phone them and they said that they would like this. I did not see them again until New Years Eve. The couple came out to greet me and said "thank you" for linking them with the reading program coordinator.

This illustration highlights how these connections are made. Importantly it also shows the significance of the emerging trust between the program manager and service users.

In summary then, the data shows that the mobile family resource centre works to increase awareness and use of services by a) making connections between individuals and community organisations, and b) facilitating networks between service providers. While we do not want to dismiss the importance of the information resources distributed, it seems that from an outcomes perspective the greatest impact is demonstrated in terms of network formation. The mobile family resource centre therefore acts as a kind of catalyst for the creation of new—and development of existing—social networks that contribute to community well-being.

DISCUSSION

We now return to the question posed earlier in the paper: What does this evaluation and its findings mean for the measurement of program impact, particularly in the context of promoting health and well-being to the broader community?

The methodology used to measure impact of mid-level outcomes in this evaluation is not limited by constraints of experimental designs where for example results are based on the use of control and treatment groups and a comparison of the two. Such methods often test a hypothesis and use deductive methods to draw conclusions about the hypothesis. The approach used in this evaluation uses qualitative methods and inductive methods to generate a model that may be tested in ongoing evaluation activities or in other settings. As noted in the literature (1,5,14), this approach is important in terms of generating theories or models and for informing and understanding of the context in which the program takes place. The literature shows that it has been widely used in the evaluation of health programs.

There may be a temptation to evaluate programs such as the mobile family resource centre only using data about the number of events attended, the number of contacts made and the quantity of resources distributed. We noted at the outset of this chapter that the purpose of the evaluation of the mobile family resource centre was largely to measure impact. However, none of these numeric measures assess impact—what kind of difference it made. The challenge faced here then was to find appropriate methods that did measure impact.

The data shows definitively that it does make a difference. While impact can be assessed quantitatively in terms of the uptake of information provided, a perhaps more important finding from this evaluation relates to the way the mobile family resource centre works. The model illustrated in figure 2 represents this. What we can say from an analysis of the data is that the success of the model is dependent on the catalytic nature of the program manager's work at events and activities. Further, we may also induce that a factor that contributes to the success is the trust built up between the program manager and representatives of other organisations as well as the public more generally. In terms of reaching 'hard to engage' members of the community, the identification of the centre as a neutral point of contact is also important. In addition, the data shows that an important outcome—not initially envisaged—is the extent to which networks in the community are supported and facilitated through this service. While the aim of the program initially was to promote awareness and use of services that promote health and well-being for parents of young children an equally important outcome has been the facilitation of networks and collaboration among service providers. Impact can therefore be seen in a number of ways:

- Increased availability of information for parents of young children;
- Increasing use or uptake of information and services;
- Increasing community engagement of parents including those who are 'hard to engage'; and
- Improved interagency networks.

While it is not possible using this methodology to track down individuals and examine case by case the impact on individuals, the methodology does allow on overall assessment of the program's impact to be made. The journaling approach captures a series of stories that offer insight into the program's impact at a variety of levels. Its effectiveness as an evaluation tool depends to some extent on the meticulous recording of observations by the program manager. Analysis by an independent evaluator to some extent objectifies what could otherwise be criticised as purely subjective findings.

Conclusions

This chapter has examined the case of an evaluation of a program's impact where clients are unknown, and yet where impact was expected in terms of changing awareness and increasing service use of health and community services for parents of young children. The evaluation used a combination of tools and methods to assess impact. By recording and quantifying resources that are being distributed the evaluation has been able to establish a framework whereby demand for health and parenting information can be measured and monitored for changes over time. Use of a comprehensive journaling tool enables program impact to be assessed in terms of contacts' referral to service providers; connections made between the program manager and other local services; and in terms of formation of new social networks.

The mobile family resource centre is not a unique program. There are many examples in the literature of this kind of activity with its goal of getting information out to people and then expecting them to use that to access services in their community. What is different about this program though is that it has been shown—with sound evidence—to make a difference. This raises the possibility that other programs faced with similar evaluation challenges, can also be effectively measured in terms of impact. The challenge for funding bodies also, is to develop performance indicators that not only reflect program activity and service delivery, but also program impact for individuals and communities.

REFERENCES

[1] Stufflebeam D, Shinkfield A. Evaluation theory, models and applications. San Francisco: Jossey-Bass, 2007.

[2] Blamey A, Mackenzie M. Theories of change and realistic evaluation: Peas in a pod or apples and oranges? Evaluation 2007;13(4):439-55.

[3] Pawson R. Nothing as practical as a good theory. Evaluation 2003;9(4):471-90.

[4] WK Kellogg Foundation. Logic Model Development Guide. 2004 [cited August 2005]; Available from: http://www.wkkf.org/Pubs/Tools/Evaluation/Pub3669.pdf

[5] Patton M. Qualitative research and evaluation methods. Thousand Oaks, CA: Sage, 2002.

[6] Pawson R. Evidence-based policy: The promise of 'realist synthesis'. Evaluation 2002;8(3):340-58.

[7] Mitchell P. Building capacity for life promotion: Technical report volume 1: Australian Institute of Family Studies; 2000.

[8] Judge K, Bauld B. Strong theory, flexible methods: evaluating complex community-based initiatives. Critical Public Health 2001;11(1):19-38.

[9] Mason P, Barnes M. Constructing theories of change: Methods and sources. Evaluation 2007;13(2):151-70.

[10] Hansen HF. Choosing evaluation models: A discussion on evaluation design. Evaluation 2005;11(4):447-62.

[11] McKenzie R, Naccarella L, Stewart A, Thompson C. Targeting what matters in health promotion evaluation: Using the RE-AIM approach to identify success in real-world settings. Evaluation J Australasia 2007;7(1):19-26.

[12] Katz I. Using secondary data for evaluating community programs–opportunities and challenges. Australasian Evaluation Society International Conference. Holiday Inn Esplanade, Darwin: Australasian Evaluation Society, 2006.

[13] Johnson B, Christensen L. Educational research: Quantitative, qualitative and mixed approaches, second ed.Boston, MA: Pearson Educ, 2004.

[14] Stevenson J, Thomas D. Intellectual contexts. In: Shaw I, Greene J, Mark M, eds. The Sage handbook of evaluation. London: Sage, 2006:200-24.

In: Rural child health: International aspects
Editors: Erica Bell and Joav Merrick

ISBN: 978-1-60876-357-3

Chapter 12

TRANSLATING CHRONIC CONDITION SELF-MANAGEMENT PROGRAMMES (CCSM) INTO LIFESTYLE MANAGEMENT PROGRAMMES FOR YOUNG PEOPLE

Peter W Harvey*[*], *BEd, Dip T, PhD and Jessica Staker
School of Population Health and Clinical Practice and School of Medicine,
The University of Adelaide, North Terrace, Adelaide, South Australia

The techniques applied in chronic condition self-management programmes (CCSM) to support patients with chronic conditions are basic counselling and communication strategies that would benefit people at all stages of life and wellness. The question being explored here is why, as a society, we wait until people develop essentially preventable chronic conditions before helping them to develop the life skills they need to manage their lives and their human interactions better rather than working to avoid or prevent many chronic conditions that develop as a result of people lacking such skills? If we were to teach coping and managing skills to everyone in a supportive and structured way, using the peer-led teaching and learning strategies and basic counselling and education processes that have been shown to be successful for other older groups with chronic illness, the overall population impact would be more significant. Therefore why wait until people have chronic conditions before empowering them with basic life management techniques? Do people need to be sick before they can be motivated to live more effective lives? Is sickness the main stimulus for triggering health-related behaviour change or can other factors in people's lives serve to inform and motivate lifestyle change?

---

* Correspondence: Peter Harvey, BEd, Dip T, PhD, Senior lecturer and manager, State-wide Gambling Therapy Service, Margaret Tobin Centre, Flinders University, Flinders Drive, Bedford Park, 5042 Australia. Tel: 08 8404 2609; Fax: 08 8404 2101; E-mail: peter.harvey@flinders.edu.au

Introduction

More and more attention is being devoted, through private health fund initiatives and government supported programmes and interventions, to the idea that the adverse impacts of illness and disease represent a cost and burden to society that we do not need to carry to the extent that is the case currently. Such illnesses, especially lifestyle related diseases such as many chronic health conditions, can be mitigated successfully through individuals assuming more responsible and healthy approaches to their lives and to the management of their health and wellbeing. That is, we can improve wellbeing and reduce the financial impact of illness upon the health system through educating people in approaches to healthy living and by developing their skills for participating positively and constructively in the management of their health earlier in life (1-5).

> "Many things designed to make life easier, from remote control to non-iron sheets, have really only made us more sedentary. Studies show that the Amish are much less likely to get fat than other Americans. If you stop seeing repetitive chores as drudge work and instead look at them as a meditative form of mild exertion, you will be helping the weight loss and wellness cause in a big way (6, p213)"

Indeed, creating and sustaining such behaviour change in our population in relation to lifestyle choices is crucial to effective health service management and to securing the future of subsequent generations in both developed and developing countries (7-9).

Such efforts, however, remain focused on people with existing chronic illness and are yet to grapple with longer-term earlier intervention and prevention of illness that will be necessary if we are to improve population based health and wellbeing. We cannot simply wait until chronic illness occurs and then learn to manage it. Rather, we need to prevent much of this illness burden from occurring in the first instance and put more resources into managing actual cases after diagnosis. It is postulated here that components of the chronic illness self-management approach deployed with patients who have chronic and complex illness might also be deployed advantageously with younger people to prevent or delay onset of chronic conditions in this population (6, p233).

Researchers have been developing and testing care planning and patient-centred education processes through programmes like the Sharing Health Care SA (SHCSA) demonstration project (10-13) as well as encouraging community partnerships and the formation of volunteer and self-help groups to support patients to manage their chronic conditions. Peer-led self-management programmes are designed to draw on the knowledge and skills of patients who have learnt to manage their condition through paying attention to early warning signs, managing symptoms and dealing more effectively with the social and physical impacts of their illness (14-16). Two-hour sessions for around twelve to fourteen participants are typically run once a week for six weeks. Topics discussed range from sharing experiences of living with chronic illness, learning to manage pain and depression, goal setting and planning positive consumer oriented strategies for living a more active life. Participants indicated that they felt more comfortable in these sessions if they were led by trained peer-educators rather than by professionals per se. Each session begins with a review of activities from the previous week and with discussion about participants' progress towards achieving their life goals. Variations of this process have also been developed and implemented for Aboriginal people (17).

Whilst not all self-management programmes have demonstrated long-term and sustainable benefits for all participants involved or for all categories of chronic illness, significant numbers of studies and meta-analyses suggest that major benefits do generally accrue to patients involved in these processes (1,13,18). Consequently, this approach to prevention and management of chronic conditions, whilst not the total answer to chronic condition management, now appears set to continue in Australia through collaboration between health service agencies, GPs and community volunteer groups across (19).

At the same time, however, we also need to be doing more for younger people to ensure that their lifestyle choices leave them with the best chance of optimising their health and wellbeing for the future. The current crisis in relation to confirmed cases of chronic illness is now being addressed through major government and private health system initiatives in this area, but we still need to develop more preventive approaches as well as working to improve quality of life for existing chronic illness sufferers (7, p5). As we have seen:

> "Recent developments in primary health care, preventive care, early intervention programmes, population health constructs and coordinated care trials in Australia have explored the idea of changing our emphasis in health care from responsive acute care to more integrated, whole population community wellbeing management. This idea suggests that much illness and even trauma experienced by individuals in our communities can be prevented or managed in a more constructive and positive manner than has been the case to date. Much disabling illness need not occur at all and can be avoided through better community based management models, education programmes, and lifestyle changes that contribute to more healthy communities (20)"

Communities are now becoming more cognisant of the fact that prevention is not only an appealing idea in terms of achieving improved health outcomes and quality of life, but that it is also good for business. It can help to moderate demand for costly health care, assist consumers to understand how to live healthier and more fulfilling lives and help to sustain much more dynamic communities generally. The alternative to such approaches to health care is to continue to respond, at great expense, to health problems as they occur and in a reactive manner. This also implies an acceptance of the fact that we will need to spend an increasing proportion of our economic wealth (GDP) on end point health care in the future if we continue to allow the degradation of our living space and our lifestyles to affect our wellbeing adversely…'prevention in all things starts in childhood.' (6, p235)

Communities are now in a good position to improve health management opportunities for younger people by adapting the principles of chronic illness self-management, currently being developed for patients with chronic conditions. Such earlier intervention and self-management training approaches for younger people may serve to inform their lifestyle choices, which if left uninformed and un-managed, could result in significant expansion of the numbers of people with preventable chronic conditions in the future (7).

Much chronic illness currently manifesting in society can be prevented and if not prevented outright, can be delayed effectively to allow people to live longer more effective lives free of disease. Indeed, in the US, 'Sixty percent of over-weight 5-10 year old children already have one biochemical or clinical cardiovascular risk factor such as hyperlipidemia, elevated blood pressure or increased insulin levels, and 25% have two or more (21). Australia is following these American trends closely, but the trend is not inevitable. Improvements in this alarming situation might be made through adopting an approach to education and preventive health that is based on person centred goal setting and lifestyle planning and which is informed through the application of effective life skills education in relation to healthy diet, exercise and improved self-management for healthier living and quality of life.

It is clear, given the earlier onset of conditions such as diabetes in our community today, the tendency for more young people to be overweight and more sedentary in their behaviour and our growing fascination with electronic media, that there is much we could be doing to avoid the early onset of chronic illness. A preventive approach is one possible strategy to achieve the objective of improved quality of life for our entire populations. The relatively insignificant cost of early intervention strategies when compared to the social, emotional and financial costs of creating a society that will otherwise be overwhelmed by preventable chronic disease in the future is a cogent argument for beginning this work as soon as possible. Booth notes that:

> "A large majority of chronic diseases are preventable by engaging in low-risk lifestyles. Low-risk behaviour was defined as a combination of five variables; BMI less than 25; a diet high in serial fibre and polyunsaturated fat and low in trans fat and glycemic load (which reflects the effect of diet on the blood glucose level); engagement in moderate to vigorous physical activity for at least half an hour per day; no current smoking; and the consumption of on average of at least half a drink of an alcoholic beverage per day (22) sited in (7)"

THE COHORT

The focus of such a programme would be students in schools where recent work has highlighted alarming trends in increased obesity levels.

> "Secular trends in Australian children's body fatness are continuing. Further, the rates of change in girls are affected by the socio-demographic milieu (23)"

Post-school environments and other contexts in which organised learning takes place might also be targeted. A preventive health and life planning process could be integrated into all facets of living and learning.

It is true that, to some extent, aspects of this kind of programme are already in place through some teaching programmes in schools, churches and youth groups and in some family structures in which young people are coached and mentored effectively to optimal health and wellbeing. For the vast majority of people, however, there is little formal support offered through which they are able to aspire to optimal health or even begin to grasp what such a concept means today.

ECONOMIC DETERMINISM

In many communities and for many individuals the material conditions (24-29) of life are major impediments to good health (30). We know that socio-economic status can predict health outcomes in some situations (31-33), but in our current climate of indulgence and lethargy even economically well off communities are prone to the risk of high levels of chronic, but preventable illness. Economic factors are, therefore, not the only predictors of health status we might need to be cognisant of in relation to the future management of chronic illness. It is, however, possible to structure approaches to learning and living that support people at all levels of the community and assist them to develop life skills to optimise their health related opportunities rather than feeling alienated and oppressed by daily events over which they have little or no control. It is not necessary to have a 'revolution' (25,34,35) to give people better access to quality of life; we can work with what we have! Indeed, this is all we are able to do!

What is needed to ensure better management of lifestyle and health-related opportunities in the community is wider access to knowledge and communication processes through formal programmes of support for learners of all ages and at all levels of the culture. Peer education appears to be a useful strategy in this regard.

THE PROGRAMME

Local research in this area could begin with the collection of baseline data across a range of school communities and age groups to obtain a sample of BMI, activity rates and dietary patterns of young people as is currently being gathered by local researchers (23,36). This baseline data could then be used to construct intervention programmes leading to the development of a range of school-based curricula and activities around peer-led training, role play and behaviour reinforcement approaches creating and sustaining behaviour change in young people towards lowering lifestyle risk factors in the population. The focus of this type of research, as in CCSM programmes, would be on determining the optimal conditions for participation in lifestyle programmes rather than measuring clinical outcomes per se. We know the key elements of successful lifestyle options, but what we have not yet achieved is the engagement of young people in a sustained way to achieve lowered lifestyle related health risks in this population generally. A similar paradigm has been observed in relation to the treatment and management of diabetes and other chronic conditions (37).

Once pilot work is completed, an intervention study over 12 months or more to document the impact of student participation in self-help and peer-led programmes would be implemented. Ultimately a longer-term study could be established into the health outcomes resulting from student participation in the programme. Such approaches bring a major challenge for health care workers and schools. Our initial approaches to implementing and testing the model in State Department schools in rural South Australia highlighted a crowded curriculum where competing subject content and limited time for new courses made it very difficult to get such a strategy into a curriculum structure; much like the current difficulty being experienced in getting training about self-management into medical and health science curricula in Australia.

The proposed strategy could, however, be linked to health and personal development programmes or run through the student counselling programmes operating in most Australian schools today. Peer-led programmes such as the student representative council meetings in schools are known to stimulate student interest and participation along with other approaches that empower young people to be actively involved in the life of their school.

Peer-led education and student centred learning approaches engender an active and participatory environment for young people, which also creates a dynamic learning environment that offers more potential learning opportunities than traditional didactic approaches to teaching. Students listen to and learn very effectively from each other; their peers. This process is a proven strategy for engaging with and capturing the interest and active participation of students and is a key element in the successful engagement of older people diagnosed with chronic conditions.

CONCLUSIONS

To date we have been persuaded by the burgeoning rates of chronic illness in our community that strategies need to be implemented to manage the impact of chronic disease, improve patient health status and reduce the inevitable burden that these trends will place upon the health care system. However, whilst the management of existing chronic illness problems is now becoming a more important priority for governments and private insurers, we appear to be ignoring a looming crisis in regard to the health status of our younger populations, which will fuel an even faster acceleration of chronic illness rates as this group, in turn, ages and becomes prematurely and adversely affected by essentially preventable chronic health problems.

Given that existing health programmes for young people are not addressing these new problems to the extent that is needed, it is proposed that education and support strategies that have been adopted for adult populations to assist in the management of the effects of chronic illness might also be adopted with younger populations as an overall preventative health and lifestyle education strategy. As we move increasingly to population-based approaches to the management of health (20,38,39) and implementation of preventative health care strategies (40), it will be essential that communities develop ways of relating to and working with young people that can mitigate the deleterious effects of new and emerging lifestyle related threats to overall community health status and wellbeing.

Peer education appears to be successful among older population groups, with participants indicating that they prefer such approaches to the traditional health-professional-led programmes and with early outcomes indicating significant improvements in knowledge, self-management skill and health status of participants. Adaptation of this model may be the next logical step in the process of building more effective and pro-active self-managing communities (12).

References

[1] Bodenheimer T, Lorig K, Holman H, Grumbach K. Patient self-management of chronic disease in primary care. JAMA 2002;288(19):2469-75.

[2] Fries J, Carey C, McShane D. Patient education in arthritis: randomised controlled trial of a mail-delivered program. J Rheumatol 1997;24:1378-83.

[3] Norris SL, Engelgau MM, Narayan KM. Effectiveness of self-management training in type 2 diabetes: a systematic review of randomized controlled trials. Diabetes Care 2001;24(3):561-87.

[4] Flower J. Why some people get sick and others don't - a conversation with J. Frazer Mustard, MD. Healthcare Forum J 1997;40(6):12-8.

[5] McCain MN, Mustard JF. The early years study - three years later. Toronto: Can Inst Adv Res, 2002.

[6] Guiliano M. French women don't get fat. New York: Random House, 2005.

[7] Booth FW, Chakravarthy MV. Cost and Consequences of Sedentary Living: New Battleground for an Old Enemy. Res Digest 2002;3(16):8.

[8] Fries J, McShane D. Reducing need and demand for medical services in high-risk persons: A health education approach. West J Med 1998;169(4):201-7.

[9] Fries J, Koop C, Sokolov J, Carson E, Wright D. Beyond health promotion: reducing need and demand for medical care. Health Affairs 1998;17(2):70-84.

[10] Fuller J. Sharing health care. SA qualitative impact evaluation, final report. Adelaide: Univ Adelaide, 2004.

[11] Fuller J, Harvey PW, Misan G. Is client centred care planning for chronic disease sustainable? Experience from rural South Australia. Health Soc Care Community 2004;12(4):318-26.

[12] Harvey PW, Petkov J, Misan G, Warren K, Fuller J, Battersby M et al. Self-management support and training for patients with chronic and complex conditions improves health related behaviour and health outcomes! Aust Health Rev, accepted.

[13] PricewaterhouseCoopers. National evaluation of the sharing health care initiative. Final report and executive summary. Sydney: Aust Governm Dept Health Ageing, 2005.

[14] Battersby M, Reece M, Markwick M. The Partners in Health Handbook - a guide to help you become an active partner in the management of your health. Adelaide: Flinders Univ South Aust, Coordinated Care Training Unit, 2000.

[15] Lorig K, Holman H, Sobel D, Laurent D, Gonzales V, Minor M. Living a healthy life with chronic conditions. Palo Alto, CA: Bull Publishing, 2000.

[16] Von Korff M, Gruman J, Schaefer J, Curry S, Wagner E. Collaborative management of chronic illness. Ann Int Med 1997;127:1097-1102.

[17] Warren K, Lorig K, Coulthard F. LIFE: living improvements for everyone - a course in chronic condition self-management for Aboriginal people, 3rd ed. Whyalla: Spencer Gulf Rural Health School, Pika Wiya Health Service, 2006.

[18] Lorig K, Sobel DS, Ritter PL, Hobbs M. Effect of self-management programs on patients with chronic disease. Effect Clin Pract 2001;4(6):256-62.

[19] Commonwealth of Australia. Australian Better Health Initiative (ABHI). 2006 [cited; Available from: <http://www.health.gov.au/internet/wcms/publishing.nsf/Content/feb2006coag03.htm>

[20] Harvey PW. Sustainable population health: a pressing priority for community wellbeing. Environ Health 2002;2(3):66-74.

[21] Koplan JP, Dietz WH. Caloric imbalance and public health policy. JAMA 1999;282:1579-81.

[22] Hu FB, Manson JE, Stampfer MJ, Colditz G, Liu S, Solomon CG, et al. Diet, lifestyle and the risk of type 2 diabetes mellitus in women. New Engl J Med 2001;345:790-7.

[23] Dollman J, Pilgrim A. Changes in body composition between 1997 and 2002 among South Australian children: influences of socio-economic status and location of residence. Aust NZ J Public Health 2005;29(2):166-70.

[24] Heilbroner R. The worldly philosophers - the lives, times and ideas of the great economic thinkers, 6th ed. New York: Simon Schuster, 1986.

[25] Marx K, Engels F. The German ideology - part one (trans). New York: Int Publishers, 1978.

[26] Sartre J-P. Essays in existentialism. New York: Citadel Press, 1965.

[27] Weber M. The Protestant ethic and the spirit of capitalism. London: Unwin Univ Books, 1958.
[28] Flannery T. The future eaters. Melbourne, Victoria: Reed Books, 1994.
[29] Smith A. An inquiry into the nature and causes of the wealth of nations. London: William Benton, 1776.
[30] Smith JD. Australia's rural and remote health - a social justice perspective. Melbourne: Tertiary Press, 2004.
[31] Marmot M. Social determinants of health: from observation to policy. Med J Aust 2000;172:379-82.
[32] Marmot MG, Smith GD. Health inequalities among British civil servants: the Whitehall 2 study. Lancet 1991;337:1387-93.
[33] Syme L. Social and economic disparities in health: thoughts about intervention. Milbank Q 1998;76(4):493-506.
[34] Engels F. Dialectics of nature. London: Lawrence Wishart, 1941.
[35] Plamenatz J. Marx's philosophy of man. Oxford: Clarendon Press, 1975.
[36] Booth ML, Chey T, Wake M, Norton K, Hesketh K, Dollman J et al. Change in the prevalence of overweight and obesity among young Australians, 1969-1997. Am J Clin Nutr 2003;77(1):29-36.
[37] Mills PD, Harvey PW. Beyond community-based diabetes management and the COAG Coordinated Care Trial. Aust J Rural Health 2003;11(3).
[38] Harvey PW. Approaches to Population Health Care - the emerging context! Aust J Prim Health 2005;11(2):45-53.
[39] Kindig DA. Understanding population health. Milbank Q 2007;85(1):139-61.
[40] South Australian DHS. The Generational Health Review. Adelaide: Dept Human Serv, 2003.

In: Rural Child Health: International Aspects
Editors: Erica Bell and Joav Merrick
ISBN: 978-1-60876-357-3

Chapter 13

CONSULTATION LIAISON CHILD PSYCHIATRY FOR RURAL AREAS

Helen J Stain*[*], *BA(Hons), MPsych, PhD, MAPS and Brian Kelly, BMed, PhD, FRANZCP, FAChPM
Centre for Rural and Remote Mental Health, University of Newcastle, Orange, Australia

The lack of specialist mental health care in rural areas necessitates an innovative approach to service delivery. Consultation liaison (CL) psychiatry has evolved to address the high rate of mental health problems presenting in primary health care for both adults and children. The CL model has particular application in rural areas where general health services (either primary or secondary level services) rather than specialist mental health services are more likely than urban areas to be the setting for treatment of children with mental health problems and their families. However traditional CL models deliver discrete services to specific age populations rather than encompassing the whole life span. This paper describes a model of CL child psychiatry designed to break down such barriers in order to meet the needs of children and adolescents in rural general health care settings. Recommendations are proposed to facilitate the roll out of the model to address much needed health services for smaller communities.

INTRODUCTION

Mental health service delivery in rural areas often falls to the responsibility of primary care providers. In comparison to urban areas, rural residents have greater difficulty accessing mental health services due to vast distances to travel and a lack of a full range of specialist mental health services. Rates of service utilisation are influenced by issues of stigma and confidentiality in some rural areas as well as concern regarding the perceived effectiveness of services (1). In recent years there has been a surge in the development of new models of service delivery to address the specific needs of rural areas. These models have focussed on target groups (such as elderly, youth) or on phases of intervention (early psychosis,

* Correspondence: Helen J Stain, Centre for Rural and Remote Mental Health, University of Newcastle, Bloomfield Hospital, Forest Road, Orange, NSW, Australia 2800. E-mail: Helen.Stain@newcastle.edu.au

rehabilitation), or specific levels of care (eg primary care) (2,3). While evaluations of the programs have been positive a lot more work is needed to achieve service wide benefits and greater equity for rural areas. The National Health Service (NHS) of the United Kingdom has been criticised for the lack of a rural premium for health service funding in recognition of higher service costs associated with rurality (4). The NHS model based on service utilisation to demonstrate need for services and therefore funding is flawed in that rurality has been linked to lower utilisation rates. Increased costs for rural service delivery include access to staff training and need for multi skilling of staff, travel time for staff to delivery services, patient transport and mental health support for general health care staff. Rural areas in the USA have also been cited as having reduced mental health services, poorer mental health outcomes and clinicians with a more limited range of clinical skills compared to urban areas (5).

Difficulty in recruitment and retention of mental health clinicians is a well recognised problem in rural areas. Clinicians describe feeling professionally isolated and lacking clinical supervision and professional development. Methods of addressing these issues have included telepsychiatry, "fly in" specialists and urban-rural staff exchanges (6,7). General hospitals and health services play a critical role in rural areas given these are often the first point of contact for mental health problems (8). These general health services are also often the sole providers of health care in rural areas due to an absence of a broader range of specialist mental health services. There is a need for rural models of service delivery that link mental health services to the general health setting. Consultation liaison (CL) psychiatry is a service that operates between and within both mental and general health services. It is also a service that can facilitate skill development and maintenance in rural clinicians. This paper explores the ability of a CL service to address the mental health needs of children and adolescents in rural areas.

In the United Kingdom, early intervention services for mental health problems in adolescence have progressed beyond simple linkages with youth related services (such as educational and vocational services) to that of integration of these within the mental health team (9). This holistic approach to intervention will facilitate better outcomes including greater likelihood of youth re-joining their developmental trajectory following illness interruption. It is critical that intervention acknowledges the systems within which children and adolescents are positioned, such as the family, peers and school, as well as the interplay of physical and mental health.

CHILDREN AND ADOLESCENTS IN GENERAL HEALTH CARE SETTING

For an adolescent or child, admission to a general hospital can be a traumatic experience and even a time of crisis for the family. A CL service provides not only for children and adolescents, who have pre-existing mental health problems, but also for those who develop mental health problems as a result of presence or treatment of physical health conditions. Other factors that can contribute to child and adolescent mental health problems in hospital include separation from family, ongoing family dysfunction, pain, a fear of procedures or illness outcome, environmental change and past experience with hospitalisation. The young person's ability to cope with hospitalisation may be affected by their cognitive capacity and is influenced by past experience, psycho-social development, cultural factors, parental influences, and personal defence mechanisms. For example, a 14 year old with cognitive difficulties may react like an eight year old, when faced with the anxiety of prolonged painful treatment. It is important to also recognise the systemic nature of childhood and adolescence whereby young people are intricately embedded in a system or series of systems – family, school, friends and community. The hospital adds another and often unfamiliar layer to these systems, It is not uncommon for young people to perceive a lack of power or control over their environments and this adds to their anxiety particularly in the hospital setting.

Children with chronic physical conditions are also an important group to consider, whose mental health needs can be substantial but often under-recognised in the clinical setting with studies suggesting rates of emotional and behavioural problems as high as 20% in children with chronic illness (10). Particularly in rural areas, children with primary mental health problems (such as deliberate self harm, severe behavioural disturbance) requiring hospital admission may be treated chiefly within the general hospital, whether within paediatric units or in smaller facilities within a general hospital ward (11). The interaction of disease related effects (eg on biological development) and behavioural sequelae with the psychosocial impacts at varying stages of childhood development are important considerations. Providing advice and an appraisal of these issues within the assessment and management plan is a key contribution of CL Psychiatry, in line with the related tasks in adult CL practice (12). A review of CL for children identified four major changes in research for this area, namely a focus on: (i) psychosocial morbidity and functional adaptation across illness groups rather than disorder specific; (ii) child positioned within the family rather than child alone; (iii) functioning and adaptation rather than simple symptom or deficit measurement; and (iv) risk and protective factors (13). A review of research on correlates of psychosocial adjustment to chronic physical illness in childhood found that child or family variables were better predictors of adjustment than disease variables. The authors criticised models for a lack of attention to child adjustment variables such as coping, self concept and temperament (13).

Consultation liaison psychiatry affords the opportunity to address mental health needs within a general health care setting such as a rural general hospital or primary care services.. While much has been done to improve primary care mental health services there has been limited attention to secondary level services, such as general hospitals. This is a critical service given that children with psychological problems are more likely to present to primary care services with somatic symptoms rather than attend mental health services (14). For primary care presentations, 10-25% of children and more than 30% of adolescents are likely to have associated psychological problems while for 2-5% of children and adolescents it will be the main presentation (15). It is well known that children and adolescents with psychosomatic presentations have high rates of service utilisation.. While 25-50% of adults attending primary care have psychological problems, these are not well identified (15). Primary care clinicians welcome the opportunity to work closely with mental health clinicians to increase the ability to identify mental health problems and therefore improve pathways to care for these clients (16).

CONSULTATION LIASON PSYCHIATRY

The role of CL is to assist general health care clinicians with the management of patients with mental health problems in this care setting. In rural areas there is a greater likelihood of admissions for mental health problems to non psychiatric hospitals compared to urban areas for several reasons (8). There is a lack of psychiatric inpatient facilities and a preference to avoid separation of children and adolescents from their families as would arise if admitted to a psychiatric unit. In the central west region of rural New South Wales this could incur a journey of 800 km from home for admission to an adult inpatient unit or a further 300 km for a child unit, even if such a service were appropriate for the clinical problem (17). There is also a lack of bed availability should the clinician seek admission to the child mental health unit located 1,100 km from home. It is therefore essential that (i) primary care clinicians be supported in the management of mental health problems, and (ii) children and adolescents have access to mental health expertise within the general health care paediatric ward, or smaller rural hospitals. A CL service also provides formal and informal education and collaborative management for patients with mental health problems.

Given the paucity of mental health clinicians and the high rate of psychological problems in children and adolescents in primary care, a small CL team could be a cost effective means for child and adolescent psychiatry in rural areas. A review of 48 consultation liaison child psychiatry (CLCP) in the US showed services had average full time rates of 0.44 psychiatrist, 0.27 psychologist, 0.44 trainee psychiatrist, 0.25 trainee psychologist and 0.15 nurse for services with an average of 236 beds (range 10-700 beds) (18). A Norwegian review examined the availability and type of CL services provided by 39 psychiatric units in general hospitals (19). The review showed for an average of 240 beds (range 20-850 beds), 60% of hospitals were staffed by a psychiatric resident, 20% by a CL team member and 20% by a senior psychiatrist during the day. The consultations were conducted by a senior psychiatrist 40% of the time, psychiatric resident 20%, a psychologist 15%, psychiatric nurse 15% and a social worker 10% of the time. The study reported that the majority of CL teams in Norway have only one psychiatrist. The US study showed 65% of CLCP services were directed by a child psychiatrist and 10% by a psychologist with the remainder being jointly administered by psychiatry and psychology (18). By contrast a review of CL services at Geneva University Hospital referred only to the activities of psychiatrists both qualified and in training, namely one chief psychiatrist, three senior psychiatrists, three registrars and six residents (20). This level of staffing is not attainable in non urban areas such as rural Australia.

A RURAL CHILD PSYCIATRY SERVICE

In the central west of rural NSW a small CL service has been developed. The service comprises a consultant psychiatrist (0.2 full time rate), a senior clinical psychologist (0.2) and a clinical nurse consultant (CNC) with mental health training (1.0). A unique and necessary adaptation of the CL service is the need for flexibility and for general psychiatric staff to provide services for children and adolescents as well as adults rather than parallel services as recommended by others (21). The CL services two rural general hospitals with a 1.0 CNC at each of the hospitals to coordinate mental health patient care. The service works closely with paediatricians and with back up from child psychiatrists. The significant lack of child psychiatry coverage for the area requires management by adult psychiatry with input from child psychiatry via telepsychiatry consults and where possible referral to follow up care.

Although a small team, the CL service has been able to engage in each of the CL related activities listed in table 1. The CL service is a stepped care model in that a screening assessment is followed by a more detailed clinical assessment and then consultation with the wider CL team if required. Two child CL models previously described in the literature have been that of (i) the psychiatrist as the key provider of services and fulfilling a triage role or (ii) any member of the CL team responding to the referral (22). While these models appear to have been successful in a large paediatric hospital, it would be difficult to implement or maintain such models in a rural setting. Given reduced availability of clinicians, the proposed rural CL model is that of a CNC in the triage role with subsequent assessment, intervention and case consultation the psychiatrist or psychologist as required. An evaluation of the CL service at the urban Australian paediatric hospital resulted in the change to the use of the CL team in the initial assessment rather than reliance on the psychiatrist to triage. The evaluation showed greater referral rates for adolescents when allied health and nursing were involved in the initial process (23). When comparing these models to CL services in rural areas it is important to note that only 4% of referrals were through the emergency department of the hospital. With the CNC in a triage role the point of intake is very clear to the referring clinicians and the CNC has the opportunity to forge strong working relationships with hospital staff. A model that shares the triage role across the CL team could lessen the engagement of referrers in the service.

Table 1. Rural consultation liaison child psychiatry (CLCP) in practice

CLCP activity
Specialist assessment
Joint consultation
Treatment recommendations
Case management
Feedback loop – CLCP and general health / paediatric clinicians
Case debrief
Family issues
Case review
Within ward management of patient
General health care clinician professional development and treatment guidelines

For the proposed CL model, intervention such as brief psycho-education occurs during assessment and for some cases is sufficient intervention. An important focus has been to increase the confidence and competency of general health and paediatric clinicians in managing mental health problems in the paediatric ward. An inherent aspect of CL practice is the translation of different individuals' points of view to each other. On the paediatric ward this involves the views of child, parent, general health care staff and the CL team. Each interaction on the ward is an educational opportunity by the CL team either by direct exchange of information or by role modelling. Nurses caring for a child who has had a sudden physical trauma may be vicariously traumatised. The CL team can assist staff to resolve their own reactions to child trauma. Research has shown the CL nurse can have a role in changing attitudes of general health care nurses towards patients with mental health problems (24). This issue has even greater importance in smaller communities whereby stigma and confidentiality are cited by youth as limiting help seeking behaviour for mental health problems (25).

The CL model emphasises education and capacity building among the rural nurses, GPs and other staff in order to facilitate collaborative care with clear referral pathways for the assessment and care of patients with more complex problems. This approach has been associated with improved health outcomes in rural areas elsewhere (26). The aim is for general clinicians to remain actively involved in the management plan and its implementation with varying levels of involvement of the specialist mental health team as required.

While this small team model of CL for child and adolescent mental health needs has been successful in these two rural general hospitals, there is a need for further adaptation of the model for smaller rural communities. In smaller facilities it is important for CL to focus on both increasing the skills of general staff and improving access to specialist mental health services when required. A viable model requires a creative approach to staffing to overcome difficulties in recruitment of specialist mental health staff to rural areas. Although it is essential to have a CL clinician on site at the general health care setting, the model could retain the small CL team but have other CL clinicians located at different sites. Thus a network CL team could provide a CL service with coverage for adult, child and adolescent patient care. The CL team could be linked for service delivery through telepsychiatry and some fly in consultations. Telepsychiatry for child and adolescent mental health service delivery has already been shown to be effective for rural areas (27, 28). Critical to the rural small team model is the on site CL clinician who would require specialist training as well as reliable ongoing clinical supervision and support. In some settings the on site CL clinician would be a full time dedicated position while other settings would necessitate the CL clinician work across other areas as well. The CLCP rural model relies heavily on clear communication pathways between paediatric clinicians and the CL team. There is often a reticence by general psychiatric staff to engage in the mental health care of children and adolescents.

Conclusions

It is critical that CL child psychiatry take a lead role in promoting clinical services, training, research and education of the broader health care community in order to enhance mental health care for rural children and adolescents in general health care settings. Recruitment of clinicians to rural CL services could be improved by university placements in rural CL and by professional bodies encouraging integrated service delivery across populations (eg child and adult) rather than parallel services. The value of rural placements using a mentorship model in encouraging role socialisation into the profession has been demonstrated using rural – urban collaborations (29) and should be pursued for the development of rural CL child psychiatry services. Consistently across rural areas both within Australia and internationally there is the need for innovation in mental health service delivery. This paper invites rural practitioners to consider a CL model for the delivery of child and adolescent mental health services. Increased access to appropriate services, particularly for children and adolescents, requires coordination of services (mental health, health, social welfare, education), broadening the skill base of front line workers, provision of outreach services (for example, mobile or fly in teams), access to clinical consultation for staff (telepsychiatry) and greater community education.

REFERENCES

[1] Komiti A, Judd F, Jackson H. The influence of stigma and attitudes on seeking help from a GP for mental health problems. A rural context. Soc Psychiatr Psychiatric Epidemiol 2006;41:738-45.

[2] Welch M, Welch T. Early psychosis in rural areas. Aust NZ J Psychiatry 2007;41:485-94.

[3] Blashki G, Selzer R, Judd F, Hodgins G, Ciechomski L. Primary care psychiatry: Taking Consultation-Liaison psychiatry to the community. Australas Psychiatry 2005;13(3):302-6.

[4] Asthana S, Gibson A, Moon G, Brigham P. Allocating resources for health and social care: The significance of rurality. Health Soc Care Community 2003;11(6):486-93.

[5] Hilty DM, Yellowlees PM, Cobb HC, Bourgeois JA, Neufeld JD, Nesbitt TS. Models of telepsychiatric consultation-liaison service to rural primary care. Psychosomatics 2006;47(2):152-7.

[6] Kowalenko N, Bartik W, Whitefield K, Wignall A. Rural workforce development and staff support: Remodelling service provision for early intervention in child and adolescent mental health. Australas Psychiatry 2003;11(suppl 1):S110-6.

[7] Greenberg N, Boydell K, Volpe T. Pediatric telepsychiatry in Ontario: Caregiver and service provider perspectives. J Behav Health Serv Res 2006;33(1):105-11.

[8] Hungerford C. Treating acute mental illness in rural general hospitals: Necessity or choice? Aust J Rural Health 2006;14:139-43.

[9] Joseph R, Birchwood M. The national policy reforms for mental health services and the story of early intervention services in the United Kingdom. J Psychiatr Neurosci 2005;30(5):362-5.

[10] Knapp PK, Harris ES. Consultation-Liaison in child psychiatry: A review of the past 10 years. Part I: Clinical findings. J Am Acad Child Adolesc Psychiatry 1998;37(1):17-25.

[11] Gillig P. An adolescent crisis service in a rural area. Psychiatric Services 2004;55(12):1363-5.

[12] Smith G. The future of Consultation-Liaison Psychiatry. Aust NZ J Psychiatry 2003;37:150-9.

[13] Knapp PK, Harris ES. Consultation-Liaison in child psychiatry: A review of the past 10 years. Part II: Research on treatment approaches and outcomes. J Am Acad Child Adolesc Psychiatry 1998;37(2):139-46.

[14] Rauch P, Jellinek M. Paediatric consultation. In: Rutter M, Taylor E, eds. Child and adolescent psychiatry. Oxford: Blackwell, 2005:1051-66.

[15] Garralda ME. Primary health care psychiatry. In: Rutter M, Taylor E, eds. Child and adolescent psychiatry. Oxford: Blackwell, 2005:1090-100.

[16] Stain HJ, Kisely S, Miller K, Tait A, Bostwick R. Pathways to care for psychological problems in primary care.[see comment]. Aust Fam Physician 2003;32(11):955-6.

[17] Stain HJ, Sartore G, Blinkhorn S, Kelly B. Improving outcomes for child and adolescent schizophrenia in rural and remote communities of Australia. Schizophrenia Bull 2005;31:193.

[18] Shaw RJ, Wamboldt M, Bursch B, Stuber M. Practice patterns in pediatric Consultation-Liaison psychiatry. Psychosomatics 2006;47:43-9.

[19] Ekeberg O. Consultation liaison psychiatry in Norway. J Psychosom Res 2006;60(6):651-2.

[20] Archinard M, Dumont P, De Tonnac N. Guidelines and evaluation: Improving the quality of Consultation-Liaison Psychiatry. Psychosomatics 2005;46:425-30.

[21] Mayou R. Are psychological skills necessary in treating all physical disorders? Aust NZ J Psychiatry 2005;39:880-96.

[22] Harden S, Stathis S, Wagner I. Redevelopment of a consultation-liaison service at a tertiary paediatric hospital. Australas Psychiatry 2005;13(2):169-72.

[23] Wagner I, Stathis S, Harden S, Crimmins J. Models and patterns of service in child and youth consultation-liaison services. Australas Psychiatry 2005;13(3):273-8.

[24] Sharrock J, Grigg M, Happell B, Keeble-Devlin B, Jennings S. The mental health nurse: A valuable addition to the Consultation-Liaison team. Int J Ment Health Nurs 2006;15:35-43.

[25] Aisbett DL, Boyd CP, Francis KJ, Newnham K, Newnham K. Understanding barriers to mental health service utilization for adolescents in rural Australia. Rural Remote Health 2007;7:624.

[26] Hilty D, Yellowlees P, Nesbitt T. Evolution of telepsychiatry to rural sites: Changes over time in types of referral and in primary care providers' knowledge, skills and satisfaction. Gen Hosp Psychiatry 2006;28:367-73.

[27] Hilty D, Yellowlees P, Cobb H, Bourgeois J, Neufeld J, Nesbitt T. Models of telepsychiatric consultation-liaison service and rural primary care. Psychosomatics 2006;47:152-7.

[28] Dossetor DR, Nunn KP, Fairley M, Eggleton D. A child and adolescent psychiatric outreach service for rural New South Wales: A telemedicine pilot study. J Paediatr Child Health 1999;35:525-9.

[29] Charleston R, Goodwin V. Effective collaboration enhances rural preceptorship training. Int J Ment Health Nurs 2004;13:225-31.

In: Rural child health: International aspects
Editors: Erica Bell and Joav Merrick

ISBN: 978-1-60876-357-3

Chapter 14

EDUCATING ADOLESCENTS ABOUT PBERTY: ARE WE MISSING SOMETHING?

Hatim A Omar*[*]*, MD
Section of Adolescent Medicine, Department of Pediatrics,
University of Kentucky, Lexington, Kentucky, United States of America

Adolescents undergo significant physical and cognitive changes during their pubertal development. These changes contribute to and impact their future development. Educating adolescents at an early age about their expected development decreases the possible anxiety associated with this period of life and also helps adolescents make better choices in regards to their sexuality. In order to assess the degree of education regarding pubertal development and sexuality, we conducted a survey of late adolescents (median age 19 years) and parents of adolescents. A total of 409 adolescents (237 females, 172 males) and 124 parents completed the survey. 14.4% of teens (36.6% of males and 2% of females) reported that no one spoke to them prior or during puberty about pubertal development or sexuality issues. Teens receiving some form of puberty/sexuality education did so at a median age of 13 for girls and 15 for boys. More than one source of information was the most common (49%) followed by mother only (20%). 85% of parents reported talking to their teens about pubertal development and sexuality. There were several differences between areas reported covered by parents but not by teens, for example 72% of parents reported talking to their teens about gender differences in growth but only 31% of teens reported being spoken to about that. Areas that are very poorly covered are breast development in boys and sexual assault/date rape in girls at 5% and 26% respectively. In summary, it appears that we continue to do a relatively poor job in educating our kids about their development and sexuality and we do it late. Boys are even less likely than girls to be talked to about many areas of pubertal development and sexuality and when that is done, it is done at a later age.

* Correspondence: Hatim Omar, MD, Director, Adolescent Medicine, Dept. of Pediatrics, Room J422, KY Clinic, University of Kentucky Medical Center, Lexington, KY 40536-0284, United States. Tel: 859 323-5643, Fax: 859 257-7706. E-mail: haomar2@uky.edu

Introduction

The medical literature is consistent on the importance of educating adolescents about sex and pubertal development (1-7). By the twelfth grade, greater than 60% of adolescents have had sex, with 45.6% of high school age students reporting having ever been sexually active (8). Nationally, 6.8% of teens report initiation of sexual intercourse prior to 13 years of age (8). Medical literature also supports the finding that we need to improve our communication to teens about puberty and sexuality (6,9-11).

During puberty, adolescents undergo many physical and psychosocial changes in a relatively short period of time. They double their weight and gain approximately 25% in height, a growth spurt only exceeded in infancy (12). Most teens develop the ability for sequential logical thinking, the final adult stage of cognitive development, by age 16 years (13). They can reproduce and cause injury to self and others. They struggle to establish independence from their parents, to establish relationships with peers and significant others, to establish sexual identity, to finish school, and to prepare for a job or career. It is a time of intense idealism and extreme self-centeredness (12). It is a time when the peer group is valued over all others and a critical attitude is adopted towards established social norms. Being armed with appropriate information about expected changes in their body during puberty and about sexual topics could help to ease their transition through this period. In this study, we investigated the extent of pubertal development and sexuality education as seen by adolescents and parents.

Our study

We conducted a survey of young college students (late adolescents) between the ages of 18 and 22 years. Students were asked to fill in a written questionnaire that asked about education regarding pubertal development and sexuality with help available for those who found any question unclear. Subjects were also asked about their demographic data, but they were kept anonymous to allow privacy. A total of 600 surveys were distributed equally between male (M) and female (F) subjects and 409 (172 M and 237 F) were returned for a response rate of 68.2%.

Median age for both M and F was 19 years. 65% of M and 61% of F respondents lived with both parents at the start of their pubertal development and the rest lived with a single parent. 30% of M and 24% of F respondents had one or more older siblings. We also surveyed parents of adolescents who were patients in our clinic. A total of 200 surveys were distributed to parents and they were asked about their demographic data and then the same questions that the adolescents were asked. A total of 124 parents (56% F and 44% M) completed the survey for a response rate of 62%. The median age for parents was 39 years. Percentages were calculated from both surveys in regards to most aspects of pubertal development and sexuality.

Our findings

85% of parents reported talking to their adolescents about puberty and sexuality and that the age at which that was done was a median of 13 years for F and 15 years for M. In contrast, 83% of teens said that someone had spoken to them about these issues. Strikingly only 63% of males said they were educated on puberty and sexuality while 98% of females said they were. Adolescents agreed with parents that the median age at which they were educated on puberty was 15 years for boys and 13 years for girls. According to the adolescents the most common way of obtaining information on puberty/sexuality was from multiple sources (49%) followed by mother 20% (see table 1).

Table 1. Who spoke to teen about puberty?

	% Teens	% Males	% Females
Father	3	10	0
Mother	20	2	29
Sibling	9	14	7
Teacher	6	12	3
Doctor	2	1	3
Friends	5	10	3
Other	5	4	4
More than one	49	43	51

Male adolescents

A very poorly covered area in male adolescents was that of breast development (gynecomastia) where no parents reported mentioning that and only 5% of male adolescents said that someone had mentioned it to them (see Table 2). Many areas were also poorly covered such as penile growth, sexually transmitted infections (STI's), pregnancy protection and same sex attraction. In other areas such as body odor, gender differences and growth spurt, more parents said that they spoke to their adolescents about these subjects, while adolescents reported a much smaller percentage (see table 2).

Female adolescents

Overall, there was more education provided to female adolescents than to their male counterparts and more agreement between what parents and adolescents reported (see Table 3). Same sex attraction and sexual abuse/date rape were among the least covered areas while breast development and menstrual periods were the most commonly covered (see table 3).

Table 2. The % of parents reporting talking to their male adolescents about puberty and sexuality and % of male adolescents who say they were educated on the same subject

	% Parents reporting talking to male teen	% Male teens reporting being talked to by parent
Breast development	0	5
Testicular size/growth	28	26
Body odor	69	38
Pubic hair	48	28
Auxiliary hair	46	15
Acne	74	15
Increase in penis size	24	9
Spontaneous erection	28	27
Growth spurt	65	31
Gender difference in growth	63	28
Pregnancy protection	22	20
Sex in general	59	48
Wet dreams	33	22
STIs	22	32
Same sex attraction	15	16
HIV/AIDS	70	58

Table 3. The % of parents reporting talking to their female adolescents about puberty and sexuality and % of female adolescents who say they were educated on the same subject

	% Parents reporting talking to female teen	% Female teens reporting beingtalked to by parent
Breast Development	91	85
Menstrual Periods	93	96
Body odor	83	43
Pubic hair	81	62
Axillary hair	78	29
Acne	86	65
Growth spurt	83	46
Wet dreams	14	14
Gender difference in growth	81	35
Pregnancy protection	59	58
Sex in general	67	50
Rape/Sexual abuse	29	26
Vaginal discharge	45	45
STIs	14	42
Same sex attraction	9	20
HIV/AIDS	70	75

Discussion

This study addresses an area of adolescent development that has the potential of improving or worsening the future of our adolescents. Pubertal development and sexuality are major parts of adolescent development and main determinants of adulthood success. For example an early teen pregnancy or a major sexually transmitted disease can have a profound negative effect on early adulthood or the entire life span of a person. Many of the negative outcomes can be improved by providing timely and comprehensive education regarding puberty and sexuality.

There are however several limitations of this study. The subjective nature of the survey, the potential for misunderstanding of the questionnaire and the anonymity of the respondents impairs our ability to match parents and adolescents. Also the study was conducted in one state rather than on a national scale, which limits the potential for generalizing the results. That being said, the results are nevertheless useful in shedding some light on the extent of pubertal development/sexuality education our adolescents receive.

The results of this study showed significant deficiencies in the education our adolescents receive prior to and during puberty on several important issues. There is almost complete absence of education in regard to male gynecomastia despite the fact that more than 50% of males have it (14). This is important because many of these adolescents are confused and sometimes depressed by gynecomastia. We had several male adolescents that had to be treated for depression and two attempted suicide because of fear that they were "turning into girls" when they noticed they were developing breasts (unpublished observations).

Very little education seems to be provided in such areas as sexual abuse and date rape, gender differences in growth, pregnancy protection, same sex attraction and STI's (except for HIV, see table 3). At a time when teen pregnancy, STI's and acquaintance rape are very common it is no wonder that many of our adolescents are not aware of these problems because of lack of or inadequate knowledge. Overall boys generally receive less attention than girls on all aspects of sexuality (table 2, 3). Although physicians may be part of the "more than one" source of education, it is still surprising that only 2% of teens said that doctors were their source of information. Pediatricians should be in the forefront of providing accurate and timely education to their patients during routine visits.

Conclusions

Based on this study, we conclude that a relatively small proportion of our adolescents are armed with adequate information about most areas of pubertal development and sexual issues. Furthermore, the age at which most adolescents receive such information, if addressed at all, is past the age of onset of puberty for many teens. More thorough and timely education on pubertal development is needed to allow our teens to make well-informed choices in regards to their sexual life and to help prevent many problems related to poor choices resulting from inadequate and late sexuality educations.

REFERENCES

[1] American Academy of Pediatrics. Committee on school health. School health assessments. Pediatrics 2000;105(4):875-7.

[2] Kirby D. Sexuality and sex education at home and school. Adolesc Med 1999;10(2):195-209.

[3] DiCenso A. Interventions to reduce unintended pregnancies among adolescents: A systematic review of randomized controlled trials. BMJ 2002;324:1426.

[4] Ogden J. The timing, format and content of school based sex education: An experience with a lasting effect? Br J Fam Plann 1999;35(3)115-8.

[5] Jemmott JB, Sweet Jemmott L, Fong GT. Abstinence and safer sex HIV risk-reduction interventions for African American adolescents: A randomized controlled trial. JAMA 1998;279(19):1529-36.

[6] DiCenso A. Completing the picture: adolescents talk about what's missing in sexual health services. Can J Public Health. 2001; 92(1):35-8.

[7] Blake SM. Effects of a parent-child communications intervention on young adolescents' risk for early onset of sexual intercourse. Fam Plan Perspect 2001;33(2):52-61.

[8] Centers for Disease Control. Youth risk behavior surveillance—United States, 2001. MMWR 2002;5:SS-4).

[9] Jordan TR, Price JH, Fitzgerald S. Rural parents' communication with their teen-agers about sexual issues. J Sch Health 2000;70(8): 338-44.

[10] Measor L, Tiffin C, Miller K. Health professionals and the sex education of adolescents. Nurs Times 1999;95(21): 48-51.

[11] Romero-de-Castilla-Gil RJ, Lora-Lerenzo MN, Canete-Estrada R. Adolescents and sources of sex information: preferences and perceived usefulness. Aten Primaria. 2001;27(1):12-7.

[12] Strasburger V. Getting teenagers to say no to sex, drugs, and violence in the new millennium. Med Clin North Am 2000;84(4):787-810.

[13] Piaget J. Intellectual evolution from adolescence to adulthood. Hum Dev 1972;15:1.

[14] Biro FM, Lucky AW, Huster GA, Morrison GA: Hormonal studies and physical maturation in adolescent gynecomastia. J Pediatr 1990;116: 450-5.

In: Rural child health: International aspects
Editors: Erica Bell and Joav Merrick

ISBN: 978-1-60876-357-3

Chapter 15

PARENTING ADOLESCENTS

Sandra L. D'Angelo, PhD and Hatim A. Omar*, MD
Section of Adolescent Medicine, Department of Pediatrics, University of Kentucky Medical Center, Lexington, Kentucky, United States of America

The period of adolescence is often thought to be one of intense stress and turmoil. Yet many parents and teens negotiate this developmental stage without extreme family conflict and without sacrificing close relationships. This review summarizes a portion of the literature on parent-adolescent relationships, focusing on monitoring and control of adolescent behavior and parenting style. Basic principles to emphasize when working with adolescents and parents are also included.

INTRODUCTION

Adolescence was once conceptualized as a period of extreme turmoil. Hall (1) referred to this developmental stage as one of "storm and stress;" and Anna Freud's (2) characterization of adolescence as a time of "sturm and drang" also reinforced the idea that the ages between twelve and twenty are inevitably riddled with extreme emotion and conflict—both internally and with the outside world. More recently, researchers have come to view adolescence as a time of transition, but not necessarily of tumultuous change. Most youth mature to adults, and negotiate the developmental tasks of adolescence, without rebellion and psychological problems. In approximately three-quarters of families, children move through adolescence without major difficulties (3). Relationships with parents remain positive and adolescents eventually adopt values more like those of their parents than different from them (4). Larson describes adolescence as a time of transition and transformation, but not disengagement, during which teens negotiate more symmetric relationships with parents—a time of independence in the context of connectedness (5).

* Correspondence: Hatim Omar, MD, Director, Adolescent Medicine, Dept. of Pediatrics, Room J422, KY Clinic, University of Kentucky Medical Center, Lexington, KY 40536-0284 United States. Tel: 859 323-5643, Fax: 859 257-7706, E-mail: haomar2@uky.edu

Just when parents feel most frustrated and powerless, their continued presence provides a stable and nurturant force in this period of rapid change. Despite cultural differences in families and social mores, research consistently demonstrates the importance of parents to adolescent development and adjustment. Studies in East and West Germany (6) and in Australia (7) found that adolescents who perceived their parents as supportive had lower levels of delinquency and depression. Studies of youth living in mainland China (8) and in Taiwan (9) demonstrated the importance of parental warmth and involvement in such varied psychological outcomes as decreased anger and defiance, and fewer psychosomatic symptoms. Conflict between parents and adolescents living in Hong Kong (10) was related to the adolescents' self-esteem, life satisfaction, and hopelessness. Adolescents in Croatia (11) had lower rates of substance use, when parental monitoring and involvement were higher. In fact, these characteristics of parental behavior (i.e., supportive, warm, and involved) have been found to be more important than the configuration of the family (e.g., single vs. dual parent) in a study of Canadian youth (12). In a study of urban adolescents in Columbia, a strong positive bond with parents mitigated against substance abuse and delinquency even in a culture in which drugs are readily available (13).

The developmental tasks of adolescence of becoming autonomous and establishing identity, inevitably lead to some degree of conflict and tension within families. Adolescents want to make independent decisions and be in charge of their lives, but often are not yet ready to assume equal responsibilities. Finding their way to a distinct identity often involves experimenting with new behaviors, questioning parents' beliefs and values, and coming to their own conclusions about social and religious issues. This does not mean that teens will reject parental values, but simply that they must come to their own decisions about what they believe and integrate these values as their own.

Early adolescence seems to be an especially critical time in the parent-teen relationship. Conflict between teens and parents is most intense and frequent during this period, and marital satisfaction is at its lowest ebb during this time (14); parents have an average of seven minutes alone together. At the same time, family time with adolescents is decreasing; time spent with parents after 13 years is one-half that spent before ten (14). In early adolescence, teens spend more time alone in their rooms; as they grow older, time in family activities continually decreases while time with peers increases (5). The physical changes associated with entry into puberty trigger changes in the parents (15). Parents often expect more mature behavior and become more upset when their children do not meet these expectations. During this time, teens' increasing sexuality may create distance even in relationships that were previously close. These are feelings teens keep to themselves or share with friends. This increasing distance may be difficult for parents to accept—both because they miss the more intimate and dependant relationship they once had, and also because they worry about experimentation with risky behaviors. Finally, the physical changes of adolescence can trigger unexpected emotions in the parent. Steinberg hypothesized that what has been labeled as "mid-life crisis" in adults may actually be prompted by the oldest child's emergence into puberty leading parents to reflect and question their progress toward life goals or to re-evaluate the goals themselves. The adolescent's physical maturity and emerging sexuality can evoke feelings of loss of youth or worry about aging as well. In this article, we examine factors associated with changes in the parent-child relationship during adolescence (15).

Monitoring adolescent behavior

Is close parental monitoring beneficial to adolescents? The answer is not as clear-cut as we might expect. Monitoring refers to parents' actions to acquire information about teens' whereabouts, activities, and companions. It includes both active supervision of activities and movement, as well as information solicited by asking questions of teens, their friends, and parents of friends.

In several studies, monitoring has been linked to positive outcomes, especially better academic achievement, and in fewer externalizing problems such as delinquency and substance abuse, and for females, less depressed mood (11,16). When the importance of communication and monitoring were contrasted in a study of Hispanic and African-American youth (14 – 16 years), monitoring was the more important variable in limiting deviant behaviors such as drug use, school suspension, and arrests (17). The beneficial effects of monitoring have been attributed to protecting the adolescent from the negative influence of unsavory peers and deterring rule breaking.

Yet, there can be adverse effects to close monitoring and supervision of teens. When teens perceive parents as controlling and intrusive, the outcome is poorer adjustment, not better. Although parents assume that higher levels of supervision will discourage risk taking behavior and limit exposure to deviant friends, once adolescents feel that they are being controlled, parents' efforts to exert control are linked to poorer adjustment. In examining the role of parental supervision, Kerr and Stattin (18) have concluded that it is an adolescent's free disclosure of information, rather than parents' active tracking, that predicts both markers of adjustment and delinquency. Voluntary self-disclosure was the strongest predictor of low norm breaking as well as positive social-emotional outcomes such as better relationships with teachers and higher self-esteem and fewer depressive symptoms and school problems.

The practical implication of these studies is that parents' efforts to guide teens by close supervision of activities, whereabouts and friendships often produce the opposite effect, largely because they drive questionable behavior underground and produce in the teen feelings of being controlled. This feeling is antithetical to the teen's strivings for autonomy and independence. Parents need to realize that although adolescents do not need the direct supervision needed by a younger child, they still benefit emotionally and intellectually from positive contact with parents (14).

Psychological control versus monitoring

When parents attempt to exert too much control of their adolescents' behavior and activities, the result is most frequently damaging to the relationship between them. This is particularly true when parents try to regulate areas teens consider personal, such as dress and friendships. Negative psychological control refers to manipulating the parent-child bond by withdrawing love, inducing guilt, negative comments of criticism, ridiculing, or shaming, and over protectiveness. Adolescents are striving to develop their own ideas and to have greater ownership of decisions affecting their lives. When control is exercised in a negative psychological way, the development of healthy autonomy is impeded; teens do not develop adequate means to regulate their own behavior and emotions, but rather focus on responding to parents' actions. To counter parental control, teens may purposely defy or passive-aggressively sabotage parents' efforts, and they are slow to develop a healthy sense of self-confidence. Conger and Conger (19) concluded that parents who are either unwilling or incapable of changing their behavior to accommodate the changing needs of a developing adolescent may paradoxically contribute to the child's adjustment problems.

THE RECIPROCAL NATURE OF PARENT ADOLESCENT INTERACTIONS

Parents and teens exercise a reciprocal influence one another in their interaction styles (10,19,20). Over time, many teens and parents become increasingly negative toward each other (20). Once a pattern of negative interaction is established, the cycle is difficult to break. When both adolescent and parent use coercive negative behaviors in problem solving, the interactions are likely to deteriorate and grow more negative (20). This is not only damaging to the relationship, but to the parents' goal of helping teens become effective, flexible problem solvers (19). Reciprocal influences are most prominent under conditions of adolescent negativity. Reuter (20) found that having a disruptive, inflexible young adolescent (seventh grader) in the home, parents grow less nurturant over time. Nevertheless, parent influence seems to be the more important factor (10,19,20). So much so, that when parents use coercive, harsh and inconsistent strategies, providing a teen with professional help to learn to communicate better will be ineffective, unless the parents also commit to change. The Congers maintain that "parents of a disruptive, uncooperative adolescent who maintained a nurturant approach to child-rearing could eventually break or avoid being drawn into a pattern of reciprocal negativity" (19).

THE INFLUENCE OF THE PEER GROUP

During the 1960's and 70's both popular press and scientific journals placed more weight on peer influence than that of the family in determining adolescent ideas, values, and behavior. This view evolved out of observation of similarities between teens and their friends, concluding that peers networks pressured individuals to conform. The concept of peer pressure implies that friends are pitted against parents for the loyalty and mind of the teen. Although peers do influence adolescents, the effect is stronger for daily behaviors and transient attitudes than for personality or values. Parental influence is deeper and more enduring for long-term outcomes such as occupational and educational attainment and religiosity (21). With increasing age, from adolescence to young adulthood, similarity with parents grows stronger.

The similarity between adolescents and their friends is more likely due to active selection by teens to be with others who are like them (21,22). Teens have many social groups from which to choose in both school and community settings. Parents are often tempted to forbid teens to associate with peers who they believe will lead their children astray. But exercising this level of control is most often an ineffective strategy because it is difficult to monitor, encourages deception, and worsens feelings of antipathy in the adolescent.

However, parents do play an indirect role in the choice of friends through events earlier in the child's life in which they steer children toward certain activities and groups. According to Collins and colleagues (21), parenting style in early childhood also plays a role: "The chain of events that leads some adolescents into antisocial peer groups begins at home during childhood. The links in this chain include exposure to harsh and coercive parenting, which contributes to the development of aggression and to academic difficulties in school; these problems, in late childhood, lead to the selection of antisocial peers....much of what appears to be peer influence is actually the end result of familial influence at an earlier point in the child's development." (p. 222) Thus, parents and peers exercise complementary influence on teens.

PARENTING STYLES

Just as for younger children, supportive parenting helps adolescents realize the best in themselves and construct positive relationships with others. Given teens' increased interest in their peers and drive to become independent of their parents, what constitutes supportive and effective parenting at this age? Much of the research has concentrated on specific behaviors that parents use to decrease undesirable or increase desirable behaviors in their children. However, a number of researchers posit that it is not the individual behaviors or strategies employed by the parents that matter, but rather an overall style that creates an emotional context for specific parenting behaviors (15,23). For example, the behavior of setting a curfew can be either a punitively controlling maneuver or a limit that takes into consideration the child's developmental needs. The model of Baumrind (24) was based on the idea that the job of a parent is to socialize the child to conform to the demands of others while helping the child maintain a sense of personal integrity. Within this, she identified three types of parental control that were qualitatively different: permissive, authoritarian, and authoritative. Maccoby and Martin (25) extended Baumrind's typology by characterizing parenting style along two dimensions: demandingness—the ways in which parents expect compliance and social children, and responsiveness—the parent's recognition of the child's individuality and sensitivity to the child's unique needs. This schema yields four-part typology for characterizing parenting style:

- Parents who employ an authoritative parenting style are high on both dimensions. They combine expression of love and affection with expectations for appropriate behavior and consistent enforcement of standards. These parents communicate respect for adolescent autonomy by taking into consideration the child's opinions and promoting individuality and independence.
- Parents with an authoritarian style--high on the dimension of demandingness and low on sensitivity—expect adherence to parental standards, exert control and restrict autonomy, but lacks emotional warmth. The authoritarian style has been linked to adolescents' feeling of being controlled and devalued.
- Permissive parents are responsive, and their relationships with their children are warm and accepting. However parental control, limits, and expectations are lacking.

- Neglectful parenting, which lacks both warmth and behavioral expectations, yields the most worrisome outcome of adolescents at highest risk for behavioral problems including delinquency, drug and alcohol use, and early initiation of sexual activity.

In many studies, characteristics of the authoritative parenting style has been linked to positive psychosocial outcomes such as greater autonomy, self esteem, academic achievement, and less delinquency, psychiatric morbidity, and substance abuse (5,25-28). Steinberg (15) maintains that parenting style exerts its influence by providing a context for specific parenting behaviors and interactions. Thus, it is not just what parents do, but how they do it that matters. An authoritative parenting style is beneficial, because parental nurturance and involvement make adolescents more susceptible to parental influence. The supportive relationship combined with structure facilitates development of self-regulatory skills, and the verbal give and take in parent-adolescent communication foster cognitive and social competence. In families in which an authoritative style exists, the parent-adolescent interaction is transformed, and high conflict is avoided. Authoritarian parenting, in contrast, often increases resistance to parental input, such that parent behaviors that would be considered productive on face value, like school involvement, actually result in greater conflict. Can parenting style be transformed? The following discussion on parent-adolescent conflict proposes changes in the way in which parents approach interactions with teens.

CONFLICT BETWEEN PARENTS AND ADOLESCENTS

Less than ten percent of families endure serious relationship difficulties characterized by chronic escalation of arguments over serious issues (30). Parents typically are more bothered by the negative affect generated in daily conflicts than are teens, and are likely to remain troubled far longer and take longer to recover (15). Nevertheless, in most families, conflict does not undermine the quality of attachment between parents and adolescents. In fact, a limited amount of conflict may benefit families by stimulating change that brings adolescent and parent viewpoints closer together, and by creating some emotional distance that allows adolescents to differentiate themselves from parents. Whether conflict has an adaptive function depends on how disagreements are perceived, discussed, and resolved. If parents make no adjustments and are critical, harsh, or demeaning during conflict, then difficulties are likely to become more exaggerated and adolescent adjustment is poorer. When parents use direct, arbitrary force and withdrawal of love or affection in response to undesirable behaviors, conormity to parental expectations is lower and risk for problem behaviors increases (31).

Many studies that relate parent-adolescent conflict to poor adolescent adjustment have been cross-sectional and thus unable to determine whether high conflict precedes maladjustment or is a response to a poorly adjusted adolescent in the home. In a study of adolescents in Hong Kong, Shek (10,32) found that high levels of conflict, especially with fathers, predicted greater dissatisfaction with self and life and more psychiatric symptoms one year later.

When in the midst of a disagreement with teens, Sells (33) suggests the following strategy. First, listen closely to the adolescents' perspectives. Acknowledge feelings by labeling them or with a noncommittal phrase. This does not imply that you agree with the teen or condone the disputed behavior. Resist the temptation to solve the problem for the teen. Avoid lecturing and criticizing. Anticipate that teens will try to provoke parents to lose control of the situation by "pushing their buttons;" although it is tempting to react with equal emotional intensity, when teens become inflamed, it is important for parents to remain collected and rational. If the confrontation escalates, e.g., a teen uses foul language or threatens violence, "exit" and "wait" until tempers cool. Finally, it is important to restore good feelings once the conflict is over.

Greene (34), writing about inflexible and explosive children, agrees that parents and teens may need "time out" from each other during heated disagreements. However, this is not the time-out used with younger children, such as restricting a child to a room or chair, as this is typically not useful for teens. Rather, parents' withdrawal from conflict signals that they are remaining in control of their emotions, and does not mean that they are "giving in."

Greene also recommends that parents prioritize their goals when confrontations are frequent and intense. He instructs parents to create a list of behavioral priorities, than categorizes these into three "baskets." Basket A contains a limited number of behaviors, such as those that are harmful to people or property; those that are illegal; school attendance. Basket C contains behaviors that parents would like to see but do not deserve a conflict, such as what teens wear or eat. Most behaviors belong in Basket B—they are high priorities, but ones in which parents and teens can negotiate a compromise, such as curfews and activities. Through the discussion and the negotiation process, parents are helping teens learn to handle frustrating situations, generate alternative solutions to a problem, and think through the consequences of their actions.

CONCLUSIONS

Across cultures, theoretical models, and research questions—a repeating thread accentuating the importance of the adolescent-parent relationship surfaces. Whether the issue is one of the qualities of the relationship that promote willing self-disclosure, thus facilitating parental awareness of adolescent activity or the ability of parents to be sensitive to changing needs for independence in the context of dependence, studies point to the inherent importance of the parent-child relationship as a foundation upon which healthy development is built. Although adolescents' relationships with their parents emerge from those set in earlier years, parents can effect changes in their relationships with their adolescents even as they strive toward greater individuation (3). The balance between family ties and autonomy must constantly be "recalibrated" to take into account the advances in adolescent development, changes within the family, and expectations within the society (28).

GUIDELINES FOR PARENTING AN ADOLESCENT (30,33,34)

1. Respect privacy. Do not go through rooms, backpacks, or emails. Invading privacy breaks a trusting relationship and models undesirable behavior (sneakiness). Parents

of teens who are engaging in seriously inappropriate behaviors are obvious about this, and parents will know without snooping in their rooms.

2. Allow give and take in discussions.
3. Avoid lecturing and criticism; never use sarcasm or belittling.
4. Give limited amounts of advice. Too much advice undermines teens' ability to problem solve for themselves and implies parents do not believe they are capable of finding solutions. If asked for advice, first listen, then ask the teen's ideas about possible solutions.
5. Try not to react to moodiness and ill-temper with negativity. This only sets up an escalating negative interaction. Be matter of fact when setting limits.
6. Set clear standards for behavior.
7. When behavior is inappropriate, use a step approach: First let the teen know specifically what the behavior was and that there will be a consequence on the next occasion; reach an agreement with the teen about appropriate consequence; impose consequences consistently, but without argument.

    a) A good consequence is related to the inappropriate behavior; has a limited duration that lets the teen know there is another chance; can be monitored and enforced consistently, and is one the teen has been warned will occur.
    b) Do not expect teens to understand or agree with your point of view or to admit that you are correct.
    c) When teens lie about breaking limits, focus on the behavior itself, rather than the lying.

8. Remain involved in daily life without being intrusive or overprotective.
9. Be prepared for changes in levels of involvement—teens wanting to be close or receive help, followed by wanting to be alone or only with peers and wanting to solve problems for self.
10. Continue to provide warmth and acceptance during this period of disruption and shifting relationships.

REFERENCES

[1] Hall GS: Adolescence. New York, NY: Appleton, 1904.

[2] Freud A. The psychoanalytic study of the child. Adolescence 1958; 13:255-78.

[3] Henricson C, Roker D. Support for the parents of adolescents: A review. J Adolesc 2000; 23:763-83.

[4] Paikoff RL, Brooks-Gunn J, Carlton-Ford S. Do parent-child relationships change during puberty? Psychol Bull 1991;110:47-66.

[5] Larson RW, Richards MH, Moneta G, Holmbeck G, Duckett E. Changes in adolescents' daily interactions with their families from ages 10 to 18: Disengagement and transformation. Dev Psychol 1996;32:744-54.

[6] Juang LP, Silbereisen RK. Supportive parenting and adolescent adjustment across time in former East and West Germany. J Adolesc 1999;22:719-36.

[7] Patton GC, Coffey C, Posterino M, Carlin JB, Wolfe R. Parental 'affectionless control' in adolescent depressive disorder. Soc Psychiatry Psychiatr Epidemiol 2001;36:475-80.

[8] Xia G, Qian M. The relationship of parenting style to self-reported mental health among two subcultures of Chinese. J Adolesc 2001; 24:251-60.
[9] Simons RL, Wu CI, Lin KH, Gordon L, Conger RD. A cross-cultural examination of the link between corporal punishment and adolescent antisocial behavior. Criminology 2000:38:47-60.
[10] Shek DT. A longitudinal study of the relations between parent-adolescent conflict and adolescent psychological well-being. J Genet Psychol 1998; 159:53-67.
[11] Raboteg-Saric Z, Rijavec M, Brajsa-Zganec A. The relation of parental practices and self-conceptions to young adolescent problem behaviors and substance use. Nord J Psychiatry 2001;55:203-09.
[12] McFarlane AH, Bellissimo A, Norman GR. Family structure, family functioning and adolescent well-being: The transcendent influence of parental style. J Child Psychol Psychiatry 1995;36:847-64.
[13] Brook JS, Brook DW, De La Rosa M, Whiteman M, Montoya ID. The role of parents in protecting Colombian adolescents from delinquency and marijuana use. Arch Pediatr Adolesc Med 1999; 153:457-64.
[14] Rutter V. Adolescence: Whose hell is it? Psych Today 1995: 28:54-65
[15] Steinberg, L. We know some things: parent and adolescent relationships in restrospect and prospect. J Res Adolesc 2001;11:1-20.
[16] Jacobson KC. Parental monitoring and adolescent adjustment: An ecological perspective. J Res Adolesc 2000; 10:65-98.
[17] Forehand R, Miller KS, Dutra R, Change MW. Role of parenting in adolescent deviant behavior: Replication across and within two ethnic groups. J Cons Clin Psych 1997;65: 1036-41.
[18] Kerr M, Stattin H. What parents know, how they know it, and several forms of adolescent adjustment: Further support for a reinterpretation of monitoring. Dev Psychol 2000;36: 366-80.
[19] Conger KJ, Conger RD. Parents, siblings, psychological control, and adolescent adjustment. J Adolesc Res 1997;12:113-39.
[20] Reuter MA, Conger RD. Reciprocal influences between parenting and adolescent problem-solving behavior. Dev Psychol 1998; 34:1470-82.
[21] Collins WA, Maccoby EE, Steinberg L, Hetherington EM, Bornstein MH. Contemporary research on parenting: The case for nature and nurture. Am Psychol 2000;55:218-32.
[22] Ungar MT. The myth of peer pressure. Adolesc 2000; 35:167-80.
[23] Darling N, Steinberg L. Parenting style as context: An integrative model. Psychol Bull 1993;113:487-96.
[24] Baumrind D. Parenting styles and adolescent development. In: Lerner RM, Petersen AC, Brooks-Gunn J, eds. The encyclopedia on adolescence. New York, NY: Garland, 1991:746-58.
[25] Maccoby EE, Martin JA. Socialization in the context of the family: Parent-child interaction. In: Mussen PH, ed. Handbook of child psychology, Vol.4. New York, NY: Wiley, 1983:119-38.
[26] Aunola K, Stattin H, Nurmi JE. Parenting styles and adolescents' achievement strategies. J Adolesc 2000;23:205-22.
[27] Noack P, Kerr M, Olah A. Family relations in adolescence. J Adolesc 1999;22:713-17.
[28] Noack P, Puschner B. Differential trajectories of parent-child relationship and psychosocial adjustment in adolescents. J Adolesc 1999;22:795-804.
[29] Steinberg L, Silverberg SB. The vicissitudes of autonomy in early adolescence. Child Dev 1986;57: 841-51.
[30] Holmbeck GN, Paikoff RL, Brooks-Gunn J. Parenting adolescents. In: Bornstein MH, ed. Handbook of parenting, Vol 1. Mahwah, NJ: Erlbaum, 1995:91-118.
[31] Anderson AR, Henry CS. Family system characteristics and parental behaviors as predictors of adolescent substance use. Adolesc 1994; 114: 405-21.
[32] Shek DT. Parenting characteristics and adolescent psychological well-being: A longitudinal study in a Chinese context. Genet Soc Gen Psychol Monogr 1999;125:27-44.
[33] Sells SP. Treating the tough adolescent: A family-based, step-by-step guide. New York, NY: Guilford, 1998.
[34] Greene R. The explosive child. New York, NY: Harper Collins, 1998.

In: Rural child health: International aspects
Editors: Erica Bell and Joav Merrick

ISBN: 978-1-60876-357-3

Chapter 16

YOUTH SUICIDE PREVENTION IN RURAL KENTUCKY

Hatim A Omar*, MD

Section of Adolescent Medicine, University of Kentucky, Lexington, Kentucky, United States of America

Youth suicide continues to be one of the leading causes of death in the United States. Nation wide it is the third leading cause of death in the 10-24 year old age group. The rate of suicide varies somewhat from state to state. In the state of Kentucky, youth suicide is the second leading cause of death. This article describes a grass roots, community-based program for youth suicide prevention and its impact on the community. The Stop Youth Suicide Campaign was launched in 2000 and included more than 30 local agencies. This program worked through public education, education of medical care providers, schoolteachers, school counselors, youth service center personnel and many other entities that deal with adolescents. This program utilized face-to-face encounters, website, video and other forms of media education. Over a four-year period, the program has provided several conferences and many lectures and workshops to the community. The program has responded to many e-mails and phone calls from teens and/or their parents asking for help. During these years, many of these children that were seeking help ended up receiving appropriate help that contributed to changing their lives and helping them stay alive and also utilizing them to help others in that period. Simple grass roots programs are able to help and are needed in the community to combat this epidemic that is causing significant mortality and morbidity.

INTRODUCTION

Youth suicide has been a major contributing factor to mortality and morbidity over the last thirty to forty years. It has consistently been one of the leading causes of death among teenagers 10-24 years of age and has been the third leading cause of death over all in the United States among this age group. According to the Center for Disease Control, 2003 Risk

* Correspondence: Hatim Omar, MD, Professor of Pediatrics and Obstetrics\Gynecology, Director, Adolescent Medicine, University of Kentucky, 740 South Limestone Street, Kentucky Clinic, J422, Lexington, KY 40536, USA. Tel: 859-323-5643; Fax: 859-257-7706; Email. Haomar2@uky.edu

Youth Behavior Survey, an average of 8.5 percent of youth have actually attempted suicide (1). A 21 year old longitudinal study by Ferguson reports (2) suicide ideation in 28.8% of youth and suicide attempts in 7.5% by age 21 years. Autopsies of youth successfully completing suicide have identified numerous factors more significantly associated with suicide completers than with controls. These factors include non-intact family of origin, less frequent and satisfying communication with parents, history of mood disorder in mother, history of legal problems in father, family history of suicidal behavior, recent discipline (especially school suspension and juvenile court appearance), recent break up with boyfriend or girlfriend, recent separation of parents, lack of employment or school attendance, or grade failure (3) and the presence of DSM-III diagnosis (4) especially mood disorder, anxiety disorder and disruptive disorders. According to prior studies, predictors of suicide attempts include parental depression, poor family functioning (5), large number of parental changes, poor attachment to parents, exposed to sexual abuse (6), depression, hopelessness (7), anxiety disorder and substance abuse (8). Primary reasons reported for suicide attempts when given a list to choose from include: to die, relief from state of mind, escape from a situation and to make others understand how desperate one feels (9). We have previously found that one of the most quoted reasons for attempted suicide in Central Kentucky as reported by teenagers who were admitted to emergency rooms for attempted suicide was conflict with parent followed by conflict with significant other (10).

Our program

The program was named "Stop Youth Suicide Campaign" and started officially in 2000. Campaign was started by a coalition including thirty agencies in the Central Kentucky area such as the Adolescent Medicine program at the University of Kentucky (leader of the coalition), the Coroner's Office, the heath department, several local media outlets, participants from the school system, parent groups and many others. The goal of the program was: 1) To improve community awareness of the problem of youth suicide, 2) To assess the need in the community and basic knowledge on youth suicide, 3) To start a public education campaign targeting parents, teachers and everyone who has anything to do with teens, 4) To provide for improved education of medical care providers that deal with adolescents and to improve their knowledge and comfort level in screening and assessing for depression and suicide and 5) To provide around the clock, available help to any teenagers in the area who were suicidal or need help in that regard.

To accomplish these goals, the campaign started with a media press conference and an announcement by the mayor's office in Lexington, KY to inform the people of the area about the program. This was followed by several days of media information on the government television channel in the area. The campaign then started a website (www.stopyouthsuicide.com) that is available to anyone to access information on youth suicide and to be able to contact the campaign in case help is needed. The campaign then produced a local video showing teenagers, who had attempted suicide and survived, parents of youth who committed suicide and friends or peers of youth who have completed suicide as well as experts discussing ways and means on how to understand youth suicide and work on youth suicide prevention. The next step was to offer education to providers, which was done through providing numerous lectures and workshops. From October 2000 to December 2004, a total of 60 lectures and workshops and three full day conferences devoted to youth suicide prevention training to medical care providers of all levels. The campaign has also participated in working with the state government and local agencies to build and establish a State-wide youth suicide prevention program. In addition, the Stop Youth Suicide Campaign had participated in church and school activities in multiple visits to all area middle and high schools as well as religious activities to educate parents on the problem of youth suicide.

Over the years the Stop Youth Suicide Campaign has received thousands of e-mails and phone calls from teenagers who were contemplating suicide and asking for help and e-mails and phone calls from parents of teens at risk. These patients were appropriately treated in the area and referred to appropriate people if they were out of the area. A total of thirteen teenagers who were acutely suicidal with plan and readiness to complete it at the time of contacting the program were helped to change their minds and to continue to be alive as of this date. Several of the teens helped by the program have joined the campaign to help other teens. Public awareness in the area regarding youth suicide has improved based on surveys done before the launching of the program and years after (Omar H. Unpublished observations). Also, the Stop Youth Suicide Campaign played a significant role in working with the state on establishing a state suicide program that is now ongoing.

Discussion

The leading causes of death in the adolescent age group in the United States are accidents, homicide and suicide, all preventable (1). Suicide is the 2nd leading cause of death among adolescents in Kentucky and at the time of launching the Stop Youth Suicide Campaign, no other program existed in the state. Government agencies chronically lack funding for such preventive programs. Adolescent medicine specialists are the best trained professionals in understanding adolescent development as well as risk and protective factors for morbidity and mortality in this group. It should be our role (adolescent medicine specialists) to educate other health care providers and the public and to take a leading role in serving the community and advocating for the well being of adolescents. Utilizing community resources can help alleviate lack of government funding for such preventive program. The Stop Youth Suicide Campaign was able to utilize volunteers and various community resources to develop a long lasting, helpful program for prevention of youth suicide that have contributed to helping many teens at risk of suicide and improving there lives. This article is a simple descriptive presentation, so it does not provide scientific study results. It does however show that committed medical providers can help utilize community resources and with hard work, caring and dedication, can develop useful programs to provide help to distressed teens and their parents.

References

[1] Centers for Disease Control and Prevention. Surveillance Summaries, May 21, 2004. MMWR 2004;53:25-7.

[2] Fergusson DM, Woodward LJ, Horwood LJ. Risk factors and life processes associated with the onset of suicidal behavior during adolescence and early adulthood. Psychol Med 2000;30:23-39.

[3] Gould MS, Fisher P, Parides M, Flory M, Shaffer D. Psychological risk factors of child and adolescent completed suicide. Arch General Psychiatr 1996;53:1155-62.

[4] Shaffer D, Gould MS, Fisher P, Trautman P, Moreau D, Kleinman M, Flory M. Psychiatric diagnosis in child and adolescent suicide. Arch General Psychiatr 1996;53:339-48.

[5] Garber J, Little S, Hilsman Ruth, Weaver KR. Family predictors of suicidal symptoms in young adolescents. J Adolesc 1998;21:445-57.

[6] Overholser JC, Freiheit SR, DiFilippo JM (1987), Emotional distress and substance abuse as risk factors for suicide. Can J Psychiatr 1997;42:402-8.

[7] Gould MS, King R, Greenwald S, Fisher P, Schwab-Stone M, Kramer R, Flisher AJ, Goodman S, Canino G, Shaffer D. Psychopathology associated with suicidal ideation and attempts among children and adolescents. J Am Acad Child Adolesc Psychiatr 1998;37:915-23.

[8] Boergers J, Spirito A, Donaldson D. Reasons for adolescent suicide attempts: associations with psychological functioning. J Am Acad Child Adolesc Psychiatr 1998;37:1287-93.

[9] Negron R, Placentini J, Graae F, Davies M, Shaffer D. Microanalysis of adolescent suicide attempters and ideators during the acute suicidal episode. J Am Acad Child Adolesc Psychiatr 1997;36:1512-9.

[10] Omar H, Hagedorn J. Retrospective analysis of youth evaluated for suicide attempt or suicidal ideation in an emergency room setting. Int J Adolesc Med Health 2001;14(1):55-60.

In: Rural child health: International aspects
Editors: Erica Bell and Joav Merrick
ISBN: 978-1-60876-357-3

Chapter 17

CHRONIC ILLNESS AND MENTAL HEALTH ISSUES

Marlene B Huff*, PhD, LCSW, Kimberly K McClanahan, PhD and Hatim A Omar, MD
Department of Pediatrics, Division of Adolescent Medicine,
University of Kentucky, Lexington, Kentucky, United States of America

By 2015, worldwide, 1.2 billion children aged 5-14 years will have some kind of significant chronic disease. Although scientific evidence indicates that children with chronic illness have more mental health issues than their healthy peers, many controversies and gaps in the literature exist. It is imperative that an understanding of the effects of chronic illness upon the mental health status of children and adolescent be undertaken. This article uses a biopsychosocial perspective to investigate the connection between chronic illness and mental health. The intent of the article is to suggest ways that medical and mental health professionals can provide services to chronically ill children and adolescents that foster positive mental health through the achievement of all developmental tasks with as little psychological stress as possible.

INTRODUCTION

The major tasks of childhood involve achieving healthy development and functioning in the physical, cognitive, emotional, and psychosocial domains. Past research indicates that childhood chronic illness can severely impair psychosocial functioning and impede further development in all domains of functioning (1,2). Considering the biological, psychological, and social (herein referred to as 'biopsychosocial') concerns and effects in the management of chronic illness and simultaneously fostering positive mental health includes continuous assessment and management of the biopsychosocial factors which all influence one another and are integral to the healthy emotional functioning of children and adolescents.

This article uses a biopsychosocial perspective to investigate the connection between chronic illness and mental health. The intent of the article is to suggest ways that medical and

* Correspondence: Marlene B. Huff, PhD, LCSW, Department of Pediatrics, Division of Adolescent Medicine, University of Kentucky, Lexington, KY, United States. E-mail: marlene.huff@uky.edu

mental health professionals can provide services to chronically ill children and adolescents that foster positive mental health through the achievement of all developmental tasks with as little psychological stress as possible. The medical management goal is to minimize the impact of the disease on the physical and emotional development and functioning of children and adolescents while the mental health goal is to achieve balance between disease management and positive mental health. These goals can only be met through the facilitation of interactions that occur in each of the four domains of the adaptive functioning.

A focus on the developmental and biopsychosocial domains that all chronic childhood illnesses share will assist in drawing conclusions about mental health that apply regardless of the specific illness. It should be noted, however, that tremendous complexity exists among chronic illnesses including the type, severity, and progression of the illness, the resources of the family and community to support the child or adolescent, and the capacity of the health care provider team.

Childhood chronic illness

Causes of chronic illness are discussed extensively in research involving the medical aspects of childhood chronic illness (3-5). The causes typically include genetic or hereditary dispositions, birth traumas and other conditions present at birth, accidents and injuries, disease and illnesses, and conditions associated with the aging process. Detailed discussion of these causes is beyond the scope of this article. Despite varied and complex causes of childhood and adolescent chronic illness, there are striking similarities among the effects that chronic illness has on the mental health status of this population.

Common chronic illnesses

The most common and disruptive chronic illnesses that have their onset in childhood or adolescence in the United States are respiratory allergies (9%), asthma (4%), eczema and skin allergies (3%), heart disease (2%), epilepsy (0.2%), and diabetes (0.1%) (2). These chronic illnesses often co-occur with mental illness. For instance, depression and anxiety are associated with heart disease (6), type 2 diabetes (7,8), renal disease (9), obesity (10,11) and asthma (12-14).

Effects of chronic illness

By 2015, worldwide, 1.2 billion children aged 5-14 years will have some kind of significant chronic disease (15). National population-based studies from western countries show that 20-30% of adolescents have a chronic illness, defined as one that lasts longer than six months, and 10-13% of those adolescents report having a chronic illness that substantially limits their daily life or requires extended periods of care and supervision. The increasing prevalence of chronic illness across the globe further indicates the need for research that fully explores the relationship between mental health and chronic illness.

Children with chronic illnesses have an increased risk of emotional and behavioral problems (16). This risk has been documented in epidemiological studies1 as well as in studies of clinic samples (17). The assessment and treatment of emotional and behavioral problems is recognized as an essential part of treating children and adolescents with chronic illness (17). Even though children and adolescents with chronic illness may be in regular contact with general and specialty healthcare providers, they may not have access to needed mental health support services1, and many children and adolescents do not report mental health issues to medical providers (1). Glazebrook and colleagues (17), for example, suggest that pediatricians only detect approximately 25% of psychosocial problems among their chronically ill patients.

Developmental issues and mental health

Regardless of the specific developmental stage, children and adolescents must adapt to the nature and limitations of the chronic illness with its physical and emotional sequelae as well as comply with recommended medical treatments in order to attain adult functionality. In addition, children and adolescents must fulfill normative tasks of individual growth and development. Incomplete adaptation to the chronic illness, non-adherence with medical advice and/or failure to accomplish normative developmental tasks can result in significant emotional disorders, psychosocial impairment, and developmental delay (1). While adequate adaptive functioning in the psychosocial domain promotes mental health as well as effective management of the chronic illness, inadequate adaptive functioning within this domain can become a precursor to future mental health difficulties and/or play a significant role in assessing and managing current mental health concerns.

Response to living with a chronic illness depends on several factors including but not limited to personality characteristics, the specific illness, and the family. Extremely important to the complex set of sequelae is the particular developmental stage in which the child or adolescent is operating that requires energy. Infants and toddlers, for example, are beginning to develop trust and an overall sense of security. They generally have very little understanding of their illness. Children in this stage of development experience pain, restricting of motion, and separation from parents as challenges to developing trust and security.

Preschool children are beginning to develop a sense of independence. They may understand what it means to get sick but they may not understand the cause and effect nature of illness. Being in the hospital or adjusting to a medication schedule, for example, can challenge the child's developing independence.

Early school-aged children are developing a sense of mastery over their environment. They can describe reasons for illness, but these reasons may not be entirely logical. Children this age often have "magical thinking." They may believe they caused the illness by thinking bad thoughts, by hitting their brother, or by not eating their vegetables. Children also begin to sense that they are different from their peers.

Older school aged children are beginning to focus on peer relationships. They are now more capable of understanding their illness and its treatment but they should not be expected to respond as adults do. They may feel left out when they miss school or activities with their peers as developing and maintaining peer relationships is one of the most important psychosocial developmental tasks that will continue into adolescence.

Adolescents begin to develop their own identity separate from their families. Self-image becomes extremely important during the teenage years. The perception of the peer group is of paramount importance and is an issue when the adolescent's appearance is altered by illness or medication.

MENTAL HEALTH ISSUES

As stated previously, children and adolescents with chronic illness have the same developmental needs as other same age peers. In many ways, the accomplishment of developmental tasks is made more difficult by an extra set of demands and hardships associated with the chronic illness (18). Typical developmental tasks may interact with issues related to chronic illness, producing increased demands and stress upon children and adolescents. If the additional stress is not managed effectively, the risk for mental health problems increases. Although many chronically ill children and adolescents do not experience mental health problems secondary to development-related stress, several epidemiologic studies have found indications of approximately a two-fold increase in mental health problems among this group of children (1,19).

Though chronically ill children and adolescents can develop any type of mental health problem, the following discussion illustrates some of the areas in which the chronically ill may be most vulnerable.

Body image issues

One of the major developmental tasks of childhood and adolescence is the establishment of an individual identity while major changes are also occurring physically. Chronic illness may intensify concerns about personal and sexual identities with fears or distortions related to the illness. Research during the last two decades has demonstrated variability in body size preference and in body image dissatisfaction among children and adolescents based on age, pubertal status, presence or absence of a chronic illness or disability, gender, ethnicity, body mass index (BMI) or weight, and family relationships (20). Specific body image concerns among chronically ill children or adolescents have not been investigated.

Adolescents report greater body image dissatisfaction than younger children (21). In addition, dissatisfaction with one's body image and the desire for thinness, with its perceived approval from others, increases as children approach puberty (22). Girls report greater dissatisfaction than boys (23,24) and a greater desire for thinness (21). Body mass index, at risk for overweight, or being overweight have positive associations with body image dissatisfaction among youth, according to some studies (25,26).

Children and adolescents with chronic illness may struggle with body image, especially if there is a visible difference or limitation in activity. This is especially apparent for adolescents who are concerned with membership in a particular peer group. For those adolescents who may take medication on a long-term basis to manage their illness, adherence with the drug regimen may be erratic. If the medication has undesirable side effects, such as weight gain or an increase in acne, adolescents may be acutely aware of body image issues.

Chronically ill children and adolescents may attempt to manage poor body images through the development of an eating disorder: a group of disorders that have a disturbance in eating behavior that endanger physical and mental health. Eating disorders include the following:

- Anorexia Nervosa—a condition in which a person purposely limits food intake and refuses to maintain a weight within a healthy range for height and age. People with Anorexia Nervosa may also binge and purge.
- Bulimia Nervosa—a condition that involves cycles of bingeing and behaviors that follow to prevent weight gain and can include such behaviors as vomiting, using laxatives, diuretics, or involvement in excessive exercise.
- Binge Eating Disorder—a condition in which a person binge eats but does not attempt to control weight through unhealthy purging behaviors. As many as one third of obese people may have this eating disorder but have gone undiagnosed.
- Eating Disorder NOS (not otherwise specified)—a term used with individuals who have disordered eating behaviors, dissatisfaction with body weight or shape and harmful weight control behaviors that do not meet full criteria for one of the more severe eating disorders above.

Development of independence

Chronic illness frequently interferes with the attainment of independence and autonomy. Parents may be less willing to grant autonomy to children and adolescents who have chronic illness. While children and adolescents try to function autonomously, parents or caregivers may be reluctant for this to happen because they fear that the specific child or adolescent will not manage the chronic illness effectively. Since chronic illness may delay the onset of puberty with its immense increase in growth and development, parents may be even more likely to remain protective as children and adolescents may not appear to be capable of autonomous functioning. In addition, children and adolescents may become physically dependent upon the family for companionship, friendship, and social support if there is not a strong connection to the peer group.

Relationships with peers

Chronic illness and the assessment, treatment, and management of that illness often interferes with time spent in the school setting, which is children's and adolescents' primary social environment. Self-esteem issues related to acceptance of self and concerns about acceptance by others are intensified in chronic illness. In addition, if they have limited access to the school setting or other social environments because they are ill, their ability to establish and maintain peer relationships is impaired.

Given the central role that peer relationships play in the psychological development of children and adolescents, and because peer rejection and isolation have been associated with subsequent adjustment problems, chronically ill children and adolescents are at an increased risk for difficult psychological development. Meijer et al (27) and his colleagues report that the level of psychological adjustment among chronically ill children and adolescents is variable. This variability may be due, in part, to the presence of protective factors, such as the use of adequate coping strategies.

Promoting positive mental health

Promoting positive mental health among children and adolescents with chronic illness means promoting adaptation and/or competence in living with that illness. Promoting competence requires the development and maintenance of sufficient capabilities to meet cumulative and persistent demands. It may also mean reducing demands or removing barriers to successful adaptation, such as minimizing hospital visits while encouraging family involvement, increasing opportunities for peer interaction, and maximizing independence in living.

There are four strategies to consider when promoting positive mental health: 1) encourage typical life experiences, 2) increase coping skills, 3) increase use of social support and 4) empower families.

Encouragement of typical life experiences

Children and adolescents with chronic illness have the same developmental needs as other same age peers. Activities that challenge them to develop social skills, master new approaches to social situations, build self-esteem, and form separate and healthy identities away from caregivers while engaging with others (e.g., peers, family members, other adults) promote successful accomplishment of developmental tasks as well as positive mental health. As children and adolescents with chronic illness become fully integrated into family, school, and community activities, engaging in typical life experiences will become more routine and expected. Until then, however, it is often left up to the medical and mental health treatment teams to encourage parents and other caregivers to allow active participation in diverse life experiences by children with chronic illness.

Increase coping skills

Teaching children and adolescents with chronic illness and their family members how to cope with the demands of the illness is frequently a strategy used to promote mental health. Coping is behavior directed at restoring a balance between excess demands placed on children and adolescents secondary to achieving developmental tasks and managing the chronic illness with, often, inadequate resources.

If children or adolescents and their families manage to balance these needs, then the number and use of coping skills is adequate. There are times, however, when parents, caregivers, friends, or extended kinship networks are unable or unprepared to deal with the intense emotional response of chronically ill children and adolescents. Depending upon the type and severity of the chronic illness, just understanding and managing the illness can take so much time and emotional energy that the psychological aspects of the developing person are neglected (28). The neglect of these psychological aspects may result in depression, anxiety, or other disorders requiring early treatment in order to prevent long-term negative sequelae.

Increase use of social supports

Of all the resources for promoting positive mental health, none has received more attention than social support (29). There have been many conceptualizations of social support, most of which incorporate the support that is given as well as the person who gives it. Three broad categories of support are listed below:

- emotional support that provides information that one is loved and valued, that children or adolescents matter to and are connected with others;
- informational support that helps chronically ill children and adolescents solve problems and find other tangible services and resources and can give feedback about how they are doing in managing the illness; and
- instrumental support or tangible support during times of extreme stress.

Social supports can be from formal or informal sources. Formal supports include assistance that can be accessed through the school system or the hospital setting. Informal support networks refer to family, friends, relatives, neighbors, churches, clubs, and organizations with whom a person voluntarily interacts. A combination of formal and informal supports is necessary for optimal management of the chronic illness.

Empowerment of families

The notion of empowerment of families of chronically ill children and adolescents is becoming associated with service delivery across many medical and mental health settings or professions (30). Rather than parents or caregivers doing everything for chronically ill children or adolescents, thus maintaining dependency, a process is begun whereby children or adolescents with the chronic illness discover and build on their own strengths, leading to a greater sense of mastery and control over their lives. They have confidence in their own ability to acquire and use resources to meet needs, to solve problems, and to make decisions. Empowered families of chronically ill children and adolescents are not helpless and dependent, nor are they totally independent. Rather, the goal of empowerment is interdependence between self, family, informal support, and formal service providers.

CONCLUSIONS

Growing up is a stressful developmental process even for physically healthy children and adolescents. Chronic illness further complicates the developmental process. The chronic illness, treatment requirements, hospitalization, and surgery, when necessary, all intensify concerns about physical appearance, interfere with the process of gaining independence, and disrupt changing relationships with parents and peers. In addition, developmental issues complicate the children and adolescents' transition toward taking responsibility for managing their illness and learning to comply with the medical and mental health treatment plans.

The prevalence of chronically ill children and adolescents with mental health issues, worldwide, is increasing as larger numbers of these children live until and beyond adolescence. In addition, the prevalence of certain chronic illnesses in adolescence, such as diabetes (types 1 and 2) and asthma, has increased, as have survival rates from cancer.

Although scientific evidence indicates that children with chronic illness have more mental health issues than their healthy peers, many controversies and gaps in the literature exist. A full understanding of the relationship between chronic illness and mental health is yet to be available. Second, the specific types of mental health issues associated with specific chronic illnesses continue to be delineated. Third, there is inconsistency and a paucity of data regarding the connection between mental health and social issues among specific clinical groups of chronically ill children and adolescents. As research continues to illustrate the relationship between chronic illness and mental health, appropriate services will be more available to meet the needs of children and adolescents.

REFERENCES

[1] Cadman D, Boyle M, Szatmari P, Offord DR. Chronic illness, disability and mental and social well-being: Findings of the Ontario child health study. Pediatrics 1987;79:805-13.

[2] Rolland JS. Toward a psychosocial typology of chronic and life-threatening illness. Fam Syst Med 1984;2:245-62.

[3] Bowe F. Physical, sensory, and health disabilities: An introduction. Upper Saddle River, NJ: Merrill, 2002.

[4] Eisenberg MG, Glueckauf RL, Zarensky HH, eds. Medical aspects of disability: A handbook for the rehabilitation professional. New York: Springer, 1999.

[5] Falvo D. Medical and psychosocial aspects of chronic illness and disability, 2nd ed. Gaithersburg, MD: Aspen, 1999.

[6] Muehrer P. Research on co-morbidity, contextual barriers, and stigma: A introduction to the special issue. J Psych Res 2002; 53:843-5.

[7] Hippisley-Cox J, Fielding K, Pringle M. Depression as a risk factor for ischaemic heart disease in men: Population based case-control study. BMJ 1998;316-1714-9.

[8] Strik JJ, Denollet J, Lousberg R, Honig A. Comparing symptoms of depression and anxiety as predictors of cardiac events and increased health care consumption after myocardial infarction. J Am Coll Cardiol 2003;42:1801-7.

[9] Guzman SJ, Nicassio PM. The contribution of negative and positive illness schemas to depression in patients with end-stage renal disease. J Behav Med 2003;26:517-34.

[10] Linde JA, Jeffery RW, Levy RL, Sherwood NE, Utter J, Pronk NP, Boyle RG. Binge eating disorder, weight control self-efficacy, and depression in overweight men and women. Int J Obes Relat Metab Disord 2004;28:418-25.

[11] Yanovski SZ, Nelson JE, Dubbert BK, Spitzer RL. Association of binge eating disorder and psychiatric comorbidity in obese subjects. Am J Psych 1993;150:1472-9.
[12] Ortega AN, Huertas SE, Canino G, Ramirez R, Rubio-Stippec M. Childhood asthma, chronic illness, and psychiatric disorders. J Nerv Ment Dis 2002;190:275-81.
[13] Goodwin RD, Jacobi F, Thefeld W. Mental disorders and asthma in the community. Psychol Med 2003;33:879-85.
[14] Goodwin RD, Fergusson DM, Horwood LJ. Asthma and depressive and anxiety disorders among young persons in the community. Psychol Med 2004;34:1465-74.
[15] Judson L. Global childhood chronic illness. Nurs Adm Q 2004; 28:60-6.
[16] Lavigne JV, Faier-Routman J. Psychological adjustment to pediatric physical disorders: A meta-analytic review. J Pediatr Psychol 1992; 17:133-57.
[17] Glazebrook C, Hollis C, Heussler H, Goodman R, Coates L. Detecting emotional and behavioral problems in pediatric clinics. Child Care Health Dev 2003;29:141-9.
[18] Briggs-Gowan MJ, Horwitz SM, Schwab-Stone ME, Leventhal JM, Leaf PJ. Mental health in pediatric settings: Distribution of disorders and factors related to service use. J Am Acad Child Adolesc Psychiatry 2000;39:841-9.
[19] Gortmaker SL, Walker DK, Weitzman M, Sobol AM. Chronic conditions socioeconomic risks, and behavioral problems in children and adolescents. Pediatrics 1990;85:267-76.
[20] Doll HA, Petersen SEK, Stewart-Brown SL. Obesity and physical and emotional well-being: Associations between BMI, chronic illness and the physical and mental components of the SF-36 questionnaire. Obes Res 2000;8:160-70.
[21] Cohn, LD, Adler NE. Female and male perceptions of ideal body shapes: Distorted views among Caucasian college students. Psych Women Q 1992;16:69-79.
[22] Gardner RM, Friedman BN, Jackson NA. Hispanic and white children's judgments of perceived and ideal body size in self and others. Psychol Record 1999;49.
[23] Hausenblas HA, Symons-Downs D, Fleming DS, Connaughton DP. Body image in middle school children. Eat Weight Disord 2002;7(3):244-8.
[24] Siegel J, Yancey A, Aneshensel C, Schuler R. Body image, perceived pubertal timing and adolescent mental health. J Adolesc Health 1999;25:155-65.
[25] Garner DM, Rosen LW, Barry D Eating disorders among athletes: Research and recommendations. Child Adolesc Psychiatr N Am 1998;7:839.
[26] Presnell K, Stice E. An experimental test of the effectiveness of dieting on bulimic pathology: Tipping the scales in a different direction. J Abnorm Psychol 2003;112:166-70.
[27] Meijer SA, Sinnema G, Bijstra J, Mellenbergh GJ, Wolters WHG. Coping styles and locus of control as predictors for psychological adjustment of adolescents with a chronic illness. Soc Sci Med 2002;54:1453-61.
[28] Newacheck PW, Taylor WR. Childhood chronic illness: Prevalence, severity, and impact. Am J Pub Health 1992;82:364-71.
[29] McClellan C, Cohen L. Family functioning children with chronic illness compared with healthy controls: A critical review. J Pediatrics 2007;150(3):221-3.
[30] Bauman LJ, Drotar D, Leventhal JM, Perrin EC, Pless IB. A review of psychosocial interventions for children with chronic health conditions. Pediatrics 1997;100(2):244-51.

SECTION FIVE:
CLINICAL PERSPECTIVES ON RURAL HEALTH

In: Rural child health: International aspects
Editors: Erica Bell and Joav Merrick
ISBN: 978-1-60876-357-3

Chapter 18

SUBSTANCE ABUSE AMONG ADOLESCENTS

***Abdel Salous, MSc*[1] *and Hatim A Omar, MD*[*2]**
[1]MD/PhD Program
[2]Division of Adolescent Medicine, Department of Pediatrics, University of Kentucky College of Medicine, Lexington, Kentucky, United States of America

This chapter aims to provide a global perspective on substance abuse among adolescents across different cultures, and to review appropriate strategies in communicating with the adolescent population about substance abuse. Drug abuse continues to be a major public health issue in the United States, especially among adolescents. The attitude toward and involvement in drug abuse among adolescents is a complex problem shaped by multiple psychosocial parameters. Psychosocial variables such as ethnicity, and religion, and group dynamics, while deeply intertwined in shaping the cultural identity of adolescents, also deliver their impact to substance abuse in this patient population. In a society largely composed of a diverse immigrant population, cultural sensitivity of the healthcare provider to patient culture is critical to patient centered care and effective clinical outcomes. Summary: Cultural sensitivity of healthcare providers is critical to addressing the health needs of adolescent patients in the increasingly culturally heterogeneous patient population of the United States.

INTRODUCTION

The World Health Organization defines substance abuse as: the harmful or hazardous use of psychoactive substances, including alcohol and illicit drugs (1). Substance abuse is public health care problem with global dimensions: worldwide psychoactive substance use is estimated at two billion alcohol users, 1.3 billion smokers and 185 million drug users (1). In the United States alone, drug abuse results in roughly 40 million serious illnesses or injuries (2). While statistics on drug abuse abound, the magnitude of this problem in the adolescent population remains most disturbing. In the most recent report by Johnston et al (3) "51% of America's teenagers have tried an illicit drug by the time they finish high school".

* Correspondence: Professor Hatim A Omar, MD, Department of Pediatrics, Room J422, University of Kentucky, Lexington, KY 40536-0284 United States. Tel: 859-323-5643; Fax: 859-257-7706; Email: haomar2@uky.edu

Furthermore, adolescents 12-20 years of age comprise 49.8% of all persons aged 12 or older who used illicit drugs in the in 2007, with the highest frequency in the 18-20 age group (4).

Clearly, these statistics call attention to the importance of addressing substance abuse in adolescents. Yet more importantly, cultural diversity is on the rise in the United States as a nation of immigrants. A recent report by the US Census Bureau states that in 2042, whites will no longer be a majority in the country. Moreover, as of today, 1 in every 3 Americans is a minority (5). Therefore, addressing the healthcare needs of an increasingly diverse population poses the real challenge to health care providers. In this light, the purpose of this review is to highlight the different attitudes and perceptions of various populations toward substance use/abuse and propose guidelines to help address the unique needs of these populations.

ATTITUDES TOWARD DRUG ABUSE IN ASIA

In many eastern cultures, emotional problems and substance abuse are cause for dishonor. Among traditional Asian-Indians, for example, substance use is perceived as a moral problem contributing to family shame and loss of prestige (6). However, substance abuse seems on the rise in US immigrant refugee populations from Southest Asia, suggestive of cultural influence. This is quite interesting from a historic perspective. In Asia, particularly in China, drug abuse along with its associated health problems, was brought by the British in the 17th century, but abated following independence of China from the British Empire. However, since the 1980s, the extensive modernization and westernization in China since has been associated with increasing drug abuse, suggestive again of cross-cultural influence (7). In terms of cultural views, intravenous drug abuse, commercial sex, and AIDS are associated with social stigmata. Surprisingly, AIDS was significantly less stigmatizing than either intravenous drug abuse or commercial sex. In fact, coexistence of AIDS with either commercial sex or intravenous drug use significantly decreased the stigma of either commercial sex or intravenous drug use alone, suggesting a mitigating effect of disease on social stigmata (8).

ATTITUDES TOWARD DRUG ABUSE IN AFRICAN CULTURES

Adolescent perception of drug abuse is varies and correlates with the dominant cultural norms, yet leaves many questions unanswered. For example, in a study of adolescents in South Africa, personal attributes and peer substance use correlated highly with drug abuse in adolescents. Parental factors and environmental stressors correlated less strongly with drug abuse in the same patient sample. It is interesting to notice that the adolescent lifetime rate of Marijuana in South Africa was significantly less than that in the United States (6-12% vs. 19.7%) (9). This may be due to the low availability of Marijuana compared to other drugs. For example, in Ethiopia, Somalia, Nigeria, and Yemen in the Arabian Peninsula, a common drug of abuse is an amphetamine-like substance called Cathinone, derived from a flowering plant called Khat or Catha edulis (10). Chewing Khat in Yemen is widespread due to its mild stimulant effect and deep social and cultural tradition, yet it poses significant health risks (11). While it is unclear what the motives are for adolescents to chew Khat, it has been suggested that students use it to enhance performance on examinations (11). Although initially the regulation of Khat was limited to local levels, its worldwide spread especially among immigrants from Eastern African countries has spurred classification and subsequent regulation (12).

Attitudes Toward Drug Abuse in Latin America

In contrast to Eastern cultures, the Latino culture attitude toward substance use especially drinking alcohol is on the opposite end of the spectrum. In fact, boys are introduced to "manhood" by initiation of drinking, usually by the father or the male figure in the family. Also, what is considered "underage drinking" in North America is acceptable within the Latino family (13). Refusing to drink in the family is interpreted as rejection of other family members (14). It is interesting that the family assumes the gatekeeper role with regards to drinking habits in Latino culture. This may be explained by fact that most Latino men and women continue to live with their parents after reaching 18 years of age (13). A study by Navarro et al (15) confirmed the importance of the family role in prevention of substance abuse and found that the main reason for drug consumption was "to have fun". Other Latin American cultures in Cambodia and Haiti consider narcotics as medicine rather than drugs of abuse (14).

Attitudes Toward Drug Abuse in Western Cultures

Adolescent substance use is considered deviant in most Western cultures including Europe and North America (16). The perception of drug abuse by adolescents in the United States has been well documented. Perception of harm correlated negatively with cigarette smoking, binge drinking, and illicit drug use (4). Also, adolescents who perceived a strong parental disapproval of drug use were less likely to abuse drugs. In addition, participation in religious services correlated with less incidence of drug abuse among adolescents. On the other hand, subjects engaging in fights were more likely to abuse drugs (4). Drug abuse remains a challenging public health issue in the United States. Relative to other countries, addressing drug abuse issue is complicated due to the growing ethnic diversity, especially that of immigrant populations. It is particularly interesting to notice drug abuse trends among youth immigrants. A study by Blake et al (17) revealed that recent immigrant youth reported lower substance use including alcohol and Marijuana compared to residents of the US. Yet, it seems that with time, the rates of drug use in this population were no longer significantly different from the mainstream population (18). Similar results were obtained in a group of Mexican immigrants (19).

The link between substance abuse and cultural exchange is quite dynamic. On one hand, the waxing and waning of substance abuse in China in association western influence is an example of how developing countries are influenced by the "developed" world (7). On the other hand, the spread of Khat chewing from Eastern Africa and the Arabian Peninsula to Western hemisphere through immigrants is illustrative of how cultural influence acts both ways (12). Clearly, culture plays a considerable role in shaping substance abuse through the process of acculturation as seen in youth immigrants from Asia and Mexico (18,19).

In an age where globalization is facilitating cultural exchange in our society, health care providers are posed to the challenge of becoming "culturally competent" to better serve the needs of their patients via more effective communication. Aside from the important roles of families, organizations, and programs in fighting substance use, the patient-physician trust-based relationship remains indispensable to effectively addressing this issue.

PHYSICIANS AND CULTURE COMPETENCE

Recognition of and sensitivity toward cultural differences by care providers is critical to improving clinical outcomes related to substance abuse in adolescents. From an economic standpoint, the WHO estimates that for every dollar invested in drug treatment, seven dollars are saved in health and other social costs (1). The role of the physician is to appreciate cultural relativism and treat patients in the appropriate cultural context when dealing with substance abuse.

In this regard, some investigators have pointed out that many substance abuse prevention programs were designed for a White, middleclass recipient population and influenced by mainstream American values (20). Other authors assert that such programs are inadequate to the needs of ethnic minorities (21). In support of the alternative view, Hecht et al. found that "minority youth responded more favorably to programs in which teachers or characters were members of their own group" (22). To conclude, perhaps the Institute of Medicine report on "Unequal treatment", sums it best by highlighting that "education as the best strategy to develop cultural competence among providers" (23).

REFERENCES

[1] Management of substance abuse: Facts and figures. World Health Organization 2008 [cited December 28, 2008]; Available from: http://www.who.int/topics/substance_abuse/en/.

[2] Drug abuse. National Library of Medicine-Medline 2008 15 December 2008 [cited December 28, 2008]; Available from: http://www.nlm.nih.gov/medlineplus/drugabuse.html.

[3] Johnston LD, O'Malley PM, Bachman JG, Schulenberg JE. Monitoring the future national results on adolescent drug use: Overview of key findings. Washington, DC: Natl Inst Drug Abuse, 2007.

[4] Results from the 2007 national survey on drug use and health: National findings. Washington, DC: Substance Abuse Ment Health Serv Adm, 2007. [cited December 28, 2008]; Available from: http://www.drugabusestatistics.samhsa.gov/NSDUH/2k7NSDUH/2k7results.cfm#Ch2.

[5] Bernstein R, Edwards T. An older and more diverse nation by midcentury. Washington, DC: US Census Bureau News, 2008.

[6] Bhattacharya G. Drug abuse risks for acculturating immigrant adolescents: case study of Asian Indians in the United States. Health Soc Work 2002;27(3):175-83.

[7] Lu L, Wang X. Drug addiction in China. Ann NY Acad Sci 2008;1141:304-17.

[8] Chan KY, et al. Disentangling the stigma of HIV/AIDS from the stigmas of drugs use, commercial sex and commercial blood donation - a factorial survey of medical students in China. BMC Public Health 2007;7:280.

[9] Brook JS, et al. Predictors of drug use among South African adolescents. J Adolesc Health 2006;38(1):26-34.

[10] Feyissa AM, Kelly JP. A review of the neuropharmacological properties of khat. Prog Neuropsychopharmacol Biol Psychiatry 2008;32(5):1147-66.

[11] Hassan NA, Gunaid AA, Murray-Lyon IM. Khat (Catha edulis): Health aspects of khat chewing. East Mediterr Health J 2007;13(3): 706-18.

[12] Nutt D, et al. Development of a rational scale to assess the harm of drugs of potential misuse. Lancet 2007;369(9566):1047-53.

[13] Mental Health Center of Dada County Newsletter. 2008 September 2008 [cited December 28, 2008]; Available from: http://www.mhcdc.org/Resources/newslettervol2.html.

[14] Amodeo M, Griffin M. Parental alcoholism and other family disruptions: adult outcomes among sisters. Am J Orthopsychiatry 1997;67(4):585-93.

[15] Tortajada Navarro S, et al. Drug consumption and perception among Latin American immigrants. Psicothema 2008;20(3):403-7.

[16] Swaim RC, Bates SC, Chavez EL. Structural equation socialization model of substance use among Mexican-American and white non-Hispanic school dropouts. J Adolesc Health 1998;23(3):128-38.

[17] Blake SM, et al. Receipt of school health education and school health service among adolescent immigrants in Massachusetts. J Sch Health 2001;71(3):105-13.

[18] Acculturation increases risk for substance use by foreign-born youth. SAMHSA News 2004 [cited 12 December 28, 2008]; Available from: http://www.samhsa.gov/samhsa_news/VolumeXII_1/article2.htm.

[19] Vega WA, Sribney WM, Achara-Abrahams I. Co-occurring alcohol, drug, and other psychiatric disorders among Mexican-origin people in the United States. Am J Public Health 2003;93(7):1057-64.

[20] Kumpfer KL, et al. Cultural sensitivity and adaptation in family-based prevention interventions. Prev Sci 2002;3(3):241-6.

[21] Gonzalez-Castro F, Alarcon-Hernandez E. Integrating cultural variables into drug abuse prevention and treatment with racial/ethnic minorities. J Drug Issues 2002;32(3):783-810.

[22] Hecht ML, Marsiglia FF, Elek E, Wagstaff DA, Kulis S, Dustman P, Miller-Day M. Culturally grounded substance use prevention: An evaluation of the Keepin' it R.E.A.L. curriculum. Prev Sci 2003;4(4):233-48.

[23] Smedley BD, Stith AY, Nelson AR, eds. Unequal treatment: Confronting racial and ethnic disparities in health care. Washington, DC: Natl Acad Press, 2002.

In: Rural child health: International aspects
Editors: Erica Bell and Joav Merrick
ISBN: 978-1-60876-357-3

Chapter 19

DERMATOLOGICAL DISORDERS AMONG ADOLESCENTS IN SUBURBAN RURAL SCHOOLS IN SOUTH INDIA

Ganapathy Kalaiselvan**, *MD and Kaliaperumal Karthikeyan, MD
Dermatology, Venereology and Community Medicine, Sri Manakula Vinayagar Medical College, Kalitheerthalkuppam, Pondicherry, India

Adolescents are a vulnerable group of the population susceptible to a variety of skin diseases. Our aim was to review the pattern of dermatoses in adolescent school children. A total of 1,246 adolescents were screened for skin disorders. Out of them 657 (52.7%) were girls and 589 (47.3) boys. Among the 1,246 examined, 527(42.9%) had dermatological problems. Female adolescents (288) outnumbered the males (239). Most of them belonged to age group of 15-18 year olds (63%). Acne vulgaris (16.1%) was the most common disease seen among the study group. Pediculosis was the second most common disease followed by polymorphous light eruption, fungal infections and scabies. The other disorders seen included psoriasis, seborrhea capitis, pityriasis alba, phrynoderma, neurofibromatosis, verruca vulgaris, xerosis, lichen striatus, alopecia areata and melanocytic nevus. The study helped us to identify the diseases prevalent in the adolescent community and orient the health education to suit their needs.

INTRODUCTION

Skin disorders are very common in adolescents. Adolescents are a vulnerable group of the population susceptible to a variety of skin diseases, because of the hormonal changes. In most of the school based studies, the study population was young schoolchildren with very few studies highlighting the dermatological diseases encountered by the adolescents (1- 3). Hence we undertook our study to review the pattern of dermatology problems in adolescent school children.

* Correspondence: Kaliaperumal Karthikeyan, MD, Consultant Dermatologist andVenereology, Sri Manakula Vinayagar Medical College, Kalitheerthalkuppam, Pondicherry, India. E-mail: karthikderm@yahoo.co.in

OUR STUDY

Our study was conducted in a rural higher secondary school (Pondicherry) in coastal south India. The climate of that region is typical of a tropical region with high temperature and humidity.

All the students in the age group of 12 to 18 years attending this higher secondary school in suburban Pondicherry were included in the study. The study was conducted between August 2007 and September 2007. Consent was obtained from all the students. All the students were screened for dermatological disorder by a dermatologist. The diagnosis was made based on a detailed history, clinical examination and appropriate investigations. The investigations were done in our hospital. The diseases were tabulated based on the etiology and results were analyzed.

OUR FINDINGS

A total of 1,246 adolescents were screened for skin disorders. Out of them 657 (52.7%) girls and 589 (47.3) boys (see table 1). The male to female ratio was 1:1.1.

Table 1. Age and gender distribution

Age group (yrs)	Male	Female	Total
12-13	71	74	145
13-14	59	81	140
14-15	74	102	176
15-16	95	120	215
16-17	122	132	254
17-18	168	148	316
Total	589	657	1,246

Among the 1,246 examined, 527 (42.9%) had dermatological problems. Female adolescents (288) outnumbered the males (239). Most of them belonged to age group of 15-18 years of age (63%). The diseases encountered are summarized in table 2.

Table 2 .Pattern of diseases

Age (years	Acne vulgaris	Pediculosis	Polymorphous light eruption	Fungal infections	scabies	Miscellaneous
12-13	3	34	4	2	3	6
13-14	4	21	4	5	1	2
14-15	15	20	5	10	2	4
15-16	35	20	7	4	-	5
16-17	54	31	9	7	5	6
17-18	100	21	5	10	11	6
Total	211	147	34	28	22	29

Acne vulgaris was the most common disease seen among the adolescents (see table 3). About 16.1% of the study group had acne vulgaris. About 8.5% of the males and 7.6% of the females had acne vulgaris. Acne vulgaris was most prevalent among the 17-18 age groups and accounted for 50% of the cases. Pediculosis was the second most common disease after acne vulgaris. About 12% of the adolescents had pediculosis and all of them were girls, but for one. Polymorphous light eruption was seen more commonly males (3.3%) than females (2.2%). Fungal infections such as tinea corporis, tinea cruris and tinea versicolor were seen in both males and females and scabies was seen in 2.1% of the adolescents. They were twice more common in males than in females. The other disorders seen included psoriasis, seborrhea capitis, pityriasis alba, phrynoderma, neurofibromatosis, verruca vulgaris, xerosis, lichen striatus, alopecia areata and melanocytic nevus.

Table 3. Acne vulgaris

Age group (yrs)	Male	Female	Total
12-13	-	3	3
13-14	2	2	4
14-15	5	10	15
15-16	19	16	35
16-17	27	27	54
17-18	63	37	100
Total	106	95	201

Discussion

The cutaneous disorders seen in adolescents are unique and require special attention, because they are more conscious of their 'looks'. Many disorders that occur in the adolescent age, such as acne can have a psychological effect. In our study acne vulgaris was the most common disease. Acne was seen in ninety-one percent of males and 79% of females of the females in New Zealand (4). In a study from Australia, 31.6% of the adolescents were affected. It was less prevalent among boys aged 10-12 years than girls of the same age; however, between the ages of 16 and 18 years, boys were more likely than girls to have acne (5). The higher incidence could probably due to genetic and nutritional factors. In another study from Hong Kong, acne was the most common disease among students, but it accounted for only 9.9% of the diseases (1). Though acne was the most common disease, the prevalence was less, because it included both primary and high school children. A similar high prevalence was noted in a study from Turkey, where 28.6% of the adolescents had acne (2). In our study acne occurred early in adolescent girls, when compared to boys. coinciding with the early onset of puberty in girls. Though most of the study group had grade 1 acne, grade 2 and 3 was also noted. But many of these adolescents did not seek treatment for the acne vulgaris.

Pediculosis was the second most common disease after acne vulgaris. In another study from Pondicherry, pediculosis was the most common disease among school children (personal communication). This study conducted about two decades ago, primarily constituted of school children. In a study from Chile, about 25.4% of the school children had pediculosis, while in a study from Argentina it was 81.5% (6,7). In contrast, in a Turkish study pediculosis was seen only in 6.8% of the children and in Nigeria it was only 3.7% (8,9). Pediculosis was exclusively confined to girls and prevalence was equal among all age groups. This was in stark contrast to the study conducted in the schools of Bordeaux academy, where males were also affected though in less numbers (10). This sexual preponderance is probably due to certain socio cultural reasons such as overcrowding, poor hygiene and long hair. Fungal infections such as tinea corporis, tinea cruris and tinea versicolor was seen in both males and females. The fungal infections were less prevalent in our study group, when compared to a study from Nigeria, where 15.2% of students had fungal infections and in a Hong Kong study it was 2.2% (1,11). In contrast to our study, polymorphous light eruption did not figure in the list of diseases in most studies. Polymorphous light eruption was seen more commonly in males probably due to increased outdoor activities in the form of sports and recreation. Scabies was seen in 2.1% of the adolescents, while this disease was not noted in studies from Hong Kong or Sweden (1,12). The prevalence varied between 1.8%-4.7% in various other studies (2,6,11,13). Most of these studies were conducted among school going children and not adolescents. The variation in prevalence could be due to the varied socio-economic status among the study groups. This is well illustrated by the fact that scabies was more prevalent in developing countries rather than the developed ones. Further the prevalence of scabies is less among adolescents probably due to better awareness and ability to take care of personal hygiene.

It is interesting to note diseases such as atopic dermatitis commonly seen in western studies was not encountered in our study. This correlates well with a hospital based study from the same area (personal communication). The disorders encountered in our study are primarily treatable and diseases such as pediculosis and scabies can be prevented by improving personal hygiene. Proper hair care and hygiene can easily control pediculosis. It was distressing to note that most of the students did not consider problems such as acne vulgaris and pediculosis as a disease and so they did not seek treatment for the same. It is important to increase awareness of these disorders among the adolescents, which can be easily done by health education. The education programs should ensure that adolescents understand their disease and know the treatment options that are available and from whom they should seek advice. Further the study helped us to identify the diseases prevalent in the adolescent community and orient the health education to suit their needs.

References

[1] Fung WK, Lo KK. Prevalence of skin disease among school children and adolescents in a student health service center in Hong Kong. Pediatrc Dermatol 2000;17:440-6.

[2] Tuncel AA, Erbagci Z. Prevalence of skin diseases among male adolescent and post-adolescent boarding school students in Turkey. J Dermatol 2005;32(7):557-64.

[3] Bahamdan K, Mahfouz AA, Tallab T, Badawi IA, al-Amari OM. Skin diseases among adolescent boys in Abha, Saudi Arabia. Int J Dermatol 1996;35(6):405-7.

[4] Lello J, Pearl A, Arroll B, Yallop J, Birchall NM. Prevalence of acne vulgaris in Auckland senior high school students. NZ Med J 1995;108(1004):287-9

[5] Kilkenny M, Merlin K, Plunkett A, Marks R. The prevalence of common skin conditions in Australian school students: 3. acne vulgaris. Br J Dermatol 1998;139(5):840-5.

[6] Sagua H, Rivera AM, Zamora M, Neira I, Araya J, Maluenda R.Epidemiological study of pediculosis capitis and scabies in schoolchildren from Antofagasta, Chile, 1995. Bol Chil Parasitol 1997;52(1-2):33-6.

[7] Chouela E, Abeldaño A, Cirigliano M, Ducard M, Neglia V, La Forgia M, et al .Head louse infestations: epidemiologic survey and treatment evaluation in Argentinian schoolchildren. Int J Dermatol 1997;36(11):819-25.

[8] Kokturk A, Baz K, Bugdayci R, Sasmaz T, Tursen U, Kaya TI,et al. The prevalence of pediculosis capitis in schoolchildren in Mersin, Turkey. Int J Dermatol 2003;42(9):694-8.

[9] Ebomoyi EW. Pediculosis capitis among urban school children in Ilorin, Nigeria. J Natl Med Assoc 1994;86(11):861-4.

[10] Courtiade C, Labrèze C, Fontan I, Taïeb A, Maleville J. Pediculosis capitis: a questionnaire survey in 4 schools of the Bordeaux Academy 1990-1991. Ann Dermatol Venereol 1993;120(5):363.

[11] Ogunbiyi AO, Owoaje E, Ndahi A. Prevalence of skin disorders in school children in Ibadan, Nigeria. Pediatr Dermatol 2005;22(1):6-10.

[12] Larsson PA, Lidén S. Prevalence of skin diseases among adolescents 12-16 years of age. Acta Derm Venereol 1980;60(5):415-23

[13] Dogra S, Kumar B. Epidemiology of skin diseases in school children: a study from northern India. Pediatr Dermatol 2003; 20(6):470-3.

In: Rural child health: International Aspects
Editors: Erica Bell and Joav Merrick

ISBN: 978-1-60876-357-3

Chapter 20

SICKLE CELL DISEASE IN SCHEDULED CASTE COMMUNITIES OF RURAL ORISSA, INDIA

Ranbir S Balgir*, Ph D
Division of Human Genetics, Regional Medical Research Centre (ICMR), Bhubaneswar, Orissa, India

The sickle cell disease is a genetically inherited commonly encountered hematological disorder in the state of Orissa. It causes high degree of morbidity, mortality and fetal wastage in the poor vulnerable people. For the first time, a carrier couple of sickle cell disease had delivered twin offspring with carrier as well as the homozygous sickle cell disease or homozygous sickle cell disease and normal offspring. The suspected cases of hemoglobinopathies suffering from anemia are routinely referred from different peripheral Primary Health Centres (PHCs) and hospitals in the state of Orissa to our centre for detailed investigations and genetic/marriage counseling. Out of these referral cases, two scheduled castes, i.e. Domb and Pana, families with twin children were referred from Kalahandi and Kandhamal districts of Orissa, respectively and were studied in details. The present study reports for the first time a rare occurrence of dizygotic twins (sickle cell trait and sickle cell disease in one family and sickle cell disease and normal child in another family) in a singleton pregnancy in the sickle cell carrier parents, respectively from Kalahandi and Kandhamal districts of Orissa, India. It is true that twin gestation does not change the preconception probability, but this study clearly shows co-existence of two different genotypes in a single pregnancy. It is a rare occasion when a single pregnancy carries either two or more distinct abnormal genotypes at a time in a womb in human beings. Dizygotic twins are genetically different and, thus, provide means of appraisal of the expression of different genotypes under the same environmental conditions.

* Correspondence: Ranbir S Balgir, PhD, Deputy Director (Senior Grade), Regional Medical Research Centre for Tribals (Indian Council of Medical Research), Nagpur Road (Near Medical College), P.O.Garha, Jabalpur-482003, Madhya Pradesh, Central India. E-mail: balgirrs@yahoo.co.in

Introduction

Hemoglobinopathies are a group of hereditary disorders including sickle cell disease, highly prevalent in some population groups, and pose a major public health genetics problem. The sickle cell anemia especially affects 60-70 million people all over the world, including growing children, adolescent girls and pregnant women (1,2). Inherited disorders of hemoglobin cause high degree of hemolytic anemia, painful crisis, frequent vulnerability to clinical jaundice, and high susceptible to various infections, and are responsible for high infant morbidity, mortality and fetal wastage (3-5). These disorders have become a life long social, psychological and financial burden on the society (2,6,7). There is no permanent cure of sickle cell hemoglobinopathy. Most of the cases remain undetected, undiagnosed and untreated. Due to nonavailability of basic diagnostic facilities, and absence of optimal treatment, many of these affected individuals die in infancy, childhood or with a limited span of life (3). The sickle cell hemoglobinopathy, which has an autosomal co-dominance inheritance, is not uncommon in Central-Eastern part of India. The homozygous sickle cell disease is a major cause of high infant morbidity, mortality and fetal wastage in Western Orissa (5). The frequency of sickle cell hemoglobinopathy is high in general castes (8), scheduled castes (9) and in some scheduled tribes (10, 11) in the Central Eastern India.

Since the time of Sir Francis Galton (1822-1911), who studied intelligence in twins in the later part of the nineteenth century to reveal the contribution of heredity and have provided research inputs for the appraisal of nature-nurture controversy for determining the relative effects of genetics and environment. Human twins provide the simplest and most powerful method for disentangling the influence of environmental and genetic factors on human characteristics. As the identical, monovular or monozygotic (MZ) twins are more similar with respect to same genotype or the same genes than the fraternal, binovular or dizygotic (DZ) twins, therefore, this is taken as evidence of a genetic influence on particular characteristics. Identical twins are genetic duplicates. Both types of twins share common life experiences. Identical twins differ from fraternal twins in the number of genes they have in common. By studying identical and fraternal twins and their families, we can estimate how genes and environment interact to influence characters, strengths, vulnerabilities, and values. In other words, the information collected about how alike or different members of a twin pair allow us to determine the influence of genes and environment. If a pair of identical twins are separated at birth and raised apart, then the similarities and differences between them can be very interesting. The similarities are more likely to be due to heredity, and the differences are more likely to be due to environment.

The MZ and DZ twins who are separated early in life and reared apart are a fascinating experiment of nature. The comparison of MZ with DZ twins yields information on the percentage of phenotype variance ascribable to heredity (H). If under a given environment, both members of a twin pair develop the same phenotype, the twins are said to be concordant. The comparison of MZ twins who have been reared apart gives an opportunity of nature-nurture interaction on the same genotype to the appraisal of the effects of two different environments. Thus, twin studies provide information on the relative contribution of heredity and environment in the manifestation of a trait, but the mode of inheritance could not be known by multiple births.

To the best of our knowledge, there are a few reports pertaining to monozygotic twin studies in sickle cell anemia (12,13), sickle β-thalassemia (14), and hemoglobinopathies. No study has ever reported the occurrence of dizygotic twins in sickle cell carrier parents. This study reports two families of scheduled caste communities (Domb and Pana) with a rare dizygotic twin pair with sickle cell disorders born to sickle cell disease carrier parents in Orissa, India.

OUR STUDY

The suspected cases of hemoglobinopathies suffering from anemia are routinely referred from different peripheral Primary Health Centres (PHCs) and hospitals in the state of Orissa to our centre for detailed investigations and genetic/marriage counseling. Out of these referral cases, two scheduled caste (Domb and Pana) families with twin children were referred from Kalahandi and Kandhamal districts, respectively to our centre for detailed laboratory investigations. Background information for these two families such as name, age, sex, caste, native place, reproductive history, family pedigree, and clinical signs and symptoms was also recorded. The index case and other available family members such as parents, brother/sister after taking informed/written consent were also subjected to clinical examination and laboratory investigations for confirmation of the diagnosis. They were also imparted genetic/marriage counseling accordingly as a measure to prevent further spread of the disease in the community.

About 2-3 ml intravenous blood samples were collected using sodium salt of ethylene diamine tetra acetic acid (EDTA) as anticoagulant by disposable syringes and needles from each individual under aseptic conditions after obtaining the informed consent. All the signs and symptoms related to sickle cell disease were recorded on the pre-designed proforma after clinical examination. Laboratory investigations were carried out following the standard procedures. Hematological parameters were studied by using an automated Blood Cell Counter (Model- MS4, Melet Schloesing Laboratories, Cergy-Pontoise Cedex, France).

The sickling test was performed by using freshly prepared sodium metabisulphite solution as reducing agent for the presence or absence of sickle cell hemoglobin (15). The routine hemoglobin lysate electrophoresis was carried out on cellulose acetate membrane (CAM) in Tris-EDTA-Borate buffer at pH 8.6 and quantification of A_2 fraction of hemoglobin was done by elution method (16); the value more than 3.5% of A_2 fraction of adult hemoglobin was taken as cut off point for determining the β-thalassemia trait. Estimation of fetal hemoglobin was done as described by Weatherall (16). All the blood samples were further subjected to confirmation by doing the hemoglobin variant analysis (made for Bio-Rad Diagnostics, Hercules California, USA).

OUR FINDINGS

Both parents (father and mother) were clinically examined by a medical doctor for signs and symptoms of sickle cell disease, irrespective of laboratory findings. They did not complain of any health problem. They were healthy young (husband aged 30 years and wife 25 years in case of Domb; and Pana husband was 35 years and wife 32 years) couples having non-consanguineous marriage and belonged to scheduled caste, i.e. Domb and Pana of Kalahandi and Kandhamal district, respectively in Orissa, India. They had neither taken any blood transfusion nor suffered from clinical jaundice or respiratory problems. Laboratory investigations showed the sickling test positive for both parents. Both parents had normal hematological (red cell) indices as well as red cell morphology. Alkaline (pH 8.6) electrophoresis of blood lysate on cellulose acetate membrane (CAM) showed both parents as the carriers of sickle cell disease, with other constituent hemoglobins (A_2 and fetal) falling in the normal range in both the families (see table 1).

Table 1. Two scheduled caste (Domb and Pana) sickle cell disease carrier families with dizygotic twin offsprings from Orissa, India.

	FAMILY-1				FAMILY-2			
	Parents		Dizygotic Twins		Parents		Dizygotic Twins	
Parameters	Father	Mother	Daughter	Son*	Father	Mother	Son-1	Son-2*
Age (in years)	25	20	3	3	35	32	3 ½	3 ½
Sex	M	F	F	M	M	F	M	M
Hb (g/dl)	12.5	11.2	9.2	7.6	14.6	12.5	10.2	10.7
RBC ($x10^6/\mu l$)	5.0	4.5	4.8	3.5	5.3	5.6	5.2	4.7
HCT (%)	38.7	36.7	30.3	24.2	37.5	38.4	37.2	35.4
MVC (fl)	77.8	82.3	63.2	69.2	75.5	81.7	82.4	72.3
MCH (pg)	25.1	25.1	19.1	21.7	27.4	26.8	28.2	25.3
MCHC (g/dl)	32.2	30.5	30.3	31.4	31.6	32.6	32.7	31.4
RDW (%)	9.0	7.6	10.2	9.7	10.2	10.5	9.8	9.3
WBC ($x10^3/\mu l$)	6.8	8.4	10.7	9.5	5.9	6.1	5.7	5.2
Sickling Test	+ve	+ve	+ve	+ve	+ve	+ve	-ve	+ve
Electrophoresis (pH 8.6)	$A+S+A_2$	$A+S+A_2$	$A+S+A_2$	$S+F+A_2$	$A+S+A_2$	$A+S+A_2$	$A+A_2$	$S+F+A_2$
Hb A_2 (%)	2.5	2.0	2.1	2.8	1.9	2.2	2.8	1.2
Hb F (%)	0.2	0.6	0.3	13.7	0.7	1.0	0.7	7.1
Hb S (%)	34.4	26.0	24.9	83.5	24.4	30.6	0.0	91.7
Hb A (%)	62.9	71.4	72.7	-	73.0	66.2	96.5	-
Diagnosis	SCT	SCT	SCT	SCD	SCT	SCT	Normal	SCD

SCT= Sickle Cell Trait; SCD= Sickle Cell Disease
*Proband.

CASE STORY 1

The quantification of the sickle (Hb S) bands revealed 34.4% and 26%, respectively for father and mother, the low percentage of Hb S indicated the probability of interaction of sickle gene with α-thalassemia at least in the mother.

Out of a full-term son and daughter twin pair aged 3 years born to these parents, the elder daughter had usual fever, cough and cold occasionally in the winter season. She had no other complaints or complications, although her hemoglobin level was low (9.2 g/dl). Her hemogram or red cell indices were also low (see table1). Her sickling test was recorded to be positive. On electrophoresis, she was identified to be a case of sickle cell trait, with hemoglobin S constituting 24.9%; the low percentage of Hb S suggested the involvement of α-thalassemia in the sickle cell disease.

The index case, the son who was born with low birth weight (as told by parents) having protruded abdomen, suffered from dactylitis in infancy. He started walking late indicating retarded growth and development, had cough and cold (upper respiratory tract infections) frequently, suffered from fever every month, and already had two times whole blood (200ml each time) transfusions after hospitalization with a gap of one year. At the time of presentation, he had recurrent fever, moderate anemia with splenomegaly (4 cm). All his hematological indices showed low values (Table1). The sickling test was found to be positive. The alkaline (pH 8.6) hemolysate electrophoresis on CAM revealed a thick band at the position of S band (83.5%), trailing towards anode. His fetal hemoglobin was detected raised (13.7%) with normal hemoglobin A_2 level (see table 1). Thus, this proband was diagnosed as a case of sickle cell disease.

Since both the proband brother (sickle cell disease) and sister (sickle cell trait) had different sickle cell genotypes under similar environmental conditions with different clinical manifestations and hematological profile, they were probably the dizygotic twins.

CASE STORY 2

Both parents were detected to be sickle cell trait. Low percentage of Hb S in father indicated the probability of interaction with α-thalassemia gene in this family also.

Both children were born full-term and had no problem. However, at the age of 2 years the younger son (son-2) manifested clinical symptoms of fever with cough and cold frequently. Both brothers had no other complaints or complications, although their hemoglobin levels were slightly lower: 10.2 (son-1) and 10.7 g/dl (son-2), respectively. Red cell indices of 2nd son were also low (Table1). The sickling test of son-1 was negative, whereas, that of son-2 was recorded to be positive. On electrophoresis, he was identified to be a case of homozygous sickle cell disease, with hemoglobin S constituting 91.7%. His fetal hemoglobin was detected raised (7.1%) with lower hemoglobin A_2 level (Table 1). At the time of referring to our Centre, the son-2 had recurrent fever, irritability, fatigue, abdominal pains, palpable spleen and joint pains, but with no jaundice and history of blood transfusion. Out of the two sons, elder (son-1) had normal adult, fetal as well as A_2 hemoglobin (see table 1). Hence, he was declared normal.

As both these brothers (one was sickle cell disease patient and other was normal) had different genotypes under similar environmental conditions with different manifestations and hematological profiles, so they were probably the dizygotic twins also.

DISCUSSION

The most striking rare finding in the present study is the carrier couples of sickle cell disease have born twin offsprings with carrier status as well as the homozygous sickle cell disease or sickle cell disease and normal progeny (see table 1). There was an equal probability in every singleton pregnancy that a carrier couple of the sickle cell disease would either bear normal, carrier or sickle cell disease offspring, but not the two of these conditions (genotypes) together. Twin gestation does not change the preconception probability, but this study clearly shows co-existence of two different genotypes in a singleton pregnancy. It is a rare occasion when a single pregnancy carries either two or more distinct (abnormal) genotypes at a time in a womb in human beings. The present study reports for the first time the occurrence of dizygotic twins in a singleton pregnancy in the sickle cell carrier parents from Kalahandi and Kandhamal districts of Orissa, India.

The nature-nurture debate may overlook the most important forces that shape human life. It is well established that identical twins—who develop from a single egg that splits after fertilization and, therefore, have the same genes—to learn how genes influence traits or predispose people to disease. Identical twins who grew up in the same household (and presumably ate the same foods, went to the same schools and so forth) share a particular trait more strongly than do fraternal twins, who come from two, separately fertilized eggs and whose genes are no more alike than those of any other siblings, it would be interesting that the similarity is due to genes rather than environment.

It is the Nature rather than the nurture. In other words, dizygotic twins are genetically different and, thus, provide means of appraisal of the expression of different genotypes under the same environment. Fraternal or dizygotic twins share 50% of their genes. Dizygotic twins are no closer than siblings and the main interest in distinguishing the roles of genetic and environmental factors in expression of disease lies with monozygotic twins. The present study points to the above ideological and conceptual debate. Even, identical (monozygotic) twin studies have shown the differences in clinical severity and frequency of crisis, implicating the nongenetic factors influencing course of the disease (12,14).

Tests for prenatal diagnosis such as amniocentesis, cord blood or chorionic villi sampling, fetal biopsy, non-invasive technology, etc. already exist to check a fetus for sickle cell during pregnancy. But some couples have strong personal objections to abortion when a pregnancy is already established. Pre-implantation genetic diagnosis (PGD) could provide couples with another way to avoid passing on sickle cell disease. A couple who is carrier of sickle cell disease has twin babies who are completely free of the sickle cell gene with the application of a technique called pre-implantation genetic diagnosis (PGD), in which fertilized embryos are tested for the disorder before implantation in the woman's uterus (17). Further refinement in this technology will become a powerful diagnostic tool in the assistive reproductive technology (ART) in the near future.

Individuals with the sickle cell disease have recurring episodes of intense pain; an increased susceptibility to infections, strokes and organ failure; and a lowered life expectancy. It is very imperative that predictive or preventive genetics and novel technologies can play a significant role in mitigating the sufferings of the affected persons. Further molecular studies are called for in such type of dizygotic twins that may provide new insight into this common genetic and health problem in India.

Conclusions

Both identical and fraternal twins allow us to determine the influence of genes and environment. Dizygotic twins with different sickle cell genotypes under similar environmental conditions manifest different clinical and hematological picture. It is a rare occasion, when a single pregnancy carries either two or more distinct (abnormal) genotypes at a time in a womb in human beings. Dizygotic twins are genetically different and, thus, provide means of appraisal of the expression of different genotypes under the same environment. The present study reports for the first time the occurrence of dizygotic twins (sickle cell trait and sickle cell disease or sickle cell disease and normal offspring) in a singleton pregnancy in the sickle cell carrier parents from Kalahandi and Kandhamal districts of Orissa, India.

ACKNOWLEDGMENTS

Author is grateful to Dr. VM Katoch, Secretary, Department of Health Research, Government of India and Director General, Indian Council of Medical Research, New Delhi for providing the necessary facilities. Thanks are also due to Mr. RK Mishra, Laboratory Technician for his support in the laboratory work.

REFERENCES

[1] Angastiniotis M, Modell B, Englezos P, Boulyzhenkov V. Prevention and control of hemoglobinopathies. Bull World Health Organ 1995;73:375-86.

[2] Balgir RS. Control and prevention of genetic load of hemoglobinopathies in India. Natl Med J India 1999;12:234-38.

[3] Balgir RS. Epidemiological study of sickle cell disease in western Orissa. Man India 1993;73:363-70.

[4] Balgir RS. The body mass index in sickle cell hemoglobinopathy. J Indian Anthropol Soc 1993;28:147-50.

[5] Balgir RS, Dash BP, Das RK. Fetal outcome and childhood mortality in offspring of mothers with sickle cell trait and disease. Indian J Pediatr 1997;64:79-84.

[6] Balgir RS. The burden of hemoglobinopathies in India and the challenges ahead. Curr Sci 2000;79:1536-47.

[7] Balgir RS. Health care strategies, genetic load, and prevention of hemoglobinopathies in tribal communities in India. South Asian Anthropologist 2004;4:189-98.

[8] Balgir RS. Spectrum of hemoglobinopathies in the state of Orissa, India: a ten years cohort study. J Assoc Phys India 2005;53:1021-26.

[9] Balgir RS. Genetic dimension of sickle cell hemoglobinopathy among five scheduled caste populations of Orissa, India. Indian Practr 2002;55:503-14.

[10] Balgir RS, Dash BP, Murmu B. Blood groups, hemoglobinopathy and G-6-PD deficiency investigations among fifteen major scheduled tribes of Orissa, India. Anthropologist 2004;6:69-75.

[11] Balgir RS. The spectrum of hemoglobin variants in two scheduled tribes of Sundargarh district in North-Western Orissa, India. Ann Hum Biol 2005;32:560-73.

[12] Amin BR, Bauersachs RM, Meiselman HJ, Mohandas N, Hebbel RP, Bowen PE, Schlegel RA, Williamson P, Westerman MP. Monozygotic twins with sickle cell anemia and discordant clinical courses: clinical and laboratory studies. Hemoglobin 1991;15:247-56.

[13] Weatherall MW, Higgs DR, Weiss H, Weatherall DJ, Serjeant GR. Genotype/phenotype relationships in sickle cell disease: a pilot twin study. Clin Lab Hemat 2005;27:384-90.

[14] Joishy SK, Griner PF, Rowley PT. Sickle ?-thalassemia: Identical twins differing in severity implicate nongenetic factors influencing course. Am J Hemat 1976;1:23-33.

[15] Dacie JV, Lewis SM. Practical hematology, 7th ed. Edinburgh: Churchill Livingstone, 1991:227-57.

[16] Weatherall DJ. Hematologic methods. In: Weatherall DJ, ed. Methods in hematology: Thalassemias. New York: Churchill Livingstone, 1983:27-53.

[17] Xu Kangpu, Shi Zhong Ming, Veeck Lucinda L, Hughes Mark R, Rosenwaks Zev. First unaffected pregnancy using preimplantation genetic diagnosis for sickle cell anemia. JAMA 1999;281:1701-6.

In: Rural child health: International aspects
Editors: Erica Bell and Joav Merrick

ISBN: 978-1-60876-357-3

Chapter 21

CHILDHOOD IMMUNIZATION IN UNGOGO, NORTHERN NIGERIA

Zubairu Iliyasu, MBBS, MPH, FWACP[1], Isa S Abubakar, MBBS, FWACP[1], Mohammed Kabir, MBBS, MSc, FWACP[1], Faisal Shuaib, MBBS, MPH[2] and Muktar H Aliyu, MD, DrPH[*3]

[1]Department of Community Medicine, Aminu Kano Teaching Hospital and Department of Community Medicine, Bayero University Kano, Nigeria

[2]Department of Epidemiology, University of Alabama at Birmingham, Birmingham, Alabama, United States of America

[3]Division of Preventive, Occupational and Aerospace Medicine, Mayo Clinic, Rochester Minnisota, United States of America

Childhood immunization is one of the most cost-effective public health interventions. This study assessed childhood immunization coverage and correlates for low vaccine uptake in northern Nigeria. Methods: A cluster sampling design was used to select 30 settlements from the study area. Survey data was collected using a pretested questionnaire administered to caregivers of 210 children ages 12 to 23 months. Results: Overall, 40.5% of the children were fully immunized having received a dose of BCG, three doses of OPV and DPT, and a dose of measles antigen. Thirty five percent and 24.5% of the children were partially and not immunized, respectively. The coverage rate for BCG was 64.8% in the study area. The coverage for DPT1, DPT2 and DPT3 were 47.1%, 44.8% and 41.0% respectively. The coverage for OPV0, OPV1, OPV2 and OPV3 were respectively 61.0%, 53.3%, 64.3% and 58.6%. Measles vaccine coverage was 61.4%. Significant predictors of a child's vaccination status were maternal and paternal education and place of birth. The major reasons for non-immunization included ignorance (29.2%), fear or misconceptions of side effects (16.9%), unavailability of vaccines (13.5%), travel (7.9%), and lack of awareness of the need for subsequent doses (7.5%). Conclusion: The low vaccine coverage requires innovative methods of vaccine delivery, strengthening of routine immunization and health education.

---

* Correspondence: Muktar Aliyu MD, DrPH, Division of Preventive, Occupational and Aerospace Medicine, Mayo Clinic, 200 First St., SW, Rochester MN 55905 United States. E-mail: mhaliyu@yahoo.com

INTRODUCTION

Five million children die in the developing world each year, and another five million are mentally or physically disabled due to the six-vaccine preventable diseases-namely diphtheria, pertussis, tetanus, measles, poliomyelitis and tuberculosis (1). Immunization of children is an important part of current preventive measures designed to improve child health and reduce such morbidity and mortality. It is considered to be among the most cost-effective public health interventions available (2). High levels of immunization coverage are required to prevent and control these vaccine-preventable diseases. Immunization coverage rates are considered a sensitive indicator of the health of a population and the capacity of a health system to deliver essential services (3) and their measurement is required to monitor programs and progress towards national immunization targets. If measured on an ongoing basis, coverage rates can be used to detect changes in the impact of immunization programs and identify under immunized subpopulations (3).

With a population of approximately 140 million (4) Nigeria remains Africa's most populous nation. Vaccine preventable diseases account for approximately 22% of child deaths in the country amounting to over 200,000 deaths per year (1). The Expanded Program on Immunization (EPI), responsible for routine immunization, started in the late 1970s. In 1990, DPT3 coverage in infants (<12 months of age) reached an estimated 56% (1). During the years following the global Universal Childhood Immunization efforts that culminated in 1990, immunization coverage rates in Nigeria declined significantly. In view of the critical need to reverse the decline and to reflect Federal Government ownership, the EPI program was re-named National Program on Immunization (NPI) in 1995. The Program recommends that a child should be given BCG, HBV1 and OPV0 at birth, OPV1, DPT1 at 6 weeks of age, OPV2, DPT2 and HBV2 at 10 weeks, OPV3, DPT3 at 14 weeks and Measles, Yellow fever, HBV3 and Vitamin A supplementation from 9-11 months. Preliminary results of a 2006 national coverage survey reported 36% DPT3 coverage and only 18% of children fully immunized (aged 12-23 months at survey time, using card + recall) (5). The survey results reveal significant differences across zones ranging from 0%-40% fully immunized children.

Although outstanding progress has been made towards interrupting the transmission of wild poliovirus globally, the situation in Nigeria remains a cause for serious concern because as at July 2006, Nigeria had 542 cases of wild poliovirus as compared to 302 cases for the same period in 2005, with intense transmission in northern Nigeria. The eleven northern states collectively contributed 956 (97.1 %) of the isolated viruses (5).

Kano state is located in northwest Nigeria and the state government suspended polio eradication initiative activities for a period of one year following controversies that the vaccine was contaminated with contraceptives and the human immunodeficiency virus. This led to suspicion and low uptake of childhood immunizations during routine and supplemental immunization activities. The objectives of the study were to determine childhood immunization coverage in Ungogo local government area of Kano state, Nigeria, identify reasons for non-vaccination and determine the effects of socio-demographic factors on childhood immunization uptake. Information obtained from the study will assist us in developing strategies for improving childhood immunization and hence decrease morbidity and mortality from vaccine preventable diseases.

OUR STUDY

Ungogo Local Government Area (LGA) is one of forty-four LGAs of Kano State, Nigeria. It has a projected population of 250,808 people (4). It is bounded to the north by Dawakin Tofa LGA, to the east by Minjibir, to the south by Nassarawa/Fagge and to the west by Gwale/Tofa LGAs respectively. Ungogo LGA has eleven health districts and forty-eight wards (settlements). The majority of the inhabitants are Hausa/Fulani, however other Nigerian tribes like Igbo, Yoruba and Ebira are also well represented.

The local government has eleven health centers, one each located in the eleven health districts. In addition, there is a general hospital and numerous health posts. The health facilities are fairly well staffed with nurses, midwives, community health extension workers and community health officers. The health care centers offer routine immunization services on Wednesdays and Fridays for the following antigens: BCG, DPT, OPV, TT and measles. The immunization record system comprises of tally books kept at the facilities and immunization cards, which are given to mothers.

Sampling and recruitment

We enrolled children aged 12-23 months who were resident in Ungogo LGA during the study period constituted the study population. A standard EPI cluster survey methodology (6-10) involving systematic sampling from a cumulative population list, was used for the study. The '30 × 7' cluster sampling method is recommended by WHO as a rapid, simplified and economic sampling method in assessment of vaccination coverage (11). Using this protocol, 30 clusters containing at least seven eligible children were selected in each settlement. This gave a sample size of 210 children. A listing of all the settlements in Ungogo LGA and their population was obtained, a cumulative population for the listed settlements computed, and systematic sampling technique was used to obtain 30 clusters. The settlement where a cluster fell constituted one of the sampled settlements. In each of these settlements, the center was located and balloting was used to determine the direction for the commencement of secondary sampling. All houses in this direction were listed and the first house to be surveyed was selected through balloting. Subsequently, all consecutive houses were entered to identify the presence of children between the ages of 12 to 23 months. Interviews were restricted to caregivers of children age 12-23 months to better reflect children who have reached the age by which they should be fully immunized.

Data collection

For each eligible child, information was obtained about vaccines received and the timeliness from immunization card when available or from mother's/caregiver's recall. Information on vaccination status was collected from vaccination cards shown to the interviewer and from mothers' verbal reports if no card was available. If the cards were available, the interviewers copied vaccination dates directly onto the questionnaire. If a vaccination card was presented but a vaccine had not been recorded on the card as having been given, the mother was asked to recall whether that particular vaccine had been given. The mother was then asked whether the child had received other vaccinations that were not recorded on the card, and if so, they too were noted on the questionnaire. If the mother was not able to provide a card for the child, she was asked to recall whether the child had received BCG, polio, DPT (including the number of doses for each), and measles vaccinations. The child's arm was also examined for evidence of BCG scar. Reasons for incomplete immunization were also elicited. This was done until at least seven eligible children were studied in each of the 30 sampled clusters.

According to the World Health Organization (WHO) (12) to be considered fully immunized, a child should receive a dose of BCG vaccine against tuberculosis at birth or soon after; three doses of DPT for the prevention of diphtheria, pertussis (whooping cough), and tetanus; at least three doses of polio vaccine; and a vaccination against measles. Regarding timeliness, DPT and polio vaccinations should be given at approximately 4, 8, and 12 weeks of age; there is also a dose of polio vaccine that should be given at birth. Measles vaccine should be given at or soon after the child reaches nine months. WHO further recommends that children receive the complete schedule of vaccinations before 12 months of age and that the vaccinations be recorded on a health card given to the parents or caretaker.

The Infant Immunization questionnaire was administered to mothers or caregivers of children in their second year of life i.e. between 12 and 23 completed months. This questionnaire was derived from the WHO EPI checklist (7). It covered enquiries about all antigens and times of administration. It used both recall and card as sources of information. In addition, it included items on payment for immunization services, immunization decision-making process as well as reasons for immunization failure.

Interviewers were twelve Hausa speaking medical students. They were divided into six teams of two students-one male and one female to facilitate access to mothers. Data collection took place over five days from the 7th through 13th September 2006. The principal author supervised the fieldwork. The supervisor scrutinized all questionnaires generated during the fieldwork and any discrepancies were clarified with the interviewers immediately.

Statistical analysis

Analyses were conducted using Epi-Info (Version 6) (CDC, Atlanta Georgia)(13). Chi-square test was used for to test for significance of association between categorical variables. Content analysis for common themes was used to evaluate open-ended questions about reasons for non-vaccination. Characteristics found to be significantly associated with vaccination coverage by bivariate analyses were entered into a multivariate logistic regression model to adjust for confounders and to determine which characteristics were independent predictors of vaccination status of the child. Two-sided significance tests were used and $p < 0.05$ was accepted as the level of statistical significance. A child was considered fully immunized if he/she received doses of the "standard six" antigens – BCG, diphtheria–pertussis-tetanus (DPT) (3 doses), polio (3 doses), and measles vaccines.

Ethical considerations

The provisions of the Helsinki declaration regarding human subjects research were adhered to (14). Institutional ethical clearance was obtained from the Aminu Kano Teaching Hospital, before the commencement of the study. Each head of household was informed that participation was completely voluntary and that no adverse action of any sort will result from non-response. Consent was obtained from each prospective mother/caregiver before commencement of interviews. Where possible, linkages with the local health centre enabled teams to provide information on how to improve utilization of services in the future.

OUR FINDINGS

The respondents were predominantly mothers (n=192, 91.4%), but also included other female caregivers (n=18, 8.6%). They were predominantly Muslims (97.6%) and belong to Hausa/Fulani (87.2%) ethnic group. More than half (50.5%) of the respondents were full time housewives. The rest were either petty traders (24.8%), civil servants (9.0%) or were engaged in other trades (15.7%).

One hundred and twenty one of the sampled children were males while 89 were females giving a male: female ratio of 4:3. Their ages ranged from 12 to 23 months with a mean age of 16?3.4 months. One fifth of the participants were the first-born of their mothers. The remaining children were 2nd (24.2%), 3rd (21.9%) or higher (33.9%) order births. Majority 113 (53.8%) of the sampled children were delivered in a hospital/health centre, while 97 (46.2%) were delivered at home. The source of routine vaccination service was hospital (78.0%), Primary health care centre (19.0%) and outreach centres (3.0%). Health cards were presented for 56.7% of children.

Immunization coverage

According to information from both the vaccination records and mothers' recall, 40.5% of the children were fully immunized, having received a dose of BCG, three doses of OPV and DPT, and a dose of measles antigen. Thirty five percent and 24.5% of the children were partially and not immunized respectively. For the individual antigens, the coverage rate for BCG was 64.8% in the local government area. Out of these, 84.6% of the children had verifiable scars suggesting a vaccine failure rate of 15.4%. The coverage for DPT1, DPT2 and DPT3 were 47.1%, 44.8% and 41.0% respectively. The coverage for OPV0, OPV1, OPV2 and OPV3 were respectively 61.0%, 53.3%, 64.3% and 58.6%. Measles vaccine coverage was 61.4%. Table 1 shows the coverage rates of all antigens on the National Program on Immunization schedule. Whereas 47.1% of children received DPT1, the proportion who go on to receive the third dose trends down to 41%; the dropout rate is thus 13%, much higher than the dropout rate of 4% for polio vaccine. In contrast, 30.4% more children received measles vaccine compared to DPT1.

Table 1. Childhood immunization indices in Ungogo LGA, Kano state, Nigeria, 2006 (n=210).'

S No.	Indicators	Percentage
1	Percentage of card retention	56.7%
2	Percentage coverage of BCG	64.8%
3	Percentage of BCG scar in those vaccinated with BCG (card and history)	84.6%
4	Percentage of BCG scar in those vaccinated with BCG (card only)	87.1%
5	Percentage coverage of DPT1	47.1%
6	Percentage coverage of DPT2	44.8%
7	Percentage coverage of DPT3	41.0%
8	Percentage coverage of OPV0	61.0%
9	Percentage coverage of OPV1	53.3%
10	Percentage coverage of OPV2	64.3%
11	Percentage coverage of OPV3	58.6%
12	Percentage coverage of Measles	61.4%
13	Percentage coverage of HBV1	58.6%
14	Percentage coverage of HBV2	17.2%
15	Percentage coverage of HBV3	45.2%
16	Percentage coverage of Yellow fever vaccine	25.7%
18	*Percentage difference in coverage between DPT1 and measles	-30.4%
19	*Percentage difference in coverage between DPT1 and DPT3	13.0%
20	*Percentage difference in coverage between OPV0 and OPV3	4.0%
21	Percentage of children fully immunized	40.5%

*Dropout rate = (Dose 1 – Dose 3) * 100/Dose 1

Immunization coverage by background characteristics

Table 2 presents vaccination coverage levels among children age 12-23 months by background characteristics, to provide an indication of the success of the vaccination program in reaching all subgroups of the population. The data show that the percentage of female children age 12-23 months who were fully immunized was almost one and a half times that of their male counterparts (49.4% versus 33.9%)[χ^2=5.2, P=0.02]. There were variations in percentage of children who received specific vaccinations by level of maternal and paternal education and place of birth. The proportion of fully immunized children showed a significant positive trend with maternal education. The percentage of fully immunized children increased by two-fold from 28% among mothers without formal education to 64.7% among mothers who had secondary education [χ^2_{trend} = 19.2, P<0.01]. A similar, but less dramatic change occurred with increasing father's education as shown in table II [χ^2_{trend} =15.3, P<0.01]. In addition, a significantly higher proportion of children born in the hospital were vaccinated compared with those born at home (55.8% versus 22.7%) [χ^2= 23.7, P<0.01]. The differential by birth order was not statistically significant.

A multivariate logistic regression model with variables that were significantly associated with vaccination coverage in the bivariate analysis included educational level of mother and father, child's gender, and place of birth. From this model, the significant predictors of vaccination of a child were educational level of father and mother and place of birth as shown in table 3.

Table 2. Association between immunization status and certain socio-demographic characteristics (n=210)

Characteristics	Vaccination status Fully vaccinated No.(%)	Not fully vaccinated No.(%)	χ^2	P value
Child's gender				
Male	41 (33.9)	80 (66.1)	5.2	0.02
Female	44(49.4)	45 (50.6)		
Mother's educational status			χ^2_{trend}	
Qur'anic only	21(28.0)	54(72.0)	19.2	0.00001
Primary school	33 (35.9)	59 (64.1)		
Secondary school	22 (64.7)	12 (35.3)		
Post-secondary school*	9 (100.0)	-		
Father's educational status			χ^2_{trend}	
Qur'anic only	22 (31.9)	47 (68.1)	15.3	0.0001
Primary school	22 (36.1)	39 (63.9)		
Secondary school	13 (32.5)	27 (67.5)		
Post-secondary school	28 (80.0)	7 (20.0)		
Place of birth			χ^2	
Home	22 (22.7)	75 (77.3)	23.7	0.0001
Hospital	63 (55.8)	50 (44.2)		
Birth order			χ^2	
1st child	19 (43.2)	25 (56.8)	0.17	0.68
2nd or higher order	66 (39.8)	100 (60.2)		

*This category was merged with secondary school while testing for association

Table 3. Predictors of full immunization among children in Ungogo LGA, Kano state, Nigeria, 2006 (n=210)

Predictor	Crude OR	Adjusted OR (95% CI)	P value
Child's gender			
Male*	1.0	Referent	-
Female	1.91	1.12(0.82-3.03)	0.42
Mother's education			
Qur'anic only*	1.0	Referent	-
Primary	1.44	1.40 (1.10-1.64)	0.02
Secondary or higher	6.64	2.41(1.78-3.15)	0.01
Father's education			
Qur'anic only*	1.0	Referent	-
Primary	1.21	1.06(1.02-2.21)	0.0001
Secondary or higher	8.55	3.07(1.76-6.72)	0.034
Place of birth			
Home*	1.0	Referent	-
Hospital	4.30	3.37 (1.94-7.84)	0.0001

Reasons for non-immunization

Altogether, 75.4% of children surveyed failed to complete or even start their primary immunization series. The reason given for non-immunization or partial immunization in the majority of cases (29.2%) was lack of awareness of the immunization programs in their locality. This was followed by unavailability of vaccines (13.5%), travel out of station (7.9%) and lack of awareness of the need for subsequent doses (7.5%). Other reasons given by 16.9% of mothers/caregivers included fear of side effects and misconceptions that vaccines could cause infertility and transmit the human immunodeficiency virus. Parents were also concerned that the vaccines they need (e.g., measles and BCG) were occasionally out of stock, while the polio vaccines were always available.

Table 4. Reasons for non-immunization among children of Ungogo LGA, Kano state, Nigeria, 2006 (n=210)

Reasons	Frequency No.(%)
Lack of awareness of the immunization programs in their locality	29.2%
Misconceptions that vaccines could cause infertility/transmit HIV	14.6%
Unavailability of vaccines	13.5%
Travel out of station	7.9%
Lack of awareness of the need for subsequent doses	7.5%
Father did not allow vaccination	7.1%
Child was ill	3.9%
Fear of side effects	2.3%
Others	4%

Discussion

This study found that 40.5% of the children in Ungogo local government area (LGA) were fully immunized. This rate is higher than Nigeria's national coverage rate of 18% (15). However, it is a far cry from the universal childhood immunization goal of 80% coverage (16). The coverage rate for individual antigens were generally low except for BCG (64.8%), polio (61.0%) and measles (61.4%) vaccines. Nevertheless, these coverage rates are still better than Nigeria's national coverage rates [BCG (48.3%), OPV0 (27.8%), Measles (35.9%) respectively] (17-20). Compared with previous studies, the current rates are better than an earlier report (17) from Panshekara village on the outskirts of Kano. The latter study found only 10% of children fully immunized. Elsewhere, only 7% of children in Sokoto (18) were fully immunized, while higher coverage rates of 44.6% and 72.2% were reported from rural Uganda (19) and India (20) respectively.

Three factors may be responsible for the comparatively better immunization coverage rate in Ungogo LGA. These include the urban nature of the LGA, higher maternal literacy level and introduction of a modified strategy of supplementary immunization activities, called immunization plus days (IPDs). The latter was a strategy to accelerate childhood immunization uptake in poliomyelitis high-risk states in northern Nigeria where this study was conducted. During such IPDs, OPV and other vaccines (e.g., measles vaccine and diphtheria-tetanus-pertussis vaccine for eligible children and tetanus toxoid vaccine for pregnant women) were offered at fixed vaccination posts, in addition to house-to-house delivery of OPV and vitamin A. In the targeted northern states, local government areas (LGAs) offered other health interventions when children were brought to vaccination posts. These interventions included distribution of soap, acetaminophen, oral rehydration salts, antihelminthics, and insecticide-treated bed nets. Additional modifications implemented as part of the IPDs were 1) holding community discussions to educate caregivers and address concerns before each round; 2) enhancing detailed SIA planning through involvement of local community leaders; 3) using qualified local health workers on the vaccination teams; and 4) enhancing field supervision by local, state, and federal authorities and through partner agencies (21).

Another point worthy of discussion is the possible impact of IPD recall on our findings. Typically vaccinations during supplementary campaigns are not documented on vaccination cards. The finding that OPV2 and OPV3 were higher than OPV1 is atypical and suggests documentation problems or recall bias due to confusion about campaign doses being recalled as routine doses by parents. In addition, OPV1, OPV2, OPV3 routine coverage should track DPT1, DPT2 and DPT3 coverage. The fact that OPV coverage was higher than DPT further supports our assertion that parents were mistakenly recalling IPD doses.

This study also observed a decreasing trend in coverage from one vaccine to the next in the NPI schedule of vaccinations. The relatively high BCG coverage of 64.8% indicates the initial enthusiasm of mothers and the advantage of being the first vaccine in the primary series given to the infant before discharge from hospital. It is particularly important in predicting immunization trends since it is given at birth (3,7). The coverage rate of 47.1% for DPT 1 provides a measure of access to immunization services. It represents the rate of voluntary immunization uptake, because it is the first vaccine dose that requires independent clinic visit after receiving BCG and OPV0 at birth before mother and child leave hospital (3,7). DPT3 coverage of 41% gives a measure of the performance of the health services. The conceptual basis for this is that personal factors that inhibit initial contact have been overcome to some extent when the first independent contact (for DPT1) is made. Subsequently, maintenance factors take pre-eminence in the decision to return for subsequent visits. These later factors include vaccine availability, effective program content communication, appropriate scheduling and health worker attitudes (3,7).

Another indicator of performance health system is the drop out rate- the proportional change of coverage rate over time (3,7). Two indicators assess immunization drop out, the percentage difference between DPT1 and DPT3 (13%) coverage and less frequently, between DPT1 and measles (30.4%). The negative dropout rate for DPT1-Measles is an indication that more mothers brought their children for measles vaccination compared to DPT1. This is not surprising as measles is of particular concern in Nigeria because of the high mortality and morbidity rate associated with the disease (21). The felt need for the vaccine among mothers and caregivers may explain the high uptake of measles vaccine relative to others. Drop out rates also give an estimate of health services performance. They estimate the quality of the services and aggregate such inputs as community knowledge and perceptions (indicator for effectiveness of health education), physical, cultural and economic access to the services (indicator for appropriateness of scheduling, location of immunization centre and logistic planning) and health worker attitudes (3,7). Weaknesses in the health system regarding routine immunization and concentration on provision of polio vaccines may be responsible. However, in addition to these institutional problems, the survey data show a strong positive correlation between mother's education, father's education and immunization coverage. For instance, the percentage of fully immunized children increased by two-fold from 28% among mothers without formal education to 64.7% among mothers who had secondary education. It has been consistently demonstrated that maternal education positively influences childhood immunization (17,18). A similar, but less dramatic change occurred with increasing father's education. This is not to say that there are no educated parents who rejected childhood immunization. The data on full immunization gave a mirror image of the relationship between educational levels and childhood immunization. Whereas the children of mothers with no formal education had the lowest level of full immunization (28%), the children of those with primary, secondary and tertiary education had progressively higher levels of coverage (35.9%, 64.7% and 100%).

Besides the effect of parental education, another factor that may affect levels of immunization in the study area is the process of household decision-making as it affects healthcare including immunization. Husband's refusal of childhood immunization was the reason for non-immunization in 7.1% of children. Furthermore, the Purdah (seclusion) system practiced in northern Nigeria restricts the movement of women outside the home. This limits access to health services in some households (22,23) and may affect place of delivery and uptake of immunization services.

The study had some limitations. First, although the WHO cluster sampling methodology used in this study is the standard in countries with scattered settlements, the coverage rates from such designs are less precise-10% precision with 95% certainty. Second, combining information from immunization cards with parental recall may overestimate coverage rates due to recall errors. Nevertheless, evidence from previous evaluation shows a high agreement (83%) between parental recall and immunization records (24). Finally, for respondents without formal education, questions were asked in local (Hausa) language, which may pose translation problems. This was minimized by standardizing the translation of common names of disease conditions and vaccines during training of interviewers. In addition, interviewers were Hausa speaking medical students who had specific training on the survey methodology.

Well-designed surveys can show which subgroups of the population are not getting immunized and why. Once this is known, special activities can be planned to immunize the missed children. The unimmunized may be difficult to reach or may belong to groups who traditionally do not use health services. These groups are frequently low in literacy skills so may not respond well to conventional methods of communication and health education, and may live in severely underprivileged conditions in remote areas or urban slums. Properly instructed young people represent a potentially potent group of educators, capable of reaching all parts of the community with information about immunization services. Promotion of girl child education and educating mothers and health workers on the timing of vaccination, their side effects and management might contribute to higher immunization coverage. There is a need to improve and strengthen the routine childhood immunization services rather than concentrate on supplemental immunization activities. Tracking systems are needed to ensure that children do not drop out of the system once they have begun the vaccination series. In addition, all children who are late in beginning their vaccination series are at increased risk of not completing the recommended vaccination series on time, and these children need intensive follow-up and recall efforts.

REFERENCES

[1] Yakubu AM. Current EPI coverage. Niger J Med 1995;9:11-3.

[2] Romanow RJ. Building on values: the future of health care in Canada. 2002. http://www.hc-sc.gc.ca/english/pdf/romanow/pdfs/HCC_Final_Report.pdf Accessed 05h Dec 2006.

[3] Bos E, Batson A. Using immunization coverage rates for monitoring health sector performance. Measurement and interpretations issues. World Bank HNP Discussion Papers, 2000.

[4] National Population Commission. National Census, Federal Republic of Nigeria. Preliminary results 2006.

[5] CDC. Progress toward poliomyelitis eradication-Nigeria, 2005-2006. MMWR 2007;56:278-81.

[6] WHO. Description and comparison of the methods of cluster sampling and lot quality assurance sampling to assess immunization coverage, Geneva, WHO/V&B/01.26 2001

[7] WHO. Expanded Program on Immunization Coverage Survey Manual (WHO/EPI/MLM/91.10)

[8] Cutts FT. The use of the WHO cluster survey method for evaluating the impact of the expanded program on immunization on target disease incidence. J Trop Med Hyg 1988;91:231-9.

[9] Henderson RH, Sundaresan T. Cluster sampling to assess immunization coverage: a review of experience with a simplified method. Bull World Health Organ 1982;60:253-60.

[10] Henderson RH. Assessment of vaccination coverage, vaccination scar rates, and smallpox scarring in five areas of West Africa. Bull World Health Organ 1973;48:183-94.

[11] Brogan D. Flagg EW. Deming M. Waldman R. Increasing the accuracy of the Expanded Program on Immunization's cluster survey design. Ann Epidemiol 1994;4:302-11.

[12] National Population Commission (NPC) [Nigeria] and ORC Macro. 2004. Nigeria Demographic and Health Survey 2003. Calverton, Maryland: National Population Commission and ORC Macro. 2004:169-72.

[13] Dean AG, Burton AH, Dicker RC. Epi Info Version 6. A word processing, database and statistics program for epidemiology on microcomputers, USD Incorporated, Stone Mountain, Georgia, 1999.

[14] Declaration of Helsinki. BMJ 1996;313:1148-49.

[15] http://www.who.int/vaccines accessed 4th May 2007.

[16] Expanded Program on Immunization. The EPI coverage survey: training for mid-level managers. Geneva, World Health Organization, 1991 WHO/EPI/MLM/91.10

[17] Kabir M, Iliyasu Z, Abubakar IS, Nwosuh J. Immunization coverage among children below two years of age in Panshekara, Kano state. Niger J Basic Clin Sci 2004;1:10-3.

[18] Okolo SN. immunization and nutritional survey of children in selected rural communities of Sokoto state. Niger J Paediatr 2003;30:12-5.

[19] Tugumisirize F, Tumwine J.K, Mworozi EA. Missed opportunities and caretaker constraints to childhood vaccination in a rural area in Uganda. East Afr Med J 2002;79:347-54.

[20] Bhatia V, Swami H.M, Rai S.R, Gulati S, Verma A, Parashar A, Kumari R. Immunization status of children. Indian J Pediatr 2004;71:313-5.

[21] Ambe J.P, Omotara B.A, Mandu B.M. Perceptions, beliefs and practices of mothers in sub-urban and rural areas towards measles and measles vaccination in northern Nigeria. Trop Doct 2001;31:89-90.

[22] Harrison K.A. Childbearing, health and social priorities: A survey of 22,774 consecutive hospital births in Zaria, Northern Nigeria. Br J Obstet Gynaecol 1985;92: 1-19.

[23] Wall L.L. Death mothers and injured wives: The social context of maternal morbidity among Hausa in northern Nigeria. Stud Fam Plann 1998; 29:4.

[24] Suarez L, Simpson DM, Smith DR. Errors and correlates in parental recall of child immunizations: effects on coverage estimates. Pediatrics 1997;99:3-5.

In: Rural child health: International aspects
Editors: Erica Bell and Joav Merrick
ISBN: 978-1-60876-357-3

Chapter 22

TRAUMATIC EVENTS AND DEPRESSIVE SYMPTOMS AMONG YOUTH IN SOUTHWEST NIGERIA

Olayinka Omigbodun, MBBS, MPH, FWACP*[*1]
Kofoworola Bakare, MBBS, MSc, FWACP[2]
and Bidemi Yusuf, PhD[3]
[1]Department of Psychiatry, College of Medicine, University of Ibadan, Ibadan
[2]Department of Paediatrics, Oyo State Ministry of Health, Ibadan
[3]Department of Epidemiology and Biostatistics,
College of Medicine, University of Ibadan, Nigeria

Traumatic experiences have dire consequences for the mental health of young persons. Despite high rates of traumatic experiences in some African cities there are no reports for Nigerian youth. Objective: To investigate the pattern of traumatic events and their association with depressive symptoms among youth in Southwest Nigeria. Methods: This is a descriptive cross-sectional study of randomly selected youth in urban and rural schools in Southwest Nigeria. They completed self-reports on traumatic events and depressive symptoms using the Street Children's Project Questionnaire and the Youth DISC Predictive Scale (DPS). Results: Of the 1,768 (88.4% response rate) responses entered into the analysis, 34% reported experiencing a traumatic situation. Following interpretative phenomenological analysis, 13 themes emerged. Frequently occurring traumatic events were 'road traffic accidents' (33.0%), 'sickness' (17.1%), 'lost or trapped' (11.2%) and 'armed robbery attack' (9.7%). A bad dream was described by 3.7%. Traumatic experiences were commoner in males (36.2%) than females (31.6%) (χ^2=4.2; p=0.041). Experiencing a traumatic event was associated with depressive symptoms (χ^2=37.98; p<0.001) especially when the event directly affected the youth as in sexual assault or physical abuse. Conclusions: A third of youth in Southwest Nigeria have described an experienced traumatic event. Road traffic accidents, armed robbery attacks and communal disturbances depict the prevailing social environment, while 'bad dreams' revealed the influence of cultural beliefs. Policy makers need to be aware of social issues impacting the health of youth. Multi-agency interventions to improve the social environment and provide mental health services for traumatised young people are essential.

* Correspondence: Olayinka Omigbodun, Department of Psychiatry, University College Hospital, Ibadan, Nigeria. Tel: 234-2-7503880; E-mail: fouryinkas@yahoo.co.uk

INTRODUCTION

Experiencing traumatic events is associated with a wide variety of psychopathology such as depression, anxiety and post traumatic stress disorder (1). In addition, behavioural problems and poor school performance leading to negative effects on functioning as adults are also consequences of traumatic exposure in youth, (2).

Surveys carried out in several western countries revealed that 20-87% of young people are exposed to trauma before adulthood (2-4). High rates of traumatic experiences have been reported among youth in some African cities. Using the Children's Posttraumatic Stress Disorder Inventory, Peltzer (6), in a study of 148 rural children aged 6-16 years found that 67% had experienced traumatic events. In Cape Town, South Africa, Suliman et al (7), determined exposure to traumatic events in 54 school children aged 16-18 years by interview with the Kiddie Schedule for Affective Disorders and Schizophrenia for School Age Children and also by self report using the Child and Adolescent Trauma Survey. Based on interviews, 86% reported experiencing a traumatic event while a higher proportion (91%) indicated experiencing a traumatic event by self-report. In a comparative study of 2,014 adolescents in public and private urban schools in South Africa and Kenya who completed anonymous self-reports using the Trauma Checklist, more than 80% reported exposure to severe trauma with the rates in Kenya being slightly higher (85%) than in South Africa (83%) (8).

Gender is an important factor influencing traumatic exposure. Some studies report similar rates of violent exposure for males and females but with males being more likely to experience physical assault and females' sexual assault (2,9). Other studies report males having more exposure to violence than females, but with both genders having equal amounts of exposure to violence from family members and males having a greater exposure to violence from friends (5).

Depressive symptoms have been closely associated with traumatic experiences both as a risk for and a sequel (5). There are also suggestions that youth who experience violence against self are more likely to have depressive symptoms than those who experience violence to strangers (10).

Nigeria is a delicate union of over 250 different ethnic groups; it has a young democracy and over 70% of its peoples live in dire poverty (11). It has one of the highest road traffic accident rates in the world (12), there are daily reports of armed robbery (13), and frequent reports of religious and communal strife (11). Despite these social issues there are few reports on the mental health implications of these traumatic events and there is virtually no information on the rates or types of exposure to traumatic events in Nigerian youth.

Qualitative research had been known to be useful for the study of un- researched areas because it allows for the discovery of unexpected issues, themes and topics that would have been invisible if a fixed design or questionnaire were used. This study uses both qualitative and quantitative methods to examine the rate and pattern of traumatic exposure, the relationship between traumatic experiences, socio demographic factors and depressive symptoms in urban and rural youth in secondary schools in Southwest Nigeria. It is hoped that with the identification and documentation of the types, rates and circumstances of traumatic experiences, prevention strategies could be developed.

OUR STUDY

Ibadan and its environs, consisting of five urban and six rural districts are located in Southwest, Nigeria. The target population for this study included all students in secondary schools in the 11 rural and urban districts in Ibadan and its environs. All classes (Grade 7-12) were included in the study. This study on traumatic experiences in youth was just one aspect of a health study on adolescents in secondary schools.

Study design and population

A descriptive cross-sectional study was carried out. Based on an estimated prevalence of mental health problems of 20%, a minimum sample size of 1,345 students was required and this was increased to 2000 to accommodate for non response or incomplete questionnaires. A multistage random sampling procedure was used and five districts were selected, three urban nd two rural.

There were 101 schools from the five randomly selected districts and, using probability proportional to size, 20 schools were selected. Four rural public schools (there were no private schools in the rural districts selected), 10 urban public and six urban private schools. Public schools are government owned and tuition is free while private schools students pay fees. Based on rural-urban school population ratio, the sample of 2000 was divided into 70% urban and 30% rural which translated into 1400 students from urban schools and 600 students from rural schools. Information about the total number of students in each school, number in each class and ratio of boys to girls was used to select the students that would be involved in the study in each school.

Procedure, instruments and measures

The Ethical Committee, Oyo State Ministry of Health, Ibadan gave approval for the study. A few days before the administration of the instruments, the schools were visited and students were chosen from each class by random sampling. A consent form explaining the purpose and procedure of the study was available in both the local language (Yoruba) and English for both parent/guardian and student to sign (or thumb print) if they agreed to participate.

On the set day for administration of the instruments, the selected students assembled in classrooms and were reassured of confidentiality. All questionnaires had been translated to the local language, Yoruba using the back translation method. Every student was given the option to choose either an English or Yoruba questionnaire. However to reduce any language differences, each question was read aloud in both English and Yoruba by the researchers and the students completed questionnaires privately on their own. This process took about two hours and the youth had breaks in between for refreshments. The administration of the questionnaire was done in both languages because even though the language of instruction in secondary schools is English, Yoruba is the mother tongue and school pupils in this environment are bilingual. Data was collected between January and March 2004. The instruments were pre-tested in November 2003 on adolescents in a public school and were found to be acceptable.

For 95 pupils, consent was not obtained or they were absent from school on the day questionnaires were completed. Thirty two questionnaires was inadequately completed and removed from the analysis, while 104 pupils did not answer the questions on traumatic experiences.

Instruments and measures

The socio-demographic section of the questionnaire obtained information such as gender, age, religion, marital status of parents, occupation and level of education of parents.

World Health Organisation, Street Children Project, Major Life Events Questionnaire (14) was used to obtain information about traumatic events experienced by the youth. The students were given the opportunity to self report events and answer to the following questions in their own words: "Have you ever been in a situation when you were afraid you would lose your life or be severely harmed? Yes or No. If yes, please describe……." This method allowed unknown themes to emerge from this group of Nigerian youth in secondary schools.

DPS 432 NON-SKIP YOUTH {Diagnostic Interview Schedule for Children (DISC) Predictive Scales} (15) is a diagnostically based screening instrument administered by the youth. It is designed to give an indication of the likelihood of 14 different diagnosis using the Diagnostic and Statistical Manual (Version 4) criteria. It comprises of approximately 106 questions. The questions to identify depressive symptoms are as follows.

In the last one year:

1. Has there been a time when nothing was fun for you and you just were not interested in anything?
2. Has there been a time when you had less energy than you usually do?
3. Has there been a time when you felt you couldn't do anything well or that you weren't as good-looking or as smart as other people?
4. Has there been a time when you thought seriously about killing yourself?
5. Have you tried to kill yourself in the last year?
6. Has there been a time when doing even little things made you feel really tired?
7. Has there been a time when you couldn't think as clearly or as fast as usual?

There are seven depressive symptoms and a cut-off score of five or more positive answers is suggestive of a DSM-IV diagnosis of depression (15) or 'probable depression'. This study did not seek to make a diagnosis of a major depressive episode but to identify depressive symptoms among the youth. In this study a respondent who had five or more positive answers to the questions of depression was regarded as having Depressive Symptomatology.

Data analysis

Initial analysis of data was qualitative using interpretative phenomenological analysis (16). The statements describing the traumatic events the respondents felt put their life in danger or would cause them to be severely harmed, were read repeatedly and coded to identify emergent and recurrent themes which were discussed and agreed upon by the researchers.

The themes which emerged as traumatic experiences from interpretative phenom enological analysis were given codes and analysed with the other data using the Statistical Package for the Social Sciences (Version 10). Frequency tables and bar charts were generated for relevant variables. Descriptive statistics such as means and standard deviations were used to summarize continuous variables, while categorical variables were summarized with percentages.

OUR FINDINGS

Socio-demographic characteristics

Of the study sample, 1,768 (88.4%) responses were entered into the final analysis, 464/600 (73.8%) and 1,304/1,400 (93.1%) of the rural and urban sample respectively. There were 933 (52.8%) males and 835 (47.2%) females represented from all grades in high school (Grades 7 to 12). The mean age of the study population was 15.2 years (SD: 2.5years) and 19.4% were aged 18-24years. (See table one)

Table 1. Socio-demographic characteristics N=1,768

CHARACTERISTICS	N (%)
AGE (years)	
10-17	1425 (80.6)
18-25	343 (19.4)
GENDER	
Male	933 (52.8)
Female	835 (48.2)
RELIGION (3 missing)	
Islam	571 (32.4)
Christian	1194 (67.6)
MARITAL STATUS OF PARENTS (21 missing)	
Married	1372 (78.5)
Separated/Divorced	192 (11.0)
Father dead	146 (8.4)
Mother dead	31 (1.8)
Orphan	6 (0.3)
No formal Education	163 (9.2)
Koranic School	23 (1.3)
Primary School	323 (18.3)
Secondary School	481 (27.2)
Post-secondary Non-university	159 (9.0)
University Degree	276 (15.6)
Does not know/Did not indicate	343 (19.4)

Traumatic events

Six hundred and two youth (34%) reported being in situations where 'they were afraid they would lose their life or be severely harmed' and 545 described the specific traumatic events they had experienced. Thirteen (13) themes emerged as traumatic situations (see table 2).

Table 2. Traumatic experiences N=545

TYPE OF TRAUMATIC EXPOSURE n (%)
Car and other Road Traffic Accidents 180 (33.0) 'I was in a bus and the brake failed, I thought I had died but God took control' 'I had a very fatal car accident and I broke seven of my teeth and I was bleeding continuously'
Health Problem/ Sickness 93 (17.1) 'It was the period I came up with malaria and was not quickly treated' 'I was urinating blood'
Lost or trapped, 61 (11.2) 'I went somewhere alone and without my parents permission and I could not find my way back until eleven o 'clock in the night because of petrol scarcity' 'I went to one of my friend's place and found out the they were doing rituals to make money'
Armed robbers or Assassins 53 (9.7) 'The day thieves came into our house and placed the gun on my ear' 'When assassins wanted to kill my Dad'
Injury while working or playing 41 (7.5) 'I cut myself with a cutlass while cutting grass in school' 'When my nose cut, I thought I may lose my life'
Riots and Communal strife 32 (5.9) 'It was during the Sharia riots in Kano' 'When some cult groups were fighting and a lot of bullets were shot'
Bad thoughts and dreams 20 (3.7) 'Because my aunty died on my birthday and I had a dream that told me because of the date she died, I will also die' 'When I was sleeping, I had a very bad dream'
Water related incidents, almost drowning 19 (3.5) 'I nearly got drowned at the bar beach' 'A heavy rain fell and the drainage was blocked with refuse and so it resulted in flood disaster and property and goods were destroyed'.
Attack by dangerous animals 11 (2.0) 'A dog bit me' 'I was in danger with two wild dogs'
Death of a loved one 10 (1.8) 'That was when my father died' 'When my mother died'
Sexual assault 9 (1.7) 'The day I was raped' 'When I went to my brother's friend he tried to rape me'
Physical abuse 9 (1.7) 'My mother does not know how to deal with kids, she had a hot temper and so she once hit my head with a pestle' 'The day my grandmother stripped me naked and beat me for something I did not do'
Fire disasters 7 (1.3) 'The day my mummy's shop got burnt' 'The day our generator got fire'

Frequently occurring traumatic experiences were road traffic accidents (33.0%), sickness (17.1%), lost or trapped (11.2) and attack by armed robbers or assassins (9.7%). Others were riots and communal strife, bad thoughts or dreams, sexual assault, physical abuse and fire disasters.

Traumatic experiences and socio-demographic variables

Association between trauma, and socio demographic variables were investigated. Exposure to traumatic events was reported equally (34%) by students in urban and rural schools. More males (36.2%) than females (31.6%) reported exposure to traumatic events [χ^2=4.2; p = 0.041]. All who reported sexual assault were females (p<0.001) and a higher proportion of females reported a health problem as life threatening (p=0.013).

Table 3. Gender differences in reported traumatic experiences

Type of traumatic exposure reported	Gender Differences N=545		
	Male N=304 n %	Female N=241 n %	p
Armed robbers; Assassins n=53	30 (9.9)	23 (9.5)	0.889
Road traffic accidents n=180	103 (33.9)	77 (32.0)	0.634
Riots and Communal strife n=32	22 (7.2)	10 (4.1)	0.128
Attack by dangerous animals n=11	9 (3.0)	2 (0.8)	0.123**
Health problem; physical sickness n=93	41 (13.5)	52 (21.6)	0.013*
Injury while working or playing n=26	26 (8.6)	15 (6.2)	0.306
Lost, kidnapped, trapped n=61	37 (12.2)	24 (10.0)	0.416
Almost drowning n=19	15 (4.9)	4 (1.7)	0.038*
Death of a loved one n=10	5 (1.6)	5 (2.1)	0.756**
Bad thoughts and dreams n=20	10 (3.3)	10 (4.1)	0.596
Sexual assault n=9	--	9 (3.7)	0.001***
Physical abuse n=9	3 (1.0)	6 (2.5)	0.193**
Fire disasters n=7	3 (1.0)	4 (1.7)	0.704**

* Statistically significant at 5% level; **= fisher's exact test

Traumatic situations and depressive symptoms

Depressive symptomatology was reported in 28.1% of those who had been in traumatic situations and 15.6% who reported not being exposed to a traumatic event (χ^2 = 37.98; p < 0.001).

For respondents reporting no depressive symptoms, 24.3% reported experiencing a traumatic event. For those reporting 3 depressive symptoms, 32.7% experienced a traumatic event and this proportion increased to 44.2% and 63.2% for respondents reporting five and six depressive symptoms respectively (χ^2 =64.9; p<0.001).

Fifty percent or more of respondents who reported sexual assault, animal attack or physical abuse had depressive symptomatology while none of the respondents who reported experiencing a fire disaster had this (see figure 1).

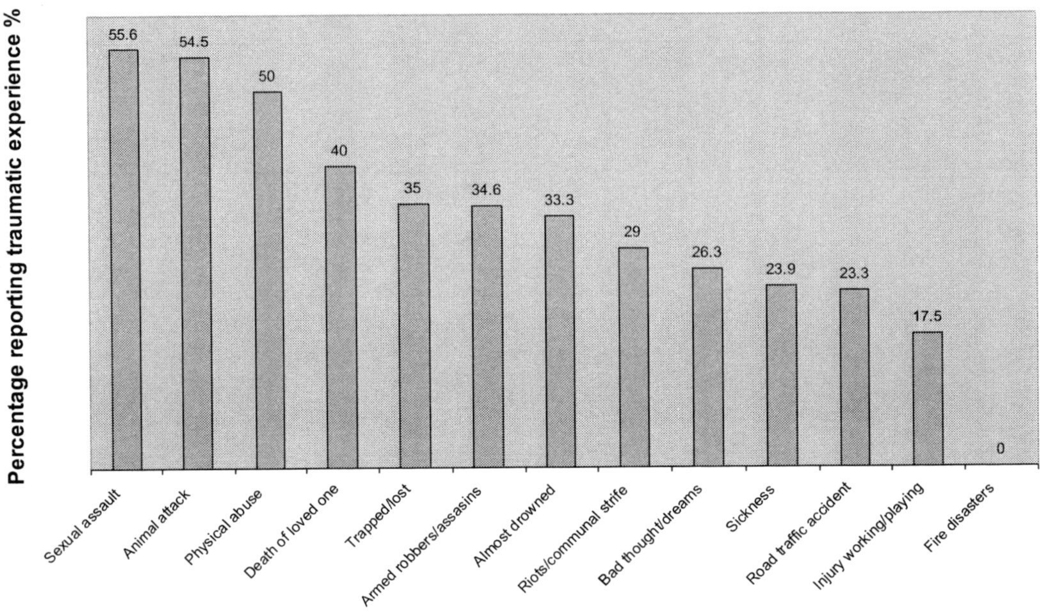

Figure 1. Proportion of students in Each Category of Traumatic Experience with Depressive Symptomatology N=545.

DISCUSSION

The rate of trauma obtained in this study (34%) was lower than rates found in other African studies (67-91%) (6-8), but falls within the range obtained in studies of traumatic experiences of adolescents and young people in the USA (20-40%). Differences in the methods used to elicit for traumatic experiences would account for this difference. In this study, situations where the youth felt they would lose their life or be severely harmed were inquired about thereby eliciting information only about 'direct' and serious traumatic experiences. No examples of traumatic experiences were given to these youth and the response depended solely to the youth's understanding of situations where they 'felt they would lose their lives or be severely harmed' and their memory for these events. This qualitative method was used to identify 'traumatic' themes within this population of Nigerian youth.

The African studies (6-8) used questionnaires to identify both 'direct' and 'indirect' traumatic experiences. A clear illustration of the differences in rates obtained by 'direct' and 'indirect' traumatic experience can be found in the South African community study (20), where all students (100%) reported exposure to indirect violence and just 56% had experienced direct trauma. The comparative study of adolescents in Nairobi, Kenya and Cape Town, South Africa (8), which found trauma exposure rates of 85% and 83% respectively utilised the Trauma Checklist which identifies direct and indirect traumatic experiences. In contrast to these studies, a rate of 35.1% similar to what was obtained in this study was found in a National telephone study of 2,000 adolescents in the USA when all that was elicited was direct traumatic experience (17). The differences in direct and indirect rates of traumatic experiences are again illustrated in a study of 337 New York public school students (5), which investigated six violent events happening to the student (direct) or to their family members, friends or strangers (indirect). The breakdown of the various violent events revealed that direct exposure rates (7.62% were shot or stabbed, 7.62% raped and 21.65% were beaten up) were much lower than indirect rates (18.29% observed violence against family, 29.29% violence against friends and 43.29% observed violence against strangers).

From the 13 themes that emerged, events that were traumatic to these Nigerian youth were depicted such as road traffic accidents, armed robbery, ethnic, political and religious riots. They were described by these young minds as traumatic and clearly portray the social environment (11). The unending battle with communicable diseases such as malaria is reflected. Physical abuse is amply illustrated by a youth, who was stripped naked by a grandmother and caned publicly. Corporal punishment is used freely and openly on youth in Nigeria both for minor violations and major misdemeanors. A study of children attending a psychiatric clinic revealed that 7.9% had experienced various forms of abuse including beatings with belts and rods with evidence on their bodies (21).

Despite these traumatic expressions which reflect the social atmosphere, the themes (car accidents, fire incidents, violent crime, physical abuse, sexual assault) are similar to the reported traumas as found in the commonly used measures such as the K-SADS, Trauma Survey and the (CATS) Child and Adolescent Trauma Survey (CATs) (6-8) with the exception of 'dreams'. In the culture of the Southwest of Nigeria where the study is carried out, dreams are regarded as a sign or symbol and a bad dream is interpreted as a bad sign (22). Should bad dreams be seen as a traumatic experience? This traumatic experience emerging from within the young person is worth investigating.

Several studies clearly illustrate gender differences in traumatic experiences as found in this study (5). Fitzpatrick and Boldizar (23) in a study of African-American youth found that males were more likely than females to be victims of and witnesses to violent acts. In the study of youth in two African cities, Nairobi and Cape Town, Seedat et al (8), also found that males had a higher mean number of trauma exposures, were more likely to be physically assaulted or threatened, witness riots and report sexual assault than girls. It is not exactly clear why this study of African youth found more of sexual assault among males because most other studies have found higher rates of sexual assault in females as found in this study (2,5,9).

In this study, the highest rates of depressive symptoms were associated with sexual assault; animal attack and physical abuse, all direct and personal attacks on the self. None of the youth who reported fire incidents had depressive symptoms. This is similar to the findings of Seedat et al (8) where sexual and physical assault by someone in the family were associated with depressive symptoms and reporting natural disasters was not associated with psychopathology. Similarly Martinez and Richters (10) explored the relationship between exposure to violence and depression among 54 early adolescents and found that violence against self or someone close to the students was significantly associated with depressive symptoms whereas witnessing violence against a stranger had no correlation with depressive symptoms. The association between traumatic experiences and depressive symptoms is further substantiated in this study with the increase in the proportion of those who suffered traumatic experience as there is an increase in the number of depressive symptoms present.

This study has demonstrated that over a third of youth in Southwest Nigeria had witnessed a direct and severe traumatic event. The types of traumatic experiences are similar to 'direct' traumatic experiences as described in other measures with the exception of 'bad dreams' which can be described as 'internally' generated traumatic experience these young people experienced.

Limitations to this study include eliciting information about life threatening experience relying solely on the youth's understanding, concept of danger and memory. If specific examples had been given to the youth, the rates may have been higher. It is also likely that the youth had experienced several traumatic experiences but would only describe the most terrifying or that which came readily to their minds. Also 5% (104/2,000) of the study population did not respond to the questions of traumatic experiences and the reasons for this were not given since the questionnaires were self-reports. No information was obtained from parents and caregivers. However previous studies suggest that parents may not be aware of all their children's traumatic experiences and that youth reported high threat life events are more valid than those reported by parents (24). This study has also relied solely on retrospective reports which are known to underestimate levels of traumatic events. These may further account for the lower rate obtained.

Nevertheless a relatively large sample of young people representing all strata of the Nigeria secondary school youth, rural, public urban and private urban was used to explore an un –researched area. In planning interventions in this environment the voices of these young people need to be heard. Improvements in the social environment should be important priorities for the policy makers to improve the health of the populace. Also in planning for mental health services, the needs of traumatised youth should be addressed.

ACKNOWLEDGMENT

We thank Drs. Yomi Esan, Folorunsho Nuhu, Kunle Adesokan, and the Oyo State Ministry of Health, School Health Nurses, for their assistance with data collection.

REFERENCES

[1] Brown ES, Fulton MK, Wilkeson A, Petty F. The psychiatric sequelae of civilian trauma. Compr Psychiatry 2000;41(1):9-23.

[2] Gwadz MV, Nish D, Leonard NR, Strauss SM. Gender differences in traumatic events and rates of post-traumatic stress disorder among homeless youth. J Adoles 2007;30(1):117-29.

[3] Amir M, Sol O. Psychological impact and prevalence of traumatic events in a student sample in Israel: the effect of multiple traumatic events and physical injury. J Trauma Stress 1999;12(1):139-54.

[4] Elklit A. Victimization and PTSD in a Danish national youth probability sample. J Am Acad Child Adolesc Psychiatry 2002; 41(2):174-81.

[5] Moses A. Exposure to violence, depression, and hostility in a sample of inner city high school youth. J Adoles 1999;22(1):21-32.

[6] Peltzer K. Posttraumatic stress symptoms in a population of rural children in South Africa. Psychol Rep 1999;85(2):646-50.

[7] Suliman S, Kaminer D, Seedat S, Stein DJ. Assessing post-traumatic stress disorder in South African adolescents: using the child and adolescent trauma survey (CATS) as a screening tool. Ann Gen Psychiatry 2005;4(1):2.

[8] Seedat S, Nyamai F, Njenga F, Vythilingum B, Stein DJ. Trauma exposure and post-traumatic stress symptoms in urban African schools. Survey in Cape Town and Nairobi. Br J Psychiatry 2004; 184:169-75.

[9] Traut A, Kaminer D, Boshoff D, Seedat S, Hawkridge S, Stein DJ. Treatment utilisation and trauma characteristics of child and adolescent inpatients with posttraumatic stress disorder. Curationis 2002;25(4):67-72.

[10] Martinez P, Richters JE. The NIMH community violence project: children's distress symptoms associated with violence exposure. Psychiatry 1993;56(1):22-35.

[11] Internal Displacement Monitoring Centre (IDMC) Nigeria: Heightened risk of violence and displacement ahead of 2007 elections. A profile of the internal displacement situation. www.internal-displacement.org (Retrieved September 21, 2007)

[12] Thanni, LOA, Kehinde, OA. Trauma at a Nigerian teaching hospital: pattern and documentation of presentation. Afr Health Sci 2006; 6(2):100-7.

[13] Ehikhamenor, EE, Ojo, MA. Comparative analysis of traumatic deaths in Nigeria. Prehos Disaster Med 2002;20(3):197-201.

[14] World Health Organisation. Programme on substance abuse, World Health Organisation, Street Children Project. Description and implementation methodology. Geneva: WHO, 1994.

[15] Lucas C P, Zhang H, Fisher P W, et al. The DISC predictive scales (DPS): Efficiently screening for diagnoses. J Am Acad Child Adolesc Psychiatry 2001;40:443-9.

[16] Shaw RL. Why use interpretative phenomenological analysis in Health Psychology? Health Psych Update 2001;10(4):48-52.

[17] Boney-McCog S, Finkelhor D. Psychosocial sequelae of victimization in a national youth sample. J Consult Clinic Psych 1995;63(5):726-36.

[18] Breslau N, Davis GC, Andreski P, Peterson E. Traumatic events and posttraumatic stress disorder in an urban population of young adults. Arch Gen Psychiatry 1991;48(3):216-22.

[19] Giaconia RM, Reinherz HZ, Silverman AB, Pakiz B, Frost AK, Cohen E. Traumas and posttraumatic stress disorder in a community population of older adolescents. J Am Acad Child Adolesc Psychiatry 1995;34(10):1369-80.

[20] Ensink K, Robertson BA, Zissis C, Leger P. Post-traumatic stress disorder in children exposed to violence. S Afr Med J 1997; 87:1526-30.

[21] Omigbodun OO. Psychosocial issues in a child and adolescent psychiatric clinic population in Nigeria. Soc Psych Psychiatr Epidemiol 2004;39(8):667-72.

[22] Fanilola K. Dreams in Yoruba Worldview. http://www.yoruba.org (Retrieved February 2 2007)

[23] Fitzpatrick KM, Boldizar JP. The prevalence and consequences of exposure to violence among African-American youth. J Am Acad Child Adolesc Psychiatry 1993;32(2):424-30.

[24] Sandberg S, Rutter M, Pickles A, McGuinness D, Angold A. Do high-threat life events really provoke the onset of psychiatric disorder in children? J Child Psychol Psychiatry 2001;42 (4):523-32.

In: Rural child health: International aspects
Editors: Erica Bell and Joav Merrick

ISBN: 978-1-60876-357-3

Chapter 23

HYPERANDROGENISM AND OBESITY

Amit M Deokar*, MD, MPH, Shawn J Smith, MD, Amanda J Goodwin, PA-C and Hatim A Omar, MD
Division of Adolescent Medicine, Department of Pediatrics, University of Kentucky, Lexington, Kentucky, United States of America

This chapter has a two-fold objective. One, it addresses the association of hyperandrogenism and obesity and the complex metabolic derangements that are part of the problem. Clinical management of these co-morbidities is challenging and complex. Second, this chapter will aid health care providers with the key features to an early diagnosis and intervention to decrease the morbidities in the short as well as long term. Method: Systematic review of articles and information on the topic of interest that were published in the last 15 years. Conclusion: Obesity and hyperandrogenism are integral parts of Metabolic Syndrome/Polycystic Ovarian Syndrome (PCOS)/Hyperandrogenism, Insulin resistance, and Acanthosis Nigricans (HAIR-AN). With the childhood obesity epidemic, the metabolic syndrome and the associated abnormalities are routinely seen in clinical practice and these have a tremendous economic burden on the society and the quality of life.

INTRODUCTION

Obesity in children and adolescents has increased at an alarming rate in the last two decades. Over the years, researchers have acquired a better understanding about the strong association of obesity in metabolic syndrome (MS, previously known as metabolic syndrome X) (1). Patients with MS have various metabolic abnormalities that can include abnormal glucose and insulin ratio, insulin resistance, high blood pressure, altered lipid profile, pro-thrombotic and pro-inflammatory state. Teenagers with MS are predisposed to long term morbidities, such as early coronary artery disease, hepatic steatosis, type 2 diabetes, and stroke (1). Evidence

* Correspondence: Assistant professor Amit M Deokar, MD, MPH, Department of Pediatrics, Room J422, University of Kentucky, Lexington, KY 40536-0284 United States. E-mail: amit-deokar@uky.edu

suggests that an overweight teenager has an 80 percent chance of continuing to be overweight in the adult life (2).

Approximately 17 percent of children aged 2-19 years are considered overweight based on a survey by National Health and Nutrition Examination Survey of 2003-2004 (3). As noted earlier, the rate of obesity has doubled in adolescents, who are in the 12-19 year age group (4). The prevalence of obese and overweight children may be different depending on the gender and ethnicity. For example, the obesity rates are higher in African Americans, Hispanic Americans, males, and those living in the southern states (2). The definition of obesity varies in adolescents when compared to adults due to different proportion of body fat in boys and girls at different ages (5). Body Mass Index (BMI) is a reliable tool to assess obesity, because it is easy to obtain and correlates well with the body fat (6). Any adolescent with a BMI of 30 kg/m2 or 95th percentile for gender and age falls in the overweight category. They are considered at risk of being overweight if their BMI is between 85th and = 95th percentile. In the US, the economic burden of direct and indirect healthcare cost due to obesity and co-morbidities is estimated to be well over $ 117 billion annually. As the obesity rates have doubled and tripled respectively in children and adolescents, so have the health care costs (7). This impacts the healthcare burden directly.

Obesity and hyperandrogenism (HA) are strongly associated in patients who have been diagnosed to have polycystic ovarian syndrome (PCOS)/HA/MS. This article addresses their relationship with one another and specific management options. A subset of (PCOS) includes hyperandrogenism, insulin resistance and acanthosis nigricans, abbreviated as HAIR-AN (8,9). Historically PCOS was described based on findings of multiple cysts in the ovaries, irregular or no menstrual periods, and hirsuitism. However, absence of ovarian cysts does not rule out this syndrome (10). Women with high androgen levels have associated HAIR-AN features in about 5-10 percent of cases (11). The onset of PCOS/HAIR-AN may occurs in adolescent years and the diagnosis is likely to be delayed until early adulthood (8,9).

PATHOPHYSIOLOGY

As PCOS/HAIR-AN is being studied more over the last two decades, different theories have been proposed to explain the features of the syndrome, including obesity. The primary problem in HA appears to be due to an altered hypothalamo-pituatary-ovarian axis. The anovulation and thus abnormal or absence of menstrual periods is from a persistent leutenizing hormone (LH) surge and its high concentration in the blood. There is also an increased GnRH surge as the negative feedback from estrogen and progesterone is ineffective due to relative hypothalamic insensitivity. The LH surge results in increased production of androgens. The level of follicle stimulating hormone (FSH) is less when compared to the LH resulting in decreased enzymatic (aromatase) conversion of androgen to estrogen and thus anovulation.

Another key association of HA is hyperinsulinsm. This is due to peripheral insulin resistance, which can result in a hyperglycemic state. The level of sex hormone binding globulin (SHBG) is decreased due to the high insulin levels and consequently there is a rise in the free testosterone level (8). Insulin also increases the androgen production by directly stimulating the theca cells (12). Both hyperinsulinism and HA predispose an individual to have an athrogenic lipid profile. Total cholesterol, triglycerides (TG) levels are also elevated. Increased activity of the enzyme lipase affects the cholesterol metabolism and could result in a decreased level of the high density lipoprotein-cholesterol (HDL-C) (13). Another postulated mechanism for HAIR-AN is a genetic mutation of the insulin receptor (tyrosine kinase domain) (9).

Effects of HA can be multi-fold. Even though increased androgen production in women is associated with obesity, one study in 2002 by Gapstur et al (14) in obese men have found to have lower testosterone and dehydroepiandroterone sulfate (DHEAS) levels. High androgen levels in children and adolescents are linked to precocious puberty, accelerated bone growth, height, features of PCOS, and are more commonly seen in obese subjects compared to non-obese. In pre-pubertal obese children the level of DHEAS is often elevated (14).

Recently, researchers have looked at the effects of proteins like adiponectin, resistin, leptin, and TNF-a on the fat metabolism, peripheral insulin resistance, and energy expenditure (15). Resistin is produced by the mature visceral and subcutaneous adipocytes and influences insulin sensitivity. Adiponectin and leptin, also secreted from the adipocytes, have similar roles (16). A recently published study by Shin et al (17) suggested obesity as an inflammatory process due to findings of increased levels of C-reactive protein (CRP) and TNF found in obese children. The adiponectin level was found to be much lower concentration in these children. Retinol Biding Protein 4 (RBP4) is present in omental and subcutaneous fat and is expressed more in women with PCOS (18). The high levels of androgen and features of metabolic syndrome have shown to normalize in post-menarche obese adolescents after weight reduction (19).

DIAGNOSTIC CRITERIA

A standard list of the diagnostic criteria for MS in children and adolescents is still lacking. However, a modified diagnostic criteria for children using the NCEP criteria and data from the National Health and Nutrition Examination Survey (NHANES, 1988-94) is widely used. The National Cholesterol Education Program (NCEP) and the Adult Treatment Panel III (ATP III) include at least 3 of 5 of the following criteria for the diagnosis of MS in adults (1,2,20,21).

- Abnormal lipid panel: Hypertriglyceridemia (>150 mg/dl) and low HDL-C (<40mg/dl in males and <50 in females).
- High fasting glucose level. Hyperglycemic state is defined as fasting glucose level of 100 mg/dl or more.
- Elevated blood pressure, systolic, diastolic, or both using reference ranges. From example, blood pressure of >135/85 mmHg is considered abnormal.
- Increased waist circumference/abdominal girth. BMI is fairly reliable in assessing obesity in children.
- High insulin resistance (criterion in children).
- The World Health Organization (WHO) criteria required elevated insulin or glucose level (>110mg/dl) in addition to at least two of the following:[2]
- Abdominal obesity

- Waist size >94 cm or waist to hip ratio of >0.9
- Triglycerides > 150 mg/dl or HDL <35 mg/dl
- Blood pressure >140/90 mmHg.

HAIR-AN is a clinical diagnosis and includes the following, in addition to criteria mentioned above (9):

a) Acne, hirsuitism, temporal balding, clitoromegaly, and deepening of voice (suggestive of high androgen level).
b) Acrochordons (skin tags), acanthosis nigricans (usually found on the neck, axillae, and back). These are suggestive of insulin resistance and altered hormonal levels.

SUGGESTED WORKUP

Anthropometric measurement, vital signs, with a complete history and physical exam (including genital) is recommended. A detailed family, past medical, and medication history should also be documented. Laboratory data that may be useful includes, fasting levels of insulin, glucose (complete metabolic panel to assess liver and renal function), lipid panel, glucose/insulin ratio, HgA1c, and AM cortisol level. Oral glucose tolerance test (2 hour) is also recommended to document hyperglycemic state. One test that has high sensitivity and specificity is the euglycemic hyperinsulinemic clamp. This may be impractical in a clinical setting due to the time consuming and complex nature of the test (9). A thorough endocrine evaluation should include thyroid function tests, serum prolactin, DHEA-S, am 17-hydroxyprogesterone (17-OHP), SHBG level, and free and total testosterone. IGF-1 level may be helpful in a suspected growth hormone producing tumor (22).

In order to establish the diagnosis of PCOS, the presence of multiple ovarian cysts is not necessary. Likewise, an abdominal/pelvic ultrasound detection of multiple ovarian cysts does not confirm that diagnosis either. Occasionally a computed tomography (CT) or an MRI of the abdomen/pelvis may be necessary in situations where there are progressive signs of hyperandrogenism (22).

OUTCOME

Metabolic syndrome (PCOS and HAIR-AN subset) in children can lead to potentially complicated short and long term medical problems. This exhaustive list includes but is not limited to the following (6):

- Distorted body image and perception
- Low self-esteem and depression
- Acne
- Obesity associated problems like snoring, obstructive sleep apnea, disordered sleep, gastro esophageal reflux disease (GERD), gall stones, joint pain, exercise intolerance, features of diabetes, coronary artery disease, and skin changes, etc.

- Amenorrhea (predisposing to subsequent inadequate bone mineralization) and possibly infertility.

TREATMENT OPTIONS

The timeframe for the diagnosis of metabolic syndrome/HAIR-AN to the outcome of the treatment varies from patient to patient and can be often protracted. A multidisciplinary approach is often required to address the metabolic as well as the psychological stressors associated with this syndrome. reatment should be geared toward specific metabolic abnormalities as well (6,9,23). It is important for the healthcare provider to be aware of the concerns that teenagers may have when it relates to cosmetic appearance. At a psychological developmental stage where bodily appearance plays an important role in a teenager's life, skin related problems such as acanthosis nigricans, acne, and hirsuitism may be quite troubling (22). This can affect their self-esteem directly. Health care providers should have a low threshold for referring these teenagers to counseling services.

LIFESTYLE MODIFICATION

Although compliance can play a big role with this approach, it is considered one of the most favored and successful mode of treatment in obese patients, who also have HA (22). Weight loss can dramatically improve the ovarian function and decrease the levels of androgens (24). Different dietary changes such as caloric restriction of carbohydrates or fat with increased protein intake have been previously studied. There is no sufficient data available if restriction of carbohydrates is better than that of fat intake. It is therefore prudent to use the expertise of a dietician or nutritionist who can work with obese/overweight individuals.

MEDICATION MANAGEMENT

Typically, in addition to the lifestyle modification, medical treatment may include a combination of one or more of these therapies such as anti androgens, insulin-sensitizing agents, combined hormonal contraceptives, bariatric surgery, and complementary and alternative medicine treatment options. As part of a multidisciplinary approach, psychological counseling is very crucial.

INSULIN-SENSITIZING AGENTS

Biguanide: Metformin (trade names such as Glugophage®, Rhiomet®), a pregnancy category B drug, has traditionally been used in type 2 diabetes mellitus (DM). From a glycemic stand point, Metformin interferes with the hepatocyte mitochondrial respiratory oxidative process and decreases gluconeogenesis. This however, is not a complete blockade of gluconeogenesis. It also facilitates the glucose transport in tissues such as the skeletal muscles, by activating the enzyme tyrosine kinase (TK) on the insulin receptors and enhancing the glucose transporter system. Some of this action is also on the adipocytes. It also acts against the gluconeogenic effects of glucagon. Metformin is particularly useful in obesity associated with HA. Due to its insulin lowering effect, there is a consequent decrease in the free and total testosterone and an increase in the estradiol level (25). This has a beneficial effect on ovulation, hirsuitism and acne.

As obesity is strongly associated with cardiovascular morbidity and mortality, metformin has an added benefit of being cardioprotective. It has shown to decrease the free fatty oxidation, which helps improve the insulin sensitivity as well. It may also help lower the total cholesterol (TC), very low density lipopoprotein cholesterol (VLDL-C), low density lipoprotein cholesterol (LDL-C), and increase the high density lipoprotein cholesterol (HDL-C). It also lowers the platelet aggregation and adhesion, and decreases the levels of tissue plasminogen inhibitor 1 and von Willebrand factor. This has a positive effect on homeostasis (26). It can induce vascular relaxation and reduce the oxidative stress (25,26). A combination of flutamide (an androgen receptor blocker) and metformin with an addition of drosperinone (a 4th generation progesterone) has shown to decrease abdominal fat (27).

Usual side effects from metformin may include gastrointestinal symptoms such as nausea, flatulence and diarrhea. These may be reduced by taking it with food. Treatment may be started with a single daily dose, preferably at a lowest possible dose. It may then be increased to a twice daily dose. It is not recommended to go over the maximum dosage of 2.25 grams/day (25). One must be aware of the potential toxicity from metfromin that includes lactic acidosis in rare situations. Metformin is fairly safe for the mother and baby during pregnancy and lactation (28).

Thiazolidinediones: Rosiglitazone is an insulin sensitizing agent, whose action on the peroxisome proliferator-activated receptor (PPAR) on the adipocytes improves glucose transport into the cell by increasing the adiponectin secretion (29). In studies done earlier on overweight women with PCOS, there was a decrease in the insulin resistance and return of ovulation as indicated by regular menses. The SHBG level also shows an increase that helps with the ovulation. Some of the side effects include weight gain and cardiac failure in susceptible individuals (30).

REGULATION OF THE HORMONAL/ANDROGEN IMBALANCE AND USE OF ORAL CONTRACEPTIVES

Combination birth control pills (BCP's) are the cornerstone in the treatment of HA. Their mechanism of action includes the following:

- Increase the SHBG production and level: This allows a reduction of free testosterone.
- Suppress LH: Decreases androgen production from the ovaries.
- Anti-minerelocorticoid activity: Certain progestins such as Drosperinone have low androgenic activity and are generally preferred in HA. The brand name contraceptives Yasmin® and Ortho-Tri-Cyclen® contain Drosperinone.

The effects of combination BCP's include normalization of menses and a decrease in acne and hirsuitism (22). In addition to the above, other pharmacologic agents have been tried in

HA states are cyproterone acetate, finastreride, glucocorticoid, such as prednisone (patients with late onset congential adrenal hyperplasia (CAH) having PCOS features), and spironolactone.

SURGICAL OPTIONS

Bariatric Surgery: A decrease in obesity-related morbidity has been well documented in individuals that have undergone Roux-en-Y gastric bypass surgery. Although this is an optional procedure that has been evaluated mostly in morbidly obese adults, the guidelines are quite conservative for the adolescent population. Morbidly obese teenagers, who have failed the non-surgical approach may be considered for a gastric bypass surgery. Other justifications in addition to the above includes a BMI of 40 kg/m2 or more, physical and psychosocial co morbidities from obesity (31). Bariatric surgery intended to result in weight loss can positively impact obesity, PCOS, and reverse anovulation. The risks from obesity during pregnancy in morbidly obese teens is also decreased by the procedure (31). A 1 to 2 year wait post operatively for becoming pregnant is usually recommended. As there can be potential complications from this surgical procedure, careful multidisciplinary evaluation for the need for surgery is needed.

COMPLEMENTARY AND ALTERNATIVE MEDICINE

Alternative approaches in the treatment of PCOS have been recently gaining popularity. In view of side effects from the traditional medical and surgical treatment, researchers have looked at the benefits of acupuncture, a traditional form of Chinese medicine. Acupuncture has been shown to modulate neuro-endocrine systems that results in lowering of the increased sympathetic tone in individuals with PCOS. By releasing ß-endorphins the technique of acupuncture can directly influence the HPA axis and lower the cortisol and LH levels (32). As a result, its beneficial effects on metabolic, ovulation, and other neuro-endocrinal endogenous systems can positively influence the features of PCOS/HA. Other forms of alternative medicine such as homeopathy, Ayurveda, diet supplements, and hypnotherapy have been tried to treat obesity in adults with some encouraging results even though some are not very convincing (33).

FEDERAL/STATE PROGRAM

The CDC (Center for Disease Control and Prevention), the Division of Nutrition and Physical Activity (DNPA) and the health departments of 28 states have established the Nutrition and Physical Activity Program to Prevent Obesity and Other Chronic Diseases (NPAO) since 1999 using the social ecological model (34). Healthcare providers are encouraged to contact their individual health departments to learn more about the program, where available.

Conclusions

Metabolic syndrome, hyperandrogenism, and PCOS are integral part of complex metabolic abnormalities that have a great impact on the health and general well-being of an individual. The diagnosis is often late and this adds to the economic burden from obesity related problems. The following key points will aid the healthcare provider with the timely diagnosis of HA/MS/PCOS and appropriate interventions.

- Healthcare provider awareness of obesity in childhood and adolescence.
- Utilizing diagnostic criteria and/or clinical diagnosis of PCOS/HA/MS. One may refer to the NCEP, NHANES, ATP III, WHO diagnostic criteria.
- A complete history, including that of the individual, family, past, and medications.
- Complete physical exam. As noted earlier, the diagnosis of HAIR-AN is clinical.
- Laboratory and radiological work up. The list includes fasting insulin, glucose (complete metabolic panel to assess liver and renal function), lipid panel, glucose/insulin ratio, HgA1c, and AM cortisol level. Oral glucose tolerance test (2 hour), thyroid function tests, serum prolactin, DHEA-S, am 17-hydroxyprogesterone (17-OHP), SHBG level, free and total testosterone, IGF-1 level are also recommended.
- Management that includes medical, surgical, lifestyle modification techniques, and appropriate referrals to other sub-specialty providers for addressing associated co morbidities. Keeping in mind that some patients may desire to utilize alternative and complimentary medicine options as well.
- Multidisciplinary approach that includes, the primary care provider, sub-specialist, social worker, nutritionist, and counselor/psychologist.

References

[1] Kranz S, Mahood LJ, Wagstaff DA. Diagnostic criteria patterns of US children with metabolic syndrome: NHANES 1999-2002. Nutrition J 2007;6:38.

[2] Strasburger VC, Braverman PK, Rogers PD, Holland-Hall CM. Adolescent medicine: A handbook for primary care, 1st ed. Philadelphia, PA: Lippincott Williams Wilkins, 2005.

[3] CDC. Prevalence of overweight among children and adolescents: United States, 2003-2004. 2007 [cited 2008 05/16/2008]; Health E-Stat. National Center for Health Statistics. Centers for Disease Control.]. http://www.cdc.gov/nchs/products/pubs/pubd/hestats/overweight/ overwght_child_03.htm

[4] National Association of Children's Hospitals and Related Institutions (NACHRI). Childhood Obesity Statistics and Facts. 2007 [cited 2008 05/16/2008]; Available from: http://www.childrenshospitals.net/ AM/Template.cfm?Section=HomepageandTEMPLATE=/CM/ContentDisplay.cfmandCONTENTID= 34357.

[5] CDC. Defining overweight and obesity, 2007 [cited 2008 05/14/2008]; Definition for children and teens]. Available from: http://www.cdc.gov/nccdphp/dnpa/obesity/defining.htm

[6] Krebs NF, Himes JH, Jacobson D, Nicklas TA, Guilday P, Styne D. Assessment of child and adolescent overweight and obesity. Pediatrics 2007;120(Suppl 4):S193-228.

[7] Stein CJ, Colditz GA. The epidemic of obesity. J Clin Endocrinol Metab 2004;89(6):2522-5.

[8] McCartney CR, Prendergast KA, Chhabra S, Eagleson CA, Yoo R, Chang RJ, et al. The association of obesity and hyperandrogenemia during the pubertal transition in girls: obesity as a potential factor in the genesis of postpubertal hyperandrogenism. J Clin Endocrinol Metab 2006;91(5):1714-22.
[9] Rager KM, Omar HA. Androgen excess disorders in women: the severe insulin-resistant hyperandrogenic syndrome, HAIR-AN. ScientificWorldJournal 2006;6:116-21.
[10] Mukhtar I Khan DMK, ,. Polycystic ovarian syndrome. 2006 [cited 2008 05/14/2008]; Available from: http://www.emedicine.com/med/topic2173.htm
[11] Barbieri RL, Hornstein MD. Hyperinsulinemia and ovarian hyperandrogenism. Cause and effect. Endocrinol Metab Clin North Am 1988;17(4):685-703.
[12] McCartney CR, Blank SK, Prendergast KA, Chhabra S, Eagleson CA, Helm KD, et al. Obesity and sex steroid changes across puberty: evidence for marked hyperandrogenemia in pre- and early pubertal obese girls. J Clin Endocrinol Metab 2007;92(2):430-6.
[13] Valkenburg O, Steegers-Theunissen RP, Smedts HP, Dallinga-Thie GM, Fauser BC, Westerveld EH, et al. A more atherogenic serum lipoprotein profile is present in women with polycystic ovary syndrome: a case-control study. J Clin Endocrinol Metab 2008;93(2):470-6.
[14] Gapstur SM, Gann PH, Kopp P, Colangelo L, Longcope C, Liu K. Serum androgen concentrations in young men: a longitudinal analysis of associations with age, obesity, and race. The CARDIA male hormone study. Cancer Epidemiol Biomarkers Prev 2002;11(10 Pt 1):1041-7.
[15] Zou CC, Liang L, Hong F. Relationship between insulin resistance and serum levels of adiponectin and resistin with childhood obesity. Indian Pediatrics 2007;44(4):275-9.
[16] Hendler I, Blackwell SC, Mehta SH, Whitty JE, Russell E, Sorokin Y, et al. The levels of leptin, adiponectin, and resistin in normal weight, overweight, and obese pregnant women with and without preeclampsia. Am J Obstet Gynecol 2005;193(3 Pt 2):979-83.
[17] Shin JY, Kim SY, Jeung MJ, Eun SH, Woo CW, Yoon SY, et al. Serum adiponectin, C-reactive protein and TNF-alpha levels in obese Korean children. J Pediatr Endocrinol Metab 2008;21(1):23-9.
[18] Stanley T, Misra M. Polycystic ovary syndrome in obese adolescents. Curr Opin Endocrinol Diabetes Obes 2008;15(1):30-6.
[19] Wabitsch M, Hauner H, Heinze E, Bockmann A, Benz R, Mayer H, et al. Body fat distribution and steroid hormone concentrations in obese adolescent girls before and after weight reduction. J Clin Endocrinol Metab 1995;80(12):3469-75.
[20] de Ferranti SD, Gauvreau K, Ludwig DS, Neufeld EJ, Newburger JW, Rifai N. Prevalence of the metabolic syndrome in American adolescents: Findings from the Third National Health and Nutrition Examination Survey. Circulation 2004;110(16):2494-7.
[21] Cook S, Weitzman M, Auinger P, Nguyen M, Dietz WH. Prevalence of a metabolic syndrome phenotype in adolescents: Findings from the third National Health and Nutrition Examination Survey, 1988-1994. Arch Pediatr Adolesc Med 2003;157(8):821-7.
[22] Harwood K, Vuguin P, DiMartino-Nardi J. Current approaches to the diagnosis and treatment of polycystic ovarian syndrome in youth. Horm Res 2007;68(5):209-17.
[23] McClanahan KK, Omar HA. Navigating adolescence with a chronic health condition: a perspective on the psychological effects of HAIR-AN syndrome on adolescent girls. ScientificWorldJournal 2006;6:1350-8.
[24] Huber-Buchholz MM, Carey DG, Norman RJ. Restoration of reproductive potential by lifestyle modification in obese polycystic ovary syndrome: role of insulin sensitivity and luteinizing hormone. J Clin Endocrinol Metab 1999;84(4):1470-4.
[25] Kirpichnikov D, McFarlane SI, Sowers JR. Metformin: an update. Ann Intern Med 2002;137(1):25-33.
[26] Bailey CJ. Metformin--an update. Gen Pharmacol 1993;24(6):1299-309.
[27] Ibanez L, De Zegher F. Flutamide-metformin plus an oral contraceptive (OC) for young women with polycystic ovary syndrome: switch from third- to fourth-generation OC reduces body adiposity. Hum Reprod 2004;19(8):1725-7.
[28] Goldenberg N, Glueck C. Medical therapy in women with polycystic ovarian syndrome before and during pregnancy and lactation. Minerva Ginecol 2008;60(1):63-75.

[29] Majuri A, Santaniemi M, Rautio K, Kunnari A, Vartiainen J, Ruokonen A, et al. Rosiglitazone treatment increases plasma levels of adiponectin and decreases levels of resistin in overweight women with PCOS: a randomized placebo-controlled study. Eur J Endocrinol 2007;156(2):263-9.

[30] Lago RM, Singh PP, Nesto RW. Congestive heart failure and cardiovascular death in patients with prediabetes and type 2 diabetes given thiazolidinediones: a meta-analysis of randomised clinical trials. Lancet 2007;370(9593):1129-36.

[31] Miller RJ, Xanthakos SA, Hillard PJ, Inge TH. Bariatric surgery and adolescent gynecology. Curr Opin Obstet Gynecol 2007;19(5):427-33.

[32] Stener-Victorin E, Jedel E, Manneras L. Acupuncture in polycystic ovary syndrome: current experimental and clinical evidence. J Neuroendocrinol 2008;20(3):290-8.

[33] Pittler MH, Ernst E. Complementary therapies for reducing body weight: a systematic review. Int Journal Obes 2005;29(9):1030-8.

[34] Hamre R, et al. CDC's state-based nutrition and physical activity program to prevent obesity and other chronic diseases. July 2006 January 17, 2008 [cited 2008 06/24/08]; Available from: http:// www. cdc.gov/nccdphp/dnpa/ obesity/state_programs/pdf/NPAO_Performance_Report_2005.pdf

In: Rural child health: International aspects
Editors: Erica Bell and Joav Merrick

ISBN: 978-1-60876-357-3

Chapter 24

MENTAL HEALTH ASPECTS OF AN ADOLESCENT MEDICINE CLINIC PATIENT POPULATION

Abdel Salous, MSci[1], Linah Al-Alem, MSci[2,3] and Hatim A Omar, MD*[4]

[1]University of Kentucky College of Medicine MD/PhD Program
[2]Department of Molecular and Biomedical Pharmacology
[3]Obstetrics and Gynecology, University of Kentucky College of Medicine
[4]Division of Adolescent Medicine, Department of Pediatrics, University of Kentucky College of Medicine, Lexington, United States of America

The correlation between exposure to forms of violence and development of mental disorders in victims is well established. The purpose of this chapter was to identify mental health problems in an adolescent medicine clinic population in Lexington, KY and to investigate potential correlation of mental disorders with psychosocial factors. Data were gathered from the charts of 169 adolescent clinic patients (age 10-22) seen in the clinic for mental health care and analyzed using Excel. 68% of the patient population was urban, while 32% was rural. In terms of gender, 40% of the patients were male and 60% were female. 80% of the patients were white, 13% black, and 7% had other racial background(s). The most prevalent mental disorders in this group were depression 32.12%, 13% with generalized anxiety disorder, 8.2% with an attention deficit disorder (including ADHD), and 5.76% with an adjustment disorder. The above mentioned demographic trends showed that depression continues to be the most common mental health problem in this population regardless of gender, ethnic origin or economic status. This also highlights the need for availability of mental health support to this patient population. Further work is needed to spotlight the most significant psychosocial factors and root causes of mental health conditions in this age group.

* Correspondence: Professor Hatim A Omar, MD, Department of Pediatrics, Room J422, University of Kentucky, Lexington, KY 40536-0284 United States. Tel: 859-323-5643; Fax: 859-257-7706; Email: haomar2@uky.edu

Introduction

By 2020, adolescents, representing individuals in the 10-22 year old age range, are expected to comprise 14% of the United States population (1). Adolescence is a challenging transition phase with physical, cognitive, and emotional changes all of which may have a significant impact on mental health (2). Epidemiological data from the World Health Organization showed that 20% of all adolescents worldwide have one or more mental or behavioral health problems (3). In addition, it has been shown that up to 50% of all adult mental disorders have their onset in adolescence (3). This early onset of disease becomes more critical when a common mental disorder such as depression, is expected to show a rising trend during the coming 20 years of their lives (3). Moreover, although the incidence of depression peaks during middle age, depression is becoming increasingly recognized during adolescence and young adulthood (4).

Approximately 20% of depressive patients end their lives by committing suicide (5). With respect to adolescents, suicide attempt rates were highest among adolescents 15 to 19 years old (6). In addition, completed suicide remains among the top three causes of death in the population aged 15–34 years in both males and females (3). Other mental disorders such as adjustment disorders, lead to psychosocial impairment, problems with the legal system, and restlessness (7). As for attention deficit and hyperactivity disorders, they in turn negatively impact scholastic performance, social relationships, and social behavior (8). Overall, the effect of mental disorders on society accounts for over 15 percent of the burden of disease in the United States, surpassing the disease burden caused by all cancers (9). In economic terms, children with mental health disorders impose a greater load on their parents to cut work hours, to quit work, and to spend more time arranging their child's care compared to children with other healthcare needs (10).

The causes of mental disorders in adolescents are complex and may evolve due to a wide variety of psychosocial stressors, physical injuries, developmental changes, exposure to various forms of abuse, genetics and cultural influences (4,11-13). To better characterize the relative impact of the various psychosocial factors on the development of mental disorders, this study examined and reported on a sample of an outpatient adolescent clinic patients in Lexington, Kentucky. The patients were recipients of either counseling or medical services for mental disorders for which they were diagnosed. Specifically, the study sought to describe retrospectively this patient population with respect to demographic profile, age, gender, racial background, socioeconomic status, marital status, educational level, and prevalent mental disorders. The descriptive analysis in this paper is deemed to give rise to further investigation of the most significant psychosocial factors that precipitate the onset of mental disorders in adolescents.

Our study

Medical chart review was conducted for 174 patients, who received counseling or therapy for diagnosed mental disorders. Patients received psychological therapy services regularly on a outpatient basis for mental health. In addition, medical services were provided for other physical conditions patients presented with at the time of the visit. Patient data was entered in a spreadsheet program for further analysis.

Patients were excluded from the study if they did not meet the age requirements (10-22 years) at the time of data collection and if their charts lacked documentation regarding mental disorders or conditions. With all exclusions, the final sample size was 169 patients.

The different variables were entered in separate columns, grouped, codified, and analyzed statistically using Excel functions.

OUR FINDINGS

The age range of the patients included in the study was 10-22 at the time of the study. The mean age was 15.6 and the median age was 16 years, while the mode value for age was 17 years (see table 1). As expected, the majority of the patient population was urban (68%). The remaining 32% came from the surrounding rural areas such as Montgomery, Anderson, and Jessamine counties in addition to others (table 2). In terms of gender, 40% of the patients were male and 60% were female (see table 2).

Table 1. Age profile of subjects in the study (n=169)

Age Range	**Minimum** 10	**Maximum** 22	
Age Distribution	Mean 15.6	Median 16	Mode 17

Table 2. Demographic characteristics of subjects in the study (n=169). *The insurance plan was documented as an indicator of socioeconomic status (SES). High SES patients were carriers of a private insurance plan while low SES patients were carriers of other non-private insurance plans such as state medical assistance or no insurance. **Other includes Hispanic, mixed racial origin and unspecified racial origin. ***Other includes dropouts, home schooling and other educational arrangements

Geographic Distribution	Urban 68%	Rural 32%		
Gender Distribution	Female 60%	Male 40%		
Socioeconomic Status*	High 61%	Low 39%		
Ethnic Background**	White 80%	Black 13%	Other 7%	
Marital Status	Single 98%	Married 1%	Other 1%	
Educational Level***	High School 67%	Middle School 23%	College 5%	Other 5%

Insurance plan was documented as an indicator of socioeconomic status either as high or low. 61% of all patients had private insurance reflecting a high socioeconomic status. The remaining 39% reflected a low socioeconomic status. These patients received financial assistance, or were carriers of other non-private insurance.

Ethnic background showed that 80% of the patients were white, 13% black, and 7% had other racial backgrounds including Hispanic and mixed racial background (see table 2). With regards to marital status, 98% of the patients reported their status as single, 1% as married, and 1% as other (see table 2). The educational profile of the patients showed that 67% were in high school, 23% in middle school, and 5% in college. The remainder 5% includes dropouts and patients with other educational arrangements including home schooling (see table 2).

Mental disorders

The most prevalent mental disorders in this group were depression, generalized anxiety, ADHD, and adjustment disorders in the listed order. 32.1% of the patients were diagnosed with a depression disorder, while 13.0% of the patients were diagnosed with a generalized anxiety disorder. 8.2% of patients had attention deficit disorder (including ADHD) and 5.8% of patients had an adjustment disorder. Eating disorders, including both bulimia and anorexia nervosa 3.9%, Insomnia accounted for 2.7%. The rest of mental disorders grouped under "other" included: anger management, Asperger's syndrome, bipolar disorder, conversion disorder, obsessive-compulsive disorder, pain disorder, panic disorder, post-traumatic stress disorder, and trichitillomania (see figure 1).

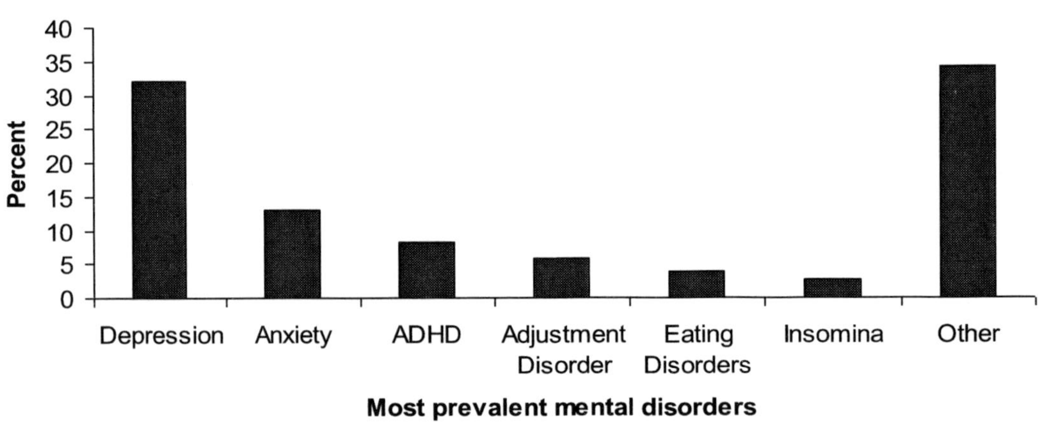

Figure 1. Prevalence Mental Disorders (n=169).

Discussion

The goal of this study was to characterize a representative outpatient adolescent population receiving treatment for mental health. The age range of the patients was 10-22 years at the time of the study. The mean, median, and mode values for age were indicative of a higher incidence of mental health disorders during high school (see table 1).

The incidence of mental health disorders seemed higher in urban areas as represented by two thirds of the patients (see table 2). This may reflect the additional stressors of urban life as compared with rural settings. Alternatively, proximity of urban dwellers to the urban healthcare facility may play a role in this distribution. In turn, this may indicate a greater need for mental health services to this sector of the adolescent population. This demographic trend may be also attributed to insufficiency of medical services in rural areas.

Approximately 60% of all patients were female while 40% were males (see table 2). These results point to a higher prevalence of mental disorders among women versus men. This trend is in agreement with mood disorder rates of 5%-12% for men and 10%-25% for women ages 15 and older (14). An alternative explanation for this trend is that women have higher susceptibility to psychosocial factors. For example, violence, socioeconomic disadvantage, low income, low or subordinate social status and rank are all psychosocial factors that affect women disproportionately compared with men (15). In addition, women are more vulnerable to forms of abuse and associated development of mental disorders (15,16). Also, according to the National Survey on Drug Use and Health, women with substance abuse disorders were more likely than men to seek treatment (17).

As for the socioeconomic status, 61% of patients had private insurance plans while low SES patients were carriers of medical assistance plans or no insurance. The potential correlation between the socioeconomic status and the types of mental disorders poses an interesting question to be explored in future studies.

With regards to race distribution, 80% of the patients were white, 13% black, and 7% had other racial backgrounds (see table 2). This breakdown roughly paralleled the national distribution with 75% white, 12% African American, 3.6% Asian, and 2.4% with mixed racial backgrounds (18). Although racial diversity closely matched the national averages, it is important to recognize the wider variation that may exist in other communities. For example, rural communities and inner city communities may deviate significantly from these trends. In terms of educational profile it clearly showed that high school students were major recipients of mental health services in this clinic.

The most prevalent mental disorder in this group was depression followed by anxiety disorders. Unfortunately, the prevalence of mental disorders in adolescents has not been as well documented as that for adults (2).

This study sought to provide a brief description of an adolescent patient population receiving mental health care services in an outpatient clinic. This goal was accomplished by reporting on the demographic characteristics and the most prevalent mental disorders in this patient sample. We conclude that mental health issues were a significant problem in adolescents with depression as the most common disorder. Access to mental health care is therefore crucial to help prevent consequences (such as suicide) and to help teens grow into healthy adults.

ACKNOWLEDGMENTS

The authors would like to thank Dr. Marlene Huff, Dr. Kimberly McClanahan, Ms. Elizabeth Johnson, and Ms. Heidi Smith for their help in data collection and advice.

REFERENCES

[1] Kolbe L. Adolescent health: population as patient. Adolescent health leadership forum. Elm Groove, IL: Am Acad Pediatrics, 2003. http://www.aap.org/advocacy/ahproject/AHLPopulationasPatientLKolbe.pps. Accessed May 5, 2008.

[2] Satcher D. Mental health: A report of the surgeon general. Prof Psychol Res Pr 2000;31(1):5-13.

[3] The World Health Organization. The world health report. Mental health: New understanding, new hope. Geneva: WHO, 2001:19-41.

[4] Lewinsohn PM, Hops H, Roberts RE, Seeley JR, Andrews JA. Adolescent psychopathology: I. Prevalence and incidence of depression and other DSM-III-R disorders in high school students. J Abnorm Psychol 1993;102(1):133-44.

[5] Goodwin FK, Jamison KR. Suicide. Manic-depressive illness. New York: Oxford Univ Press, 1990:227-46.

[6] Suicide Prevention Resource Center (2004). United States Suicide Fact Sheet. http://www.sprc.org/stateinformation/PDF/statedatasheets/sprc_national_data.pdf. Accessed May 5, 2008.

[7] Pelkonen M, Marttunen M, Henriksson M, Lonnqvist J. Adolescent adjustment disorder: precipitant stressors and distress symptoms of 89 outpatients. Eur Psychiatry 2007;22(5):288-95.

[8] Lauth GW, Heubeck BG, Mackowiak K. Observation of children with attention-deficit hyperactivity (ADHD) problems in three natural classroom contexts. Br J Educ Psychol 2006;6(Pt 2):385-404.

[9] National Institute of Mental Health (2008). Mental health statistics. http://www.nimh.nih.gov/health/statistics/index.shtml. Accessed May 5, 2008.

[10] Busch SH, Barry CL. Mental health disorders in childhood: assessing the burden on families. Health Aff 2007;26(4):1088-95.

[11] Fischer T, Koch P, Saager C, Kohut GN. The radio-radial external fixator in the treatment of fractures of the distal radius. J Hand Surg [Br] 1999;24(5):604-9.

[12] Kessler RC, Davis CG, Kendler KS. Childhood adversity and adult psychiatric disorder in the US National Comorbidity Survey. Psychol Med 1997;27(5):1101-19.

[13] MacMillan HL et al. Childhood abuse and lifetime psychopathology in a community sample. Am J Psychiatry 2001;158(11):1878-83.

[14] Waraich P, Goldner EM, Somers JM, Hsu L. Prevalence and incidence studies of mood disorders: a systematic review of the literature. Can J Psychiatry 2004;49(2):124-38.

[15] The World Health Organization. Gender and women's mental health: Gender disparities and mental health: The facts. http://www.who.int/mental_health/prevention/genderwomen/en/. Accessed May 5, 2008.

[16] Sanci L, Coffey C, Olsson C, Reid S, Carlin JB, Patton G. Childhood sexual abuse and eating disorders in females: findings from the victorian adolescent health cohort study. Arch Pediatr Adolesc Med 2008;162(3):261-7.

[17] Substance Abuse and Mental Health Services Administration. National survey on drug use and health, 2004. http://www.oas.samhsa.gov/NSDUH/2k4nsduh/2k4Results/2k4 Results.pdf. Accessed May 5, 2008.

[18] US Census Bureau, 2000). http://www.census.gov/. Accessed May 5, 2008.

SECTION SIX: ACKNOWLEDGMENTS

In: Rural child health: International aspects
Editors: Erica Bell and Joav Merrick
ISBN: 978-1-60876-357-3

Chapter 25

About the Editors

Erica Bell, PhD, is deputy director of the University of Tasmania's Department of Rural Health. She has over thirty academic journal and conference papers and presentations in areas of interest to rural stakeholders: adolescent substance abuse, domestic violence and child health, youth crime prevention, healthy ageing and falls prevention, chronic disease, hospital error and medical education reform. Her work in small-*N* research methods for health policy and practice across these sub-disciplines is represented in her book *Research for Health Policy* published by Oxford University Press in 2010. She is also active as an international collaborator and editor in the area of rural child health, health policy and climate change. Erica also has a strong record of community engagement work, being the author of over fifty applied research reports that have developed policy and practices across health and education specialities and sectors. Prior to her employment in 2004 in rural health she was a policy research manager in the Queensland government leading a diverse multidisciplinary research team. E-mail: erica.bell Web: www.utas.edu.au/ruralhealth

Joav Merrick, MD, MMedSci, DMSc, is professor of pediatrics, child health and human development affiliated with Kentucky Children's Hospital, University of Kentucky, Lexington, United States and the Zusman Child Development Center, Division of Pediatrics, Soroka University Medical Center, Ben Gurion University, Beer-Sheva, Israel, the medical director of the Division for Mental Retardation, Ministry of Social Affairs, Jerusalem, the founder and director of the National Institute of Child Health and Human Development. Numerous publications in the field of pediatrics, child health and human development, rehabilitation, intellectual disability, disability, health, welfare, abuse, advocacy, quality of life and prevention. Received the Peter Sabroe Child Award for outstanding work on behalf of Danish Children in 1985 and the International LEGO-Prize ("The Children's Nobel Prize") for an extraordinary contribution towards improvement in child welfare and well-being in 1987. E-mail: jmerrick@zahav.net.il; Home-page: http://jmerrick50.googlepages.com/home

In: Rural child health: International aspects
Editors: Erica Bell and Joav Merrick
ISBN: 978-1-60876-357-3

Chapter 26

About the University Department of Rural Health

The University Department of Rural Health (UDRH) program is an Australian Government initiative. The UDRH Tasmania was established in 1997 and is based in Launceston, in Northern Tasmania and in Hobart, southern Tasmania. It is part of the Faculty of Health Science of the University of Tasmania. The UDRH Tasmania is part of a national network of University Departments of Rural Health - ARHEN (the Australian Rural Health Education Network). The multidisciplinary University Department of Rural Health (UDRH), Tasmania is committed to improving access to health care resources and contributing to improved health outcomes for people in rural and remote areas of Tasmania by:

- Working collaboratively to achieve an adequate, appropriately trained and stable rural health care workforce;
- Facilitating access to appropriate education and training opportunities, resources and ongoing support across the learning continuum, and
- Promoting and supporting a primary health care approach to rural health research and preventative health strategies.

Contact

Erica Bell, PhD
Deputy Director
University Department of Rural Health
University of Tasmania
Private Bag 103 Hobart
Tasmania 7000 Australia
Ph: +61 (0)3 6226 7377
Mobile: +61 (0)4 3939 4141
Facsimile: +61 (0)3 6226 1952
Email: Erica.Bell@utas.edu.au
Website: http://fcms.its.utas.edu.au/healthsci/ruralhealth/pagedetails.asp?lpersonId=2832

In: Rural child health: International aspects
Editors: Erica Bell and Joav Merrick
ISBN: 978-1-60876-357-3

Chapter 27

About the National Institute of Child Health and Human Development in Israel

The National Institute of Child Health and Human Development (NICHD) in Israel was established in 1998 as a virtual institute under the auspices of the Medical Director, Ministry of Social Affairs and Social Services in order to function as the research arm for the Office of the Medical Director. In 1998 the National Council for Child Health and Pediatrics, Ministry of Health and in 1999 the Director General and Deputy Director General of the Ministry of Health endorsed the establishment of the NICHD.

Mission

The mission of a National Institute for Child Health and Human Development in Israel is to provide an academic focal point for the scholarly interdisciplinary study of child life, health, public health, welfare, disability, rehabilitation, intellectual disability and related aspects of human development. This mission includes research, teaching, clinical work, information and public service activities in the field of child health and human development.

Service and academic activities

Over the years many activities became focused in the south of Israel due to collaboration with various professionals at the Faculty of Health Sciences (FOHS) at the Ben Gurion University of the Negev (BGU). Since 2000 an affiliation with the Zusman Child Development Center at the Pediatric Division of Soroka University Medical Center has resulted in collaboration around the establishment of the Down Syndrome Clinic at that center. In 2002 a full course on “Disability” was established at the Recanati School for Allied Professions in the Community, FOHS, BGU and in 2005 collaboration was started with the Primary Care Unit of the faculty and disability became part of the master of public health course on “Children and society”. In the academic year 2005-2006 a one semester course on “Aging with disability” was started as part of the master of science program in gerontology in our collaboration with the Center for Multidisciplinary Research in Aging.

Research activities

The affiliated staff have over the years published work from projects and research activities in this national and international collaboration. In the year 2000 the International Journal of Adolescent Medicine and Health and in 2005 the International Journal on Disability and Human development of Freund Publishing House (London and Tel Aviv), in the year 2003 the TSW-Child Health and Human Development and in 2006 the TSW-Holistic Health and Medicine of the Scientific World Journal (New York and Kirkkonummi, Finland), all peer-reviewed international journals were affiliated with the National Institute of Child Health and Human Development. From 2008 also the International Journal of Child Health and Human Development (Nova Science, New York), the International Journal of Child and Adolescent Health (Nova Science) and the Journal of Pain Management (Nova Science) affiliated and from 2009 thw International Public Health Journal (Nova Science) and Journal of Alternative Medicine Research (Nova Science).

National collaborations

Nationally the NICHD works in collaboration with the Faculty of Health Sciences, Ben Gurion University of the Negev; Department of Physical Therapy, Sackler School of Medicine, Tel Aviv University; Autism Center, Assaf HaRofeh Medical Center; National Rett and PKU Centers at Chaim Sheba Medical Center, Tel HaShomer; Department of Physiotherapy, Haifa University; Department of Education, Bar Ilan University, Ramat Gan, Faculty of Social Sciences and Health Sciences; College of Judea and Samaria in Ariel and recently also collaborations has been established with the Division of Pediatrics at Hadassah, Center for Pediatric Chronic Illness, Har HaZofim in Jerusalem.

International collaborations

Internationally with the Department of Disability and Human Development, College of Applied Health Sciences, University of Illinois at Chicago; Strong Center for Developmental Disabilities, Golisano Children's Hospital at Strong, University of Rochester School of Medicine and Dentistry, New York; Centre on Intellectual Disabilities, University of Albany, New York; Centre for Chronic Disease Prevention and Control, Health Canada, Ottawa; Chandler Medical Center and Children's Hospital, Kentucky Children's Hospital, Section of Adolescent Medicine, University of Kentucky, Lexington; Chronic Disease Prevention and Control Research Center, Baylor College of Medicine, Houston, Texas; Division of Neuroscience, Department of Psychiatry, Columbia University, New York; Institute for the Study of Disadvantage and Disability, Atlanta; Center for Autism and Related Disorders, Department Psychiatry, Children's Hospital Boston, Boston; Department of Paediatrics, Child Health and Adolescent Medicine, Children's Hospital at Westmead, Westmead, Australia; International Centre for the Study of Occupational and Mental Health, Düsseldorf, Germany; Centre for Advanced Studies in Nursing, Department of General Practice and Primary Care, University of Aberdeen, Aberdeen, United Kingdom; Quality of Life Research

Center, Copenhagen, Denmark; Nordic School of Public Health, Gottenburg, Sweden, Scandinavian Institute of Quality of Working Life, Oslo, Norway; Centre for Quality of Life of the Hong Kong Institute of Asia-Pacific Studies and School of Social Work, Chinese University, Hong Kong.

TARGETS

Our focus is on research, international collaborations, clinical work, teaching and policy in health, disability and human development and to establish the NICHD as a permanent institute at one of the residential care centers for persons with intellectual disability in Israel in order to conduct model research and together with the four university schools of public health/medicine in Israel establish a national master and doctoral program in disability and human development at the institute to secure the next generation of professionals working in this often non-prestigious/low-status field of work. For this project we need your support. We are looking for all kinds of support and eventually an endowment.

CONTACT

Joav Merrick, MD, DMSc
Professor of Pediatrics, Child Health and Human Development
Medical Director, Health Services, Division for Mental Retardation, Ministry of Social Affairs and Social Services, POB 1260, IL-91012 Jerusalem, Israel.
E-mail: jmerrick@inter.net.il

In: Rural child health: International aspects
Editors: Erica Bell and Joav Merrick
ISBN: 978-1-60876-357-3

Chapter 28

About the Book Series "Health and Human Development"

Health and human development is a book series with publications from a multidisciplinary group of researchers, practitioners and clinicians for an international professional forum interested in the broad spectrum of health and human development.

- Merrick J, Omar HA, eds. Adolescent behavior research. International perspectives. New York: Nova Science, 2007.
- Kratky KW. Complementary medicine systems: Comparison and integration. New York: Nova Science, 2008.
- Schofield P, Merrick J, eds. Pain in children and youth. New York: Nova Science, 2009.
- Greydanus DE, Patel DR, Pratt HD, Calles Jr JL, eds. Behavioral pediatrics, 3 ed. New York: Nova Science, 2009.
- Ventegodt S, Merrick J, eds. Meaningful work: Research in quality of working life. New York: Nova Science, 2009.
- Omar HA, Greydanus DE, Patel DR, Merrick J, eds. Obesity and adolescence. A public health concern. New York: Nova Science, 2009.
- Lieberman A, Merrick J, eds. Poverty and children. A public health concern. New York: Nova Science, 2009.
- Goodbread J. Living on the edge. The mythical, spiritual and philosophical roots of social marginality. New York: Nova Science, 2009.
- Bennett DL, Towns S, Elliot E, Merrick J, eds. Challenges in adolescent health: An Australian perspective. New York: Nova Science, 2009.
- Schofield P, Merrick J, eds. Children and pain. New York: Nova Science, 2009.
- Sher L, Kandel I, Merrick J. Alcohol-related cognitive disorders: Research and clinical perspectives. New York: Nova Science, 2009.
- Anyanwu EC. Advances in environmental health effects of toxigenic mold and mycotoxins. New York: Nova Science, 2009.
- Bell E, Merrick J, eds. Rural child health. International aspects. New York: Nova Science, 2009.
- Dubowitz H, Merrick J, eds. International aspects of child abuse and neglect. New York: Nova Science, 2010.

- Shahtahmasebi S, Berridge D. Conceptualizing behavior: A practical guide to data analysis. New York: Nova Science, 2010.
- Wernik U. Chance action and therapy. The playful way of changing. New York: Nova Science, 2010.
- Omar HA, Greydanus DE, Patel DR, Merrick J, eds. Adolescence and chronic illness. A public health concern. New York: Nova Science, 2010.
- Patel DR, Greydanus DE, Omar HA, Merrick J, eds. Adolescence and sports. New York: Nova Science, 2010.
- Shek DTL, Ma HK, Merrick J, eds. Positive youth development: Evaluation and future directions in a Chinese context. New York: Nova Science, 2010.
- Shek DTL, Ma HK, Merrick J, eds. Positive youth development: Implementation of a youth program in a Chinese context. New York: Nova Science, 2010.
- Omar HA, Greydanus DE, Tsitsika AK, Patel DR, Merrick J, eds. Pediatric and adolescent sexuality and gynecology: Principles for the primary care clinician. New York: Nova Science, 2010.
- Chow E, Merrick J, eds. Advanced cancer. Pain and quality of life. New York: Nova Science, 2010.

CONTACT

Professor Joav Merrick, MD, MMedSci, DMSc
Medical Director, Division for Mental Retardation
Ministry of Social Affairs, POBox 1260
IL-91012 Jerusalem, Israel
E-mail: jmerrick@internet

INDEX

D

E

I

J

K

L

M

N

O

P

Q

R

S

T

U